Meningitis and Encephalitis

Rodrigo Hasbun
Editor

Meningitis and Encephalitis

Management and Prevention Challenges

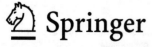 Springer

Editor
Rodrigo Hasbun
UT Health-McGovern Medical School
Houston, TX
USA

ISBN 978-3-030-06488-4   ISBN 978-3-319-92678-0   (eBook)
https://doi.org/10.1007/978-3-319-92678-0

Printed on acid-free paper

This Springer imprint is published by the registered company Springer Nature Switzerland AG
The registered company address is: Gewerbestrasse 11, 6330 Cham, Switzerland

Preface

Meningitis and encephalitis continue to be associated with high rates of mortality and neurological sequelae, and despite the availability of molecular diagnostic techniques, the majority of patients have unknown causes. The differential diagnosis is broad and includes a wide spectrum of infectious and noninfectious etiologies, some requiring urgent therapy for survival. Some of the most common challenges clinicians face include the low sensitivity of meningeal signs, overutilization of unnecessary screening cranial imaging in suspected meningitis, delays in the diagnosis of urgent treatable causes, emerging causes of meningitis and encephalitis, large proportion of unknown etiologies, low sensitivity of current microbiological techniques especially in the setting of previous antibiotic therapy, underutilization of available molecular diagnostic tests, and empiric antibiotic therapy and hospitalization for viral meningitis cases. Even though there are published guidelines, compliance with them is not optimal and physicians do not follow standardized algorithms in their empirical approach.

Due to the high rate of adverse clinical outcomes, prevention when feasible is of utmost importance. The use of conjugate vaccines for the three most common meningeal pathogens has dramatically changed the current epidemiology of bacterial meningitis, prenatal screening for Group B streptococcus in pregnancy has decreased early-onset neonatal meningitis, and vaccination for Japanese encephalitis has had a dramatic impact in the countries where it has been implemented. Adherence to protocols to prevent health-care associated meningitis and ventriculitis is effective, but compliance with them is not uniformly performed.

Finally, this book will serve to guide current and future researchers in the field to address the gaps in knowledge that currently exist in the diagnosis, management, and prevention of the most important causes of meningitis and encephalitis in the world with the ultimate goal to improve the outcomes of these devastating clinical syndromes.

Houston, TX, USA   Rodrigo Hasbun

Acknowledgments

This book represents an international collaborative effort to provide the most up-to-date evidence to help diagnose, treat, and prevent the most common central nervous system infections in the world. I want to thank all the experts for providing a thorough and insightful review of the current challenges facing clinicians. I also want to thank the Springer team (Nadina Persaud, Saanthi Shankhararaman, and G. Keerthana) for their excellent support in the organization and production of this book. I would also like to thank the Grant A Starr Foundation for our research support, my research mentor Vinny Quagliarello for the training and support, my wife for her continuous loving support, and for God for guiding my path.

Contents

List of Contributors

Ahmed Al Hammadi UT Health-McGovern Medical School, Houston, TX, USA

Linda Aurpibul, MD, MPH Research Institute for Health Sciences, Chiang Mai University, Chiang Mai, Thailand

Adarsh Bhimraj Section of Neurologic Infectious Diseases, Department of Infectious Diseases, Cleveland Clinic Foundation, Cleveland, OH, USA

Karen C. Bloch, MD, MPH Vanderbilt University Medical Center, Department of Infectious Diseases, Nashville, TN, USA

Tricia Bravo, MD Section of Neurologic Infectious Diseases, Department of Infectious Diseases, Cleveland Clinic Foundation, Cleveland, OH, USA

Rommanee Chaiwarith Division of Infectious Diseases and Tropical Medicine, Maharaj Nakorn Chiang Mai Hospital, Chiang Mai University, Chiang Mai, Thailand

Andrea T. Cruz, MD, MPH Department of Pediatrics, Baylor College of Medicine, Texas Children's Hospital, Houston, TX, USA

Mario Luis Garcia de Figueiredo Laboratory of Virology, Department of Clinical Analyses, Toxicology and Food Sciences, School of Pharmaceutical Sciences of Ribeirao Preto, University of Sao Paulo, Ribeirao Preto, Sao Paulo, Brazil

Mushira Abdulaziz Enani Department of Medicine, Section of Infectious Diseases, King Fahad Medical City, Riyadh, Saudi Arabia

Luiz Tadeu Moraes Figueiredo Virus Research Unit, School of Medicine of the University of Sao Paulo, Ribeirao Preto, Sao Paulo, Brazil

Martin Glimaker Department of Infectious Diseases, Karolinska University Hospital, Stockholm, Sweden

John J. Halperin, MD Department of Neurosciences, Overlook Medical Center, Summit, NJ, USA

Sidney Kimmel Medical College of Thomas Jefferson University, Philadelphia, PA, USA

Rodrigo Hasbun, MD, MPH UT Health-McGovern Medical School, Houston, TX, USA

Quanhathai Kaewpoowat, MD Division of Infectious Diseases and Tropical Medicine, Department of Medicine, Chiang Mai University, Chiang Mai, Thailand

Research Institute for Health Sciences, Chiang Mai University, Chiang Mai, Thailand

Prathit A. Kulkarni, MD Department of Medicine, Section of Infectious Diseases, Baylor College of Medicine, Houston, TX, USA

Megan McKenna, MD Department of Infectious Diseases, Baylor College of Medicine, Harris County Hospital District, Houston, TX, USA

Kristy O. Murray, DVM, PhD Department of Pediatrics, Baylor College of Medicine, Texas Children's Hospital, Houston, TX, USA

Melissa S. Nolan, PhD, MPH Department of Pediatrics, Baylor College of Medicine, Texas Children's Hospital, Houston, TX, USA

Luis Ostrosky-Zeichner UT Health-McGovern Medical School, Houston, TX, USA

John C. Probasco Johns Hopkins Encephalitis Center, Division of Neuro-immunology and Neuroinfectious Diseases, Department of Neurology, Johns Hopkins University School of Medicine, Baltimore, MD, USA

Shannon E. Ronca, MD, PhD Department of Pediatrics, Baylor College of Medicine, Texas Children's Hospital, Houston, TX, USA

Jose A. Serpa, MD, MS Department of Medicine, Section of Infectious Diseases, Baylor College of Medicine, Houston, TX, USA

Jeffrey R. Starke, MD Department of Pediatrics, Baylor College of Medicine, Texas Children's Hospital, Houston, TX, USA

Arun Venkatesan, MD, PhD Johns Hopkins Encephalitis Center, Division of Neuroimmunology and Neuroinfectious Diseases, Department of Neurology, Johns Hopkins University School of Medicine, Baltimore, MD, USA

Steven Paul Woods, PsyD University of Houston, Department of Psychology, Cognitive Neuropsychology of Daily Life (CNDL) Laboratory, Houston, TX, USA

Introduction

Rodrigo Hasbun

Meningitis and encephalitis may be caused by various etiologies, including viruses, bacteria, fungi, protozoa, and helminthes [1, 2]. In addition, numerous noninfectious causes may account for syndromes that mimic central nervous system (CNS) infections [1–3]. These include autoimmune disorders, neoplastic and paraneoplastic diseases, medications, collagen vascular disorders, and other systemic illnesses. CNS infections usually present with cerebrospinal fluid (CSF) pleocytosis and high CSF protein levels due to disruption of the blood brain barrier (BBB) but up to 8% may present without pleocytosis [4]. Despite the availability of microbiological tools, serologies and nucleic acid amplification tests such as single or multiplex polymerase chain reaction (PCR) for the most common infectious agents, the majority of CNS infections currently still remain with an unknown etiology [1, 3, 5]. Meningitis and encephalitis may be associated with significant morbidity and mortality, sometimes requiring emergent neurosurgical interventions or early adjunctive steroids to improve clinical outcomes [1, 3]. Furthermore, CNS infections may also have long-term neurological and neurocognitive sequelae that affect quality of life and activities of daily living. A prompt etiological diagnosis with targeted therapy can improve or prevent several of these adverse clinical outcomes in those with urgent treatable etiologies [1].

Meningitis

Patients with meningitis may have an acute (<5 days duration of symptoms), subacute (6–30 days), or chronic (>30 days) presentation [3], and the clinical manifestations may depend on the virulence of the causative agent and the location of the infection. Patients with acute meningitis usually present with fever, headache, and

R. Hasbun
UT Health-McGovern Medical School, Houston, TX, USA
e-mail: Rodrigo.Hasbun@uth.tmc.edu

© Springer International Publishing AG, part of Springer Nature 2018
R. Hasbun (ed.), *Meningitis and Encephalitis*,
https://doi.org/10.1007/978-3-319-92678-0_1

stiff neck seeking medical attention within a few hours to several days after the onset of illness [3]. The presentation may vary, depending on the age of the patient, the causative agent and due to the presence of various underlying conditions (e.g., head trauma, recent neurosurgery, presence of a cerebrospinal fluid [CSF] shunt, and immunocompromised state) [3, 6]. The most common etiologic agents of acute meningitis are unknown [3]. When a cause is identified, the most common etiologies are viruses (most often enteroviruses (children > adults), West Nile virus, and herpes simplex virus type 2 (adults) but also human immunodeficiency virus [HIV], varicella-zoster virus, and less likely mumps virus) and bacteria (e.g., *Streptococcus pneumoniae, Neisseria meningitidis*, and *Listeria monocytogenes*) [2, 3]. Less commonly, parasites (e.g., *Naegleria fowleri* and *Angiostrongylus cantonensis*) may also cause acute meningitis.

In contrast, patients with subacute or chronic meningitis typically present over weeks to months or even years [3]. These patients are more likely to be immunosuppressed, have abnormal neurological findings, have hypoglycorrhachia, and have a lower CSF pleocytosis [3]. The most common etiology is idiopathic but fungal meningitis (e.g., *Cryptococcus neoformans, Histoplasmosis* spp., and *Coccidioides* spp.); *tuberculosis* meningitis, autoimmune disorders, and neurobrucellosis are important causes [3]. Other fungi such as *Candida* spp. in neonates or in patients with ventriculoperitoneal shunts and *Aspergillus* spp. in immunosuppressed individuals are unusual causes of meningitis [2, 3].

Encephalitis

Encephalitis is caused by parenchymal brain inflammation that causes neurological dysfunction [7, 8]. A recent international consortium defined encephalitis with a combination of major and minor criteria [7]. The major criteria is altered mental status lasting >24 h without an alternative diagnosis and is a requirement for the diagnosis. The six minor criteria are (1) documented fever >38 °C (100.4 F) within 72 h before or after presentation, (2) seizures not attributable to a preexisting seizure disorder, (3) new onset focal neurological disorder, (4) CSF WBC > 5/cubic mm, (5) new or acute onset neuroimaging abnormalities consistent with encephalitis, and (6) abnormalities on electroencephalography consistent with encephalitis and not secondary to other etiologies. The presence of 2 minor criteria indicates possible encephalitis, and >3 indicates probable or confirmed encephalitis (if etiological agent is confirmed by brain biopsy, serologies, polymerase chain reaction, or antibodies in autoimmune encephalitis). A clinical overlap between encephalitis and encephalopathy may exist, the latter referring to a clinical state of altered mental status that can manifest as confusion, disorientation, or other cognitive impairment, with or without evidence of brain tissue inflammation; encephalopathy can be triggered by a number of metabolic or toxic conditions but occasionally occurs in response to certain infectious agents such as *Bartonella henselae* and influenza virus [7–9].

Of all the pathogens reported to cause encephalitis, most are viruses that may be associated with specific clinical and neuroimaging findings that suggest their diagnosis [7, 8]. Unilateral temporal lobe encephalitis is classically caused by *herpes simplex virus (HSV)* leading to clinical manifestations characterized by personality changes, altered mentation, a decreasing level of consciousness, seizures, and focal neurologic findings (e.g., dysphasia, weakness, and paresthesias) [7, 8]. Bilateral temporal lobe involvement or lesions outside the temporal lobe, insula, or cingulate are less likely caused by HSV [10]. Other herpes viruses that cause encephalitis during any season include varicella-zoster virus, cytomegalovirus, and human herpes virus 6 and are usually seen more frequently in immunosuppressed individuals. Arboviruses (e.g., West Nile, eastern equine, St. Louis, La Crosse, and Japanese encephalitis viruses) and respiratory viruses can present with thalamic and basal ganglia encephalitis presenting with tremors including Parkinsonism features [11]. Patients with West Nile typically present between June and October, while respiratory viruses usually present in children during the winter season [7, 8]. HIV can present with an encephalitis in AIDS patient without antiretroviral therapy or can present as a CD8 encephalitis in those with immune reconstitution while on antiretroviral therapy [12]. Rabies virus unfortunately is still a frequent cause of encephalitis in Asia (India especially) and in Africa [8]. Enteroviruses are rare causes of encephalitis [7, 8].

Nonviral causes of encephalitis include *Mycobacterium tuberculosis, L. monocytogenes, Rickettsia, Ehrlichia* spp., *Bartonella* spp., *Mycoplasma pneumoniae*, and *Toxoplasma gondii* (more often seen in transplant patients with *Toxoplasma* encephalitis) [7, 8]. Several free-living amebae (i.e., *Naegleria fowleri, Acanthamoeba* spp., and *Balamuthia mandrillaris*) may cause a fatal meningoencephalitis during the summer [7, 8]. Other epidemiologic clues that may be helpful in directing the investigation for an etiologic agent in patients with encephalitis include geographic locale, prevalence of disease in the local community, travel history, recreational activities, occupational exposure, insect contact, animal contact, vaccination history, and immune status of the patient [7, 8]. In many cases of encephalitis (32–75%), the etiology remains unknown, however, despite extensive diagnostic testing [7, 8]. In addition, it is important to distinguish between infectious encephalitis and autoimmune encephalitis (antibody mediated or postinfectious or postimmunization) acute disseminated encephalomyelitis (ADEM). These latter syndromes are presumed to be mediated by an immunologic response to an antecedent antigenic stimulus provided by the infecting microorganism or immunization [7, 8]. Anti-*N*-methyl-D-aspartate receptor (NMDAR) encephalitis [13, 14] is the most common cause of antibody-associated encephalitis and is typically seen in young females with an associated ovarian teratoma. Anti-NMDAR encephalitis has now been associated with both herpes simplex virus and varicella-zoster infections [15].

This book reviews the different diagnostic and management challenges that clinicians still face for the most common causes and for some of the emerging etiologies of meningitis and encephalitis in the world. The overall goal of this book is to review the current knowledge and research gaps with hopes to guide future investigators to improve the diagnosis, therapy, and outcomes for CNS infections.

References

1. Hasbun R, Bijlsma M, Brouwer MC, et al. Risk score for identifying adults with CSF pleocytosis and negative CSF Gram stain at low risk for an urgent treatable cause. J Infect. 2013;67(2):102–10.
2. Hasbun R. Cerebrospinal fluid in central nervous system infections. In: Scheld WM, Whitley RJ, Marra CM, editors. Infections of the central nervous system. 4th ed. Philadelphia: Lippincott Williams & Wilkins; 2014. p. 4–23.
3. Sulaiman T, Salazar L, Hasbun R. Acute vs. subacute community-acquired meningitis: analysis of 611 patients. Medicine. 2017;96(36):e7984.
4. Erdem H, Ozturk-Engin D, Cag Y, et al. Central nervous system infections in the absence of cerebrospinal fluid pleocytosis. Int J Infect Dis. 2017;65:107–9.
5. Leber AL, Everhart K, Balada-Llasat JM, et al. Multicenter evaluation of BioFire FilmArray meningitis/encephalitis panel for detection of bacteria, viruses, and yeast in cerebrospinal fluid specimens. J Clin Microbiol. 2016;54(9):2251–61.
6. Tunkel AR, Hasbun R, Bhimraj A, et al. Infectious Diseases Society of America's Clinical Practice Guidelines for Healthcare-associated ventriculitis and meningitis. Clin Infect Dis. 2017;64(6):e34–e65.
7. Venkatesan A, Tunkel AR, Bloch KC, Lauring AS, Sejvar J, Bitnun A, International Encephalitis Consortium, et al. Case definitions, diagnostic algorithms, and priorities in encephalitis: consensus statement of the international encephalitis consortium. Clin Infect Dis. 2013;57:1114–28.
8. Tunkel AR, Glaser CA, Bloch KC, et al. The management of encephalitis: clinical practice guidelines by the Infectious Diseases Society of America. Clin Infect Dis. 2008;47:303–27.
9. Weitkamp JH, Spring MD, Brogan T, et al. Influenza A virus-associated acute necrotizing encephalopathy in the United States. Pediatr Infect Dis J. 2004;23:259–63.
10. Chow FC, Glaser CA, Sheriff H, et al. Use of clinical and neuroimaging characteristics to distinguish temporal lobe herpes simplex encephalitis from its mimics. Clin Infect Dis. 2015;60(9):1377–83.
11. Beattie GC, Glaser CA, Sheriff H, et al. Encephalitis with thalamic and basal ganglia abnormalities: etiologies, neuroimaging, and potential role of respiratory viruses. Clin Infect Dis. 2013;56(3):825–32.
12. Lescure FX, Moulignier A, Savatovsky J, et al. CD8 encephalitis in HIV-infected patients receiving cART: a treatable entity. Clin Infect Dis. 2013;57(1):101–8.
13. Dalmau J, Lancaster E, Martinez-Hernandez E, et al. Clinical experience and laboratory investigations in patients with anti-NMDAR encephalitis. Lancet Neurol. 2011;10:63–74.
14. Gable MS, Sheriff H, Dalmau J, et al. The frequency of autoimmune N-methyl-D-aspartate receptor encephalitis surpasses that of individual viral etiologies of young individuals enrolled in the California Encephalitis Project. Clin Infect Dis. 2012;54:899–904.
15. Solis N, Salazar L, Hasbun R. Anti-NMDA receptor antibody encephalitis with concomitant detection of Varicella Zoster virus. J Clin Virol. 2016;83:26–8.

Community-Acquired Acute Bacterial Meningitis

2

Martin Glimaker

Etiology and Epidemiology

Streptococcus pneumoniae, Neisseria meningitidis, and *Haemophilus influenzae* have been the dominating bacteria for many years [1–4]. During the last decades, the incidence of bacterial meningitis has decreased from 2–4/100,000 to 1–2/100,000 in children after implementation of vaccines against *Haemophilus influenza* type B, *Streptococcus pneumonia,* and *Neisseria meningitidis* [3, 5, 6]. *Haemophilus influenzae* has almost disappeared among children, and the number of children with pneumococcal meningitis has also decreased [7]. In adults, where pneumococci is the most common meningeal pathogen, the incidence is relatively stable about 2/100,000 inhabitants. In neonates, up to an age of 4–6 weeks, group B streptococci (*Streptococcus agalactiae*), *Escherichia coli,* other enterobacteriacae, and *Listeria monocytogenes* dominate as etiological agents [8, 9]. *Listeria monocytogenes* may also cause blood stream infection and meningitis in the elderly and/or immunocompromised individuals [10, 11]. Alpha-hemolytic streptococci may be the etiological agent in a few percent of meningitis cases, especially if the infectious focus is present in the sinus, teeth, or heart valve, whereas beta-hemolytic streptococci are more seldom the etiological agent [12]. Patients with *Staphylococcus aureus* endocarditis or spondylodiscitis sometimes also suffer from meningitis [13]. Resistant gram-negative bacteria such as *Pseudomonas aeruginosa,* extended spectrum beta-lactamase (ESBL)-producing bacteria, or *Acinetobacter baumannii* are very seldom found in acute community-acquired bacterial meningitis [4]. The dominating etiologies in different patient categories are summarized in Table 2.1.

M. Glimaker
Department of Infectious Diseases, Karolinska University Hospital, Stockholm, Sweden
e-mail: martin.glimaker@sll.se

© Springer International Publishing AG, part of Springer Nature 2018
R. Hasbun (ed.), *Meningitis and Encephalitis*,
https://doi.org/10.1007/978-3-319-92678-0_2

Table 2.1 Dominating etiologies and recommended empiric antibiotic treatment in different patient categories

Patient category	Dominating etiologies	First-line empiric antibiotic treatment	Empiric antibiotic treatment if penicillin allergy	Empiric antibiotic treatment if cephalosporin/meropenem allergy
Infants up to age 4–6 weeks	S. agalactiae E. coli Enterobacteriacae L. monocytogenes	Cefotaxime or ceftriaxone + ampicillin	Meropenem	Meropenem or ampicillin + gentamycin (or other aminoglycoside)
Children older than 4–6 weeks and adults up to age 50 years	S. pneumoniae N. meningitidis H. influenzae	Cefotaxime or ceftriaxone ± vancomycin[a]	Cefotaxime or ceftriaxone[a]	Moxifloxacin + vancomycin or linezolid
Adults over 50 years old	S. pneumoniae N. meningitidis H. influenzae L. monocytogenes	Cefotaxime or ceftriaxone + ampicillin ± vancomycin[a]	meropenem[a]	Moxifloxacin + vancomycin or linezolid + trimethoprim-sulfamethoxazole
Immunocompromised patients irrespective of age	S. pneumoniae N. meningitidis H. influenzae L. monocytogenes	Cefotaxime or ceftriaxone + ampicillin ± vancomycin[a]	Meropenem[a]	Moxifloxacin + vancomycin or linezolid + trimethoprim-sulfamethoxazole

[a]Vancomycin is added if the incidence of cephalosporin resistant S. pneumoniae is >1%

Pathophysiology

Colonization of the upper respiratory tract with *Streptococcus pneumoniae*, *Neisseria meningitidis*, and *Haemophilus influenzae* is often found in healthy children. The reason why most children do not develop invasive disease whereas a few suffer a fulminant disease with meningitis is not yet well known. Meningitis cases often experience prodromal symptoms from the respiratory tract, such as otitis, sinusitis, pharyngitis, or pneumonia [4]. To cause meningitis the bacteria must break the mucosal barrier of the respiratory tract to invade the blood stream, resulting in a bacteremia, and then the bacteria also have to cross the blood-brain or blood-cerebrospinal fluid barrier [14]. A bacterial spread from a continuous source such as otitis, mastoiditis, or sinusitis may also occur. Once inside the central nervous system (CNS), the bacteria may grow rapidly because of a relative lack of immune system. Impaired mental status, neonatal or high age, comorbidity with immunocompromised state, non-meningococcal etiology, and fulminant disease are reported risk factors for poor outcome.

Acute bacterial meningitis is associated with increased intracranial pressure, which may cause a reduced cerebral blood flow resulting in ischemia or infarction, and also brain herniation [15–21]. The pathophysiological mechanisms resulting in increased intracranial pressure are multifactorial [22, 23]. The release of bacterial components in the subarachnoid space leads to an inflammatory response with a cytokine burst that contributes to (1) increased permeability of the blood-brain barrier causing cerebral extracellular edema, (2) impaired cerebrospinal fluid absorption with increased cerebrospinal fluid volume, (3) a cytotoxic intracellular brain edema, and (4) increased cerebral blood flow (hyperaemia) with microvascular leakage increasing the extracellular edema. All these events are adding to elevated intracranial pressure. Complications to acute bacterial meningitis are vasculitis, ventriculitis, subdural empyema, and brain abscess. The most important systemic complication is septic shock with multiorgan failure and disseminated intravascular coagulation, which may occur especially in meningococcal disease, a condition with very high mortality.

Clinical Picture

Acute bacterial meningitis is a fulminant condition, and the patients may deteriorate rapidly before or shortly after admission. The typical symptoms are fever, headache, neck stiffness, and impaired mental status. Two of these four symptoms are present in 90–95% of cases, whereas all these symptoms occur in only 30–40% [4]. Hence, the clinical picture is atypical in the majority. The patients often suffer from nausea and vomiting, and photophobia and hypersensitivity to sound is common. Positive Kernig's and Brudzinsky's signs may be noticed, but the sensitivity of these signs is low. Prodromal symptoms are often signs of respiratory tract infection, such as earache, rhinorrhea, and/or cough in pneumococcal meningitis or sore throat in meningococcal disease. In meningococcal cases a petechial rash is often present which may be associated with severe sepsis and septic shock with multiorgan failure. In the elderly the typical symptoms are often more absent making the diagnosis more difficult to set on clinical grounds [10]. Convulsions, as new-onset seizures, occur in about 10–15%, especially in children, and focal neurologic deficit, usually cranial nerve palsy, is observed in about 5% of patients with acute bacterial meningitis. Some patients present with psychomotor anxiety, which can be severe indicating high intracranial pressure and a risk for rapid deterioration into coma and cerebral herniation. Signs of herniation are coma combined with rigid dilated pupils, abnormal breathing pattern, increasing blood pressure combined with bradycardia, opisthotonus, or loss of all reactions.

A characteristic feature in acute bacterial meningitis is the rapid but gradual progression of cerebral symptoms over hours resulting in that the patients usually call on hospital care within 12–24 h [4]. This is in contrast to the clinical picture in patients with cerebral mass lesion, such as brain abscess, where the cerebral symptoms usually develop more slowly over several days and the patients apply hospital care after about a week of cerebral symptoms [24, 25]. The clinical findings are also different in subarachnoid bleeding where severe headache usually appears momentarily in seconds ("thunder headache") and in stroke where neurologic deficit presents suddenly. The most common differential diagnosis is viral meningitis with similar symptoms such as fever, headache, and neck stiffness, but in patients with viral meningitis, the mental status is usually not affected, and the duration of symptoms is usually longer compared to bacterial meningitis [26]. In viral encephalitis, especially herpes simplex encephalitis, the patients initially often present with severe confusion, disorientation, and/or dysphasia but often with relatively normal level of consciousness in contrast to bacterial meningitis where the level of consciousness is often decreased early in the course of disease.

In infants fever and impaired mental status indicate that acute bacterial meningitis should be suspected, but the clinical findings are often more obscured with irritability, lethargy, or weakness as the only initial symptoms [27]. Bulging fontanelle may be observed, whereas neck stiffness usually is absent. Some infants present with seizures as the only symptom, whereas others may present with temperature and color changes of the skin indicating impaired circulation associated with severe sepsis and septic shock.

Initial Diagnostic Management

Blood cultures, routine chemical and hematological analyses, and arterial blood gas with analysis of lactate should be taken immediately on admission.

Lumbar puncture and cerebrospinal fluid analyses are the mainstay in diagnosing acute bacterial meningitis because it is the only method that can confirm or refute the diagnosis [28–30]. A highly plausible diagnosis may be set "bedside" within minutes if the cerebrospinal fluid is cloudy and the spinal opening pressure is clearly elevated (>300 mmH$_2$O). The diagnosis may appear obvious within 1–2 h after cerebrospinal fluid analyses of leukocyte count (>500–1000 × 10^9/L with polynuclear predominance), glucose (cerebrospinal fluid/serum ratio <0.4), lactate level (>4–5 nmol/L), and/or protein level (>1 g/L). Furthermore, bacteria may be disclosed by direct microscopy and antigen detection in cerebrospinal fluid within a few hours. The final diagnosis is set by culture and/or polymerase chain reaction (PCR) on cerebrospinal fluid and/or blood within 1–3 days. Recently developed polymerase chain reaction (PCR) assays may disclose the diagnosis in less than 1 day from admission [31, 32]. The culture enables susceptibility testing of antibiotic resistance that makes it possible to adjust the antibiotic treatment.

A prompt lumbar puncture is the key to early diagnosis and adequate treatment. However, performing prompt lumbar puncture or computerized tomography (CT)-preceded lumbar puncture is a controversial issue. Some authorities recommended that, in certain situations with suspected increased intracranial pressure and/or cerebral mass lesion, such as brain abscess, the clinician should refrain from prompt lumbar puncture and instead first perform a CT of the brain, since it is argued that lumbar puncture may increase the risk of brain herniation [28–30]. However, firm evidence for a causal link between lumbar puncture and herniation is lacking, and the natural course of acute bacterial meningitis or a mass lesion/brain abscess may itself result in herniation [33–36]. Furthermore, it is shown that cerebral CT is poor at predicting the risk of herniation in acute bacterial meningitis [37–39] and that CT scan seldom contributes with valuable information in cases with suspected bacterial meningitis [40]. The importance of early antibiotic treatment is emphasized in all guidelines, and there is a strong recommendation that whenever lumbar puncture is delayed, e.g., due to neuroimaging, empiric antibiotics must be started immediately on clinical suspicion, even if the diagnosis has not been established [28–30]. Yet, antibiotics are started before neuroimaging in only 30–50% of the patients where lumbar puncture is done after the CT scan [1, 41, 42]. Thus, in clinical practice, adequate antibiotics are usually started at first when lumbar puncture has been performed and neuroimaging before lumbar puncture is associated with delayed adequate treatment and increased risk of mortality and unfavorable outcome [1, 42–44]. This evidently negative effect of performing CT before lumbar puncture outweighs the hypothetical risks with prompt lumbar puncture [34]. Guidelines differ as to when to perform neuroimaging before lumbar puncture in patients with suspected bacterial meningitis. There is consensus that CT should precede lumbar puncture if a mass lesion is more probable than meningitis, i.e., in cases with focal neurological deficit other than cranial nerve palsy and/or if long duration (>4 days) of cerebral symptoms is noticed. Some guidelines also recommend neuroimaging before lumbar puncture in cases with impaired mental status, new-onset seizures, immunocompromised state, or papilledema [28–30]. However, these findings may be present in acute bacterial meningitis as well as in cases with mass lesion, and adequate funduscopy is difficult to perform in the emergency room [28].

In adults, especially the elderly, acute bacterial meningitis is often one of many differential diagnoses at the emergency department and should be suspected in many cases. Patients with acute bacterial meningitis often need early treatment at an intensive care unit and some should be administered intracranial pressure-targeted therapy at a neuro-intensive care unit (see below) [21]. A highly plausible diagnosis of acute bacterial meningitis, accomplished only by lumbar puncture, is usually required to reach the decision to administer these advanced management modalities early after admission. The problem with delayed treatment due to neuroimaging before lumbar puncture is less pronounced in children because pediatricians usually start empiric treatment for bacterial meningitis on clinical grounds even without lumbar puncture and cerebrospinal fluid analyses [27]. Thus, prompt lumbar puncture is not as important in children as in adults. However, a rapid and firm diagnosis is desirable in severe cases also in children indicating early administration of corticosteroids, intensive care, and intracranial pressure-targeted treatment.

There are also difficulties associated with antibiotic treatment that is not delayed but started before cranial CT and lumbar puncture. One problem is the increased risk of cerebrospinal fluid sterilization resulting in negative culture results [45, 46], which make further secondary antibiotic choices more difficult and hinder decisions regarding length of treatment. Although blood cultures taken before treatment can help to identify the causal agent, positive blood cultures are noted in only 50–70% of ABM cases [1, 4]. Another problem with postponed lumbar puncture is the risk of delaying and further complicating differential diagnostics, i.e., for viral meningitis, herpes simplex encephalitis, tuberculosis meningitis, and various noninfectious cerebral conditions. This issue is of particular interest in adults, where differential diagnoses are more complex and symptoms less clear as compared with children beyond the neonatal period.

Delayed Lumbar Puncture

Lumbar puncture should not delay treatment with more than about 15 min. If technical problem with lumbar puncture, i.e., if the patient suffers from psychomotor anxiety and cannot lie still, adequate treatment for bacterial meningitis should be started immediately and then the patient should be transferred rapidly to the intensive care unit for sedation before lumbar puncture is performed. In cases with ongoing seizures, these must be treated and have subsided before lumbar puncture is performed.

In cases with primary suspicion of cerebral mass lesion, lumbar puncture should be delayed until after cerebral CT (see above and Fig. 2.1).

Lumbar puncture should not be performed promptly in cases with known bleeding abnormalities such as hemophilia and treatment with warfarin or direct oral anticoagulants (DOAC). In these cases lumbar puncture can be performed when the coagulation disorder is corrected to a level of INR <1.6 and a platelet count of >30 × 10^9/L [34]. In patients on treatment with clopidogrel, lumbar puncture can be performed initially only if no signs of bleeding problems, such as mucosal bleeding

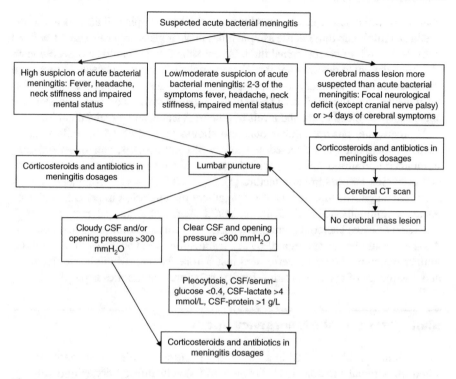

Fig. 2.1 Algorithm for diagnostic and treatment management on admission in patients with suspected community-acquired acute bacterial meningitis. *CSF* cerebrospinal fluid

from the nose, gastrointestinal or urogenital tract, or during teeth brushing, have been noticed. Patients on low molecular weight heparin can undergo lumbar puncture after 12 h (if prophylactic dose) or 24 h (if therapeutic dose) from the latest dose [28]. Lumbar puncture can be performed promptly in patients on acetylsalicylic acid or nonsteroid anti-inflammatory drugs (NSAID). Affected coagulation system associated with sepsis has not been linked with any severe risks with lumbar puncture. Thus, coagulation analyses are not required routinely before lumbar puncture in septic patients. Signs of infection at the site for spinal tap are a contraindication for lumbar puncture.

Performing Lumbar Puncture

The lumbar puncture should be performed with the patient lying horizontally on side with the back bended maximally. Funduscopy is not mandatory before lumbar puncture but should be performed if suspicion of increased intracranial pressure of long duration. The space between spinal processes L_3–L_4 or L_2–L_3 should be penetrated using a spinal tap needle with a diameter of 0.7 or 0.9 mm or with a 22 gauge needle. The opening pressure is analyzed by using a 500 mm long plastic tube that is connected to the spinal needle directly when the cerebrospinal fluid appears in the needle. At minimum three sterile sample tubes in clear glass or plastic should be filled with about 1 mL of cerebrospinal fluid. Cerebrospinal fluid should be observed visually immediately to determine if it is cloudy or clear. The first tube should be sent to the microbiology laboratory for culture, the second stored in a fridge for virus analyses if needed, and the third should be sent immediately to the chemistry laboratory for acute analyses of cell count and levels of glucose, lactate, and protein/albumin.

In aggregate, prompt lumbar puncture should be performed liberally if acute bacterial meningitis is suspected and impaired mental status, new-onset seizures, immunocompromised state, or papilledema should not be considered indications for neuroimaging before lumbar puncture [1]. Figure 2.1 shows a recommended algorithm for diagnostic and treatment management on admission in patients with suspected community-acquired acute bacterial meningitis. In patients with high suspicion of acute bacterial meningitis, corticosteroids and antibiotics in meningitis dosages should be started regardless of cerebrospinal fluid analyses. In these cases lumbar puncture should be performed just before the start of antibiotic treatment and a sequence of corticosteroids – lumbar puncture – antibiotics is proposed.

Management in the Emergency Room

The patient should be placed in a 30° sitting position in order to decrease the elevated intracranial pressure [21]. Oxygen and slowly infused crystalloid solution should be administered. A urine catheter should be placed. Patients must be continuously observed regarding mental status with Glasgow Coma Scale (GCS) or Reaction Level Scale (RLS), circulation, urine production, and respiration. A specialist in intensive care should be contacted for early referral to intensive care unit in cases with severely impaired mental status (Glasgow Coma Scale < 12/Reaction Level Scale > 2), if deterioration of mental status is noticed, if seizures have occurred, if the spinal opening pressure is very high (>400 mmH$_2$O), or if septic shock is diagnosed. In septic patients arterial lactate should be reanalyzed within 3–6 h. Adequate antibiotics and corticosteroids (when indicated) should be started within 1 h from admission to hospital. Prehospital antibiotic treatment should be given if acute bacterial meningitis is highly suspected in primary care, and the referral time to hospital is estimated to be more than 1 h [28]. Cefotaxime, ceftriaxone, or penicillin G in meningitis dosages intravenously is appropriate (see below).

Empiric Antibiotic Treatment

Initial empiric antibiotic treatment should cover the vast majority of possible bacteria that may cause acute bacterial meningitis. The drug should be bactericidal and have a good penetration of the blood-cerebrospinal fluid barrier. Since the epidemiology and the bacterial resistance pattern vary between different countries and over time, the recommendations must be flexible and should be updated continuously.

In bacterial meningitis high doses of antibiotics should be administered intravenously during the entire course of treatment because the blood-cerebrospinal fluid barrier improves after a few days of treatment, and therefore the penetration into CNS is gradually decreasing.

Several older studies of ampicillin, chloramphenicol, and cefuroxime have shown good effect but are of little value today because the susceptibility pattern has changed over time and several case reports of treatment failures with these antibiotics have been presented [47]. During recent year third-generation cephalosporins has been the mainstay in treatment of community-acquired acute bacterial meningitis [7, 28–30]. Relevant randomized clinical trials (RCTs) are presented in Table 2.2 [48–58]. Two studies have shown delayed sterilization of cerebrospinal fluid with cefuroxime compared with ceftriaxone [48, 52]. Results from experimental studies in rabbit correspond well with treatment results in humans. Animal studies have, thus, been used for development and evaluation of new antibiotic strategies [47]. The bactericidal concentrations achieved in cerebrospinal fluid have been higher for cefotaxime and ceftriaxone compared with cefuroxime. Implementation of empiric treatment with cefotaxime, ceftriaxone with or without ampicillin, and meropenem is based on a few randomized clinical trials with relatively small number of patients, and most studies are performed in children, whereas few studies have included adults (Table 2.2). Relevant randomized clinical trial of treatment of neonatal bacterial meningitis is lacking. An increasing clinical experience of, especially, cefotaxime and ceftriaxone alone or in combination with ampicillin has indicated that these antibiotics are safe and have good effect in acute bacterial meningitis.

No randomized studies have been done on treatment of resistant pneumococci, meningococci with reduced susceptibility, *Listeria monocytogenes*, or other uncommon bacteria such as streptococci, staphylococci, or enterobacteriacae. In these conditions the recommendations are based on case series and case reports supported by animal studies. The incidence of *Streptococcus pneumoniae* resistant to cephalosporins has increased in some countries, whereas a very low incidence remains in many other countries.

Meropenem has showed similar effect in vitro as cefotaxime and ceftriaxone against *Streptococcus pneumoniae*, *Neisseria meningitidis*, and *Haemophilus influenzae* including strains of pneumococci and meningococci with reduced susceptibility to penicillin. Most gram-negatives, including *Pseudomonas aeruginosa*, and *Listeria monocytogenes* are in vitro sensitive to meropenem, but the clinical experience of this treatment is limited [59]. *Streptococcus pneumoniae* that is resistant to cephalosporins is usually also resistant to meropenem. Vancomycin has good effect against cephalosporin resistant pneumococci and other resistant gram-positive bacteria, but a drawback with this drug is that the penetration of the blood-cerebrospinal fluid barrier is not as good as for cephalosporins and many other antibiotics, especially during corticosteroid treatment. Linezolid is also effective against resistant gram-positives including cephalosporin resistant pneumococci [60]. Since the bioavailability and penetration into CNS is good, linezolid is an alternative to vancomycin, but the antibacterial action is bacteriostatic rather than bactericidal, and the clinical efficacy is not as well documented as for vancomycin.

Table 2.2 Randomized controlled studies (RCTs) of empiric antibiotic treatment of community-acquired acute bacterial meningitis

References	Studied antibiotic (n)	Compared antibiotic (n)	Study population	Main results and conclusion	Comments
[48]	Ceftriaxone (174)	Cefuroxime (159)	Children[a]	Delayed sterilization and increased hearing deficit in the cefuroxime group	
[49]	1.Chloramphenicol (53) 2. Ampicillin + chloramph (46) 3. Cefotaxime (51) 4. Ceftriaxone (50)		Children[a]	No sterilization of cerebrospinal fluid in four patients in chloramphenicol group Otherwise no difference	
[50]	Ceftriaxone (39)	Ampicillin + chloramph. (42)	Children[a] and adults	No difference	
[51]	Cefotaxime (42)	Ampicillin + chloramph. (43)	Children[a]	No difference at 4 months follow-up	
[52]	Ceftriaxone (53)	Cefuroxime (53)	Children[a]	Delayed sterilization and increased hearing deficit in the cefuroxime group	
[53]	Meropenem (98)	Cefotaxime (98)	Children[a]	No difference	
[54]	Cefepime (43)	Cefotaxime (47)	Children[a]	No difference	
[55]	Meropenem (23)	Cefotaxime or ceftriaxone (22)	Adults	No difference	
[56]	Cefotaxime (38)	Ceftriaxone (44)	Children[a]	No difference	Treatment duration 4–7 days
[57]	Meropenem (129)	Cefotaxime (129)	Children[a]	No difference	
[58]	Trovafloxacin (108)	Ceftriaxone ± vancomycin (95)	Children[a]	No difference	Trovafloxacin withdrawn due to liver toxicity

Only studies with more than 40 patients are included

[a]Excluding neonatal meningitis

There is limited experience on treatment with cefepime as an alternative; besides better activity against enterobacteriacae, no advantage compared with cefotaxime or ceftriaxone has been observed [54]. The new quinolones, levofloxacin, and moxifloxacin have broad activity against most meningitis-associated bacteria (pneumococci, meningococci, *listeria monocytogenes* and *Haemophilus influenzae*), and since they are lipophilic, they penetrate the blood-cerebrospinal fluid barrier well irrespective of barrier damage [58]. A randomized clinical trial has showed similar effect of trovafloxacin as ceftriaxone in children but trovafloxacin has been withdrawn due to liver toxicity. Levofloxacin and moxifloxacin are interesting alternatives in the empiric treatment of acute bacterial meningitis, and experimental studies indicate a synergistic action between these drugs and beta-lactam antibiotics including meropenem [61]. Moxifloxacin is recommended in favor of levofloxacin in acute bacterial meningitis due to better effect on *Streptococcus pneumoniae*. However, the clinical experience of quinolones is limited, and they should be considered second-line choice, such as in cases with allergy to penicillin and/or cephalosporins. The quinolones are often active against cephalosporin resistant pneumococci, but the antibacterial activity is not as effective as for vancomycin or linezolid. Experimental animal studies have indicated that treatment with rifampicin is associated with less inflammatory response [62], and one clinical study has showed decreased mortality in pneumococcal meningitis when rifampicin was added to cephalosporin treatment [63]. However, further studies are needed before a general recommendation can be stated.

In aggregate, cefotaxime or ceftriaxone ± ampicillin must be regarded first-line empiric treatment for community-acquired acute bacterial meningitis (Table 2.1). Ampicillin should be added if *Listeria monocytogenes* can be suspected as in the newborns, in the elderly (>50 years of age), and in immunocompromised state. In cases where uncertainty whether the patient is immunocompromised or not, ampicillin should be added to the cephalosporin. Although less documented, monotherapy with meropenem is an acceptable alternative to cefotaxime or ceftriaxone with or without ampicillin, and meropenem is indicated in patients allergic to penicillin if listeriosis must be covered. Most international guidelines recommend addition of vancomycin to cover resistant pneumococci [7, 28–30]. Local epidemiological surveillance of resistance pattern is important, and the recommendations should vary depending on the actual local incidence of pneumococcal resistance to penicillin G and cephalosporins. If the incidence of cephalosporin resistance exceeds, 1% addition of vancomycin is justified. In cases with cephalosporin/meropenem allergy, a combination of moxifloxacin and vancomycin/linezolid is recommended with addition of trimethoprim-sulfamethoxazole if listeriosis is suspected. The recommendations in different age groups are summarized in Table 2.1.

Targeted Antibiotic Treatment

The antibiotic treatment for acute bacterial meningitis should be considered in three steps. The first step is to start empiric antibiotics as stated above which should be done within 1 h from admission. The second step is to adjust initial treatment according to early microbiological tests on cerebrospinal fluid such as microscopy, antigen detection, or polymerase chain reaction (PCR) results. If *Streptococcus pneumoniae* or *Haemophilus influenzae* is detected, monotherapy with cefotaxime or ceftriaxone is continued unless the *S. pneumonia*-cephalosporin resistance rate exceeds 1% in the country. If meningococci are detected, the regimen can be changed to monotherapy with penicillin G (benzylpenicillin). The third step is to determine the final antibiotic regimen after culture and susceptibility testing of cerebrospinal fluid and/or blood. The minimum inhibitory concentration (MIC) should be analyzed routinely by a disk diffusion method for penicillin G, ampicillin, cephalosporins, and meropenem. If penicillin-resistant pneumococci are noticed, further MIC-testing for vancomycin, moxifloxacin, rifampicin, and linezolid should also be analyzed. Table 2.3 summarizes the recommended treatment choices according to final diagnoses and susceptibility testing and shows proposed duration of treatment. See clinical breakpoints at https://clsi.org/blog/clsi-publishes-revised-ast-breakpoints-document/ or www.eucast.org/clinical_breakpoints/. Table 2.4 shows recommended dosages of relevant antibiotics.

Corticosteroid Treatment

Administration of the first doses of antibiotics causes bacterial lysis that is associated with release of bacterial components and endotoxins and secondary to this a massive burst of cytokines in the subarachnoid space [23]. Thus, the already activated inflammatory response accelerates further which is associated with added increase of the intracranial pressure. This inflammatory response may be modified by corticosteroids, and adjunctive therapy with corticosteroids has been supported by animal studies showing reduced inflammation in the CNS by dexamethasone [64]. The role of adjuvant corticosteroids in acute bacterial meningitis has been controversial. A Cochrane analysis has stated that corticosteroids are indicated in high-income countries, whereas the positive effect is questioned in low-income countries [65–70]. A positive effect with decreased mortality and improved long-term outcome has been shown in pneumococcal meningitis in adults [66], and decreased sequelae have been observed in *Haemophilus influenzae* meningitis in children [71]. In meningococcal meningitis no clearly positive or negative effect has been noticed, but a trend to positive effect has been reported [66, 72–75]. The only etiological agent where corticosteroids seem to result in a negative effect is *Listeria monocytogenes* [72]. In infants, low-quality data from two randomized controlled trials (RCTs) suggest that some reduction of mortality and hearing impairment may result from adding corticosteroids, but the effect is considered still unknown, and therefore this treatment is not generally recommended [76].

In aggregate, corticosteroids should be administered empirically in all adults and children over the age of 4–6 weeks with community-acquired acute bacterial meningitis. If direct microscopy of cerebrospinal fluid or if culture or polymerase chain reaction on blood and/or cerebrospinal fluid disclose *Listeria monocytogenes*, the corticosteroid treatment should be stopped. The most studied corticosteroid is dexamethasone, which should be administered in a dose of 0.15 mg/kg, maximum

Table 2.3 Targeted antibiotic treatment according to culture and susceptibility testing in cerebrospinal fluid and/or blood

Microorganism	First-line treatment	Alternative treatment	Duration of treatment[a]
Streptococcus pneumoniae			
Pc[b]-sensitive (MIC ≤ 0.06 mg/L)	Penicillin G	Cefotaxime/ceftriaxone	10–14 days
Pc-resistant (MIC[c] > 0.06 mg/L); cephalosporin-sensitive MIC < 0.5 mg/L	Cefotaxime/ceftriaxone	Meropenem	
Pc-resistant; cephalosporin-MIC 0.5–2 mg/L	Cefotaxime/ceftriaxone + vancomycin ± rifampicin	Moxifloxacin ± rifampicin	
Pc-resistant; cephalosporin-MIC >2 mg/L (resistant)	Vancomycin + rifampicin	Moxifloxacin ± rifampicin or linezolid ± rifampicin	
Neisseria meningitidis	Penicillin G	Cefotaxime/ceftriaxone	7 days
Haemophilus influenzae	Cefotaxime/ceftriaxone	Ampicillin (if beta-lactamase-negative)	10 days
Listeria monocytogenes	Ampicillin ± aminoglycoside	Penicillin G, moxifloxacin or Trimethoprim-sulfamethoxazole	14–21 days
Enterobacteriaceae (depending on resistance pattern)	Cefotaxime / Ceftazidime / Meropenem ± aminoglycoside[d]	Moxifloxacin	14–21 days
Pseudomonas aeruginosa	Ceftazidime ± aminoglycoside[d]	Meropenem ± aminoglycoside[d]	14–21 days
Staphylococcus aureus			
Methicillin-sensitive (MSSA)	Cefotaxime/ceftriaxone + rifampicin	Cloxacillin or linezolid + rifampicin	14–21 days
Methicillin-resistant (MRSA)	Linezolid or Vancomycin[d] + rifampicin	Linezolid ± rifampicin + vancomycin intrathecally	14–21 days
Streptococcus agalactiae	Penicillin G	Ampicillin / Cefotaxime/ceftriaxone	14–21 days

[a]If uncomplicated course of disease
[b]*Pc* penicillin G
[c]*MIC* minimum inhibitory concentration
[d]Can be administered intrathecally as well as intravenously

Table 2.4 Recommended dosages of antibiotics in patients with acute bacterial meningitis and normal kidney function. In patients with renal failure, reduced dosages is recommended

Antibiotic	Total daily dose in children	Number of daily doses	Dosages in adults
Ceftriaxone	100 mg/kg	1–2	2 g 12-hourly
Cefotaxime	225–300 mg/kg	4–6	3 g 6-hourly
Penicillin G	300 mg/kg	4–6	3 g 6-hourly
Ampicillin	300 mg/kg	4–6	3 g 6-hourly
Meropenem	120 mg/kg	3	2 g 8-hourly
vancomycin[a]	60 mg/kg	2–3	1 g 8-hourly
Moxifloxacin	6–8 mg/kg	1	400 mg 24-hourly
Linezolid	10 mg/kg	2	600 mg 12-hourly

[a]Aiming at a serum concentration of about 20 mg/L

10 mg, four times daily. Betamethasone is less studied but has similar anti-inflammatory effect and good penetration into CNS and seems also to have similar effect in clinical practice [72]. The adequate dosage of betamethasone is 0.12 mg/kg, maximum 8 mg, four times daily.

The first dose of corticosteroids should be given shortly before or at the same time as the first dose of antibiotics. If administration of corticosteroids is missed, initially it is considered adequate to give corticosteroids up to about 6 h after the first antibiotic dose but not later [30]. The optimal duration of corticosteroid treatment is not yet determined, but 4 days is most studied and therefore generally recommended [65]. Two days of treatment has also been shown effective [77], and especially if the patient improves rapidly, 2 days of corticosteroid treatment is probably appropriate.

Intracranial Pressure-Targeted Treatment

Despite adequate antibiotics, corticosteroids and intensive care acute bacterial meningitis still remains a challenge for the clinician, and in comatose patient's mortality rates of up to 62% have been reported [18, 36, 78, 79]. Impaired mental status is associated with increased intracranial pressure [4] and cerebral herniation and/or infarction dominate as cause of mortality and persisting neurologic deficit [15–21].

The standard of care for acute bacterial meningitis if impaired mental status or other signs of increased intracranial pressure includes intensive care with a 30° sitting position, proper analgesia and sedation, and assisted mechanical ventilation. If a severe septic syndrome is presented, the management should follow the current routines for severe sepsis and septic shock. Moderate hyperventilation and osmotherapy can be considered in a standard intensive care unit without control of intracranial pressure, but in critical cases targeted, treatment should be considered [80–83].

A neurocritical care approach using intracranial pressure-targeted treatment with favorable results has been reported in four uncontrolled studies of patients with acute bacterial meningitis presenting high intracranial pressure and severe impairment of consciousness [15–17, 84]. Promising results have also been reported in a small cohort study using lumbar drainage [82]. In one nonrandomized controlled cohort study of unconscious patients, neuro-intensive care including ventricular drainage resulted in a mortality of 10% (5/52 patients) compared with 30% (16/53 patients) if conventional intensive care was administered [21].

The following recommendations should be applied in resource-rich settings. In resource-poor settings, the treatment should be modified according to available resources. Patients with acute bacterial meningitis and impaired mental status should be centralized to hospitals where neuro-intensive care is available. In comatose patients with markedly raised spinal opening pressure (>400 mmH$_2$O), intracranial pressure-targeted treatment should be applied as soon as possible after admission. The diagnosis should be set rapidly by lumbar puncture. After a CT scan of the brain an external ventricular catheter should be applied in order to measure the intracranial pressure. Drainage of cerebrospinal fluid through this catheter should be the main intracranial pressure decreasing therapy. If an external ventricular drainage catheter cannot be applied due to technical problems or moderate coagulopathy, an intraparenchymatous pressure device should be considered for intracranial pressure control. The main goals should be intracranial pressure <20 mmHg and cerebral perfusion pressure >60 mmHg. A microdialysis catheter may be placed superficially in the brain parenchyma in order to measure the cerebral metabolism by analyzing the levels of glucose, lactate, pyruvate, and glycerol in cerebral interstitial tissue [85].

Besides drainage of cerebrospinal fluid, additional ways of achieving intracranial pressure control may also be effective. Osmotic therapy with glycerol has been suggested [69], and bolus doses of hypertonic saline aiming at a S-Na level of 150–160 mmol/L may be effective if neuroimaging shows interstitial cerebral edema. The use of mannitol for osmotic treatment is controversial because of a potential risk of rebound increase in intracranial pressure [86]. If cerebral hyperemia is detected by transcranial Doppler and/or jugular bulb, monitoring hyperventilation aiming at pCO$_2$ 4.0–4.5 kPa should be applied. The body temperature should be normal, and pyrexia should be treated aggressively with paracetamol and, if necessary, by external cooling of the patient. Induced hypothermia should be avoided because of increased risk of fatal outcome [87]. In cases with therapy-resistant increased intracranial pressure, deep sedation with Pentothal may be indicated to lower the cerebral metabolism. This latter treatment requires continuous EEG registration and microdialysis analyses. A very aggressive course of bacterial meningitis with fatal outcome within 24–72 h has been observed [36, 88–90]. In these cases the brain edema may be extremely massive risking development of compressed ventricles ("slit ventricles") when an external ventricular catheter is inserted. A few case reports suggest that a decompressive craniectomy may be considered early in the course of disease in such cases [91–93].

Follow-Up

All patients with community-acquired acute bacterial meningitis should be followed up for at least 2–6 months to assess hearing, neurologic, and neurocognitive deficits and to administer vaccination against *Streptococcus pneumoniae*.

At discharge the patients should be informed about risks for sequelae and that the convalescence period can be long but that the long-term prognosis is relatively good. At least 2–4 weeks of sick leave, or corresponding rest, should be recommended routinely. A cochlear implant should be considered within 2–3 weeks if severe hearing deficit or deafness is noticed during the hospital stay. Audiometry should be performed if any clinical signs on impaired hearing ability are noticed. At the follow-up visit, a possible immune deficiency should be considered and appropriate investigations performed accordingly. A neuropsychiatric rehabilitation may be indicated in cases with persistent fatigue, concentration disability, or other neurologic deficits.

Research Gaps and Future Directions

Community-acquired acute bacterial meningitis still remains a challenge for the physicians because of a high mortality and risk for persisting neurologic deficits despite adequate antibiotics, corticosteroids, and intensive care. At least four research fields can be considered very important for avoiding or improving outcome in bacterial meningitis: (1) immunization programs, (2) emerging resistant bacteria, (3) delayed adequate treatment, and (4) adjuvant treatment modalities.

1. Immunization programs: Implementation of vaccines against *Haemophilus influenza* type B, *Streptococcus pneumonia*, and *Neisseria meningitides* has decreased the burden of bacterial meningitis in children. The cost-effectiveness of routine immunization with the new vaccine against meningococci serotype B should be evaluated. Regarding pneumococci, the long-term effect in children and the effect in adults of routine vaccination of children are as yet unknown. The risk of serotype replacement among pneumococci must be considered, and further studies to elucidate this problem are needed.
2. Emerging resistant bacteria: During recent year multidrug-resistant pneumococci have emerged in many countries which complicates the treatment considerably. Development of new antibiotics active against these resistant bacteria is vital for improvement of the outcome in bacterial meningitis.
3. Delayed adequate treatment: Far too many cerebral CT scans are performed before lumbar puncture today which is associated with a considerable treatment delay and increased mortality. Thus, an unjustified fear of performing prompt lumbar puncture still exists which is associated with poor outcome in bacterial meningitis. Further studies, in humans as well as in animals, to elucidate the potential risks vs. safety with lumbar puncture are desirable.
4. Adjuvant treatment modalities: Further studies to evaluate different methods to decrease the raised intracranial pressure and improve the cerebral perfusion are most desirable. Cerebrospinal fluid drainage by a ventricular catheter as well as lumbar drainage, which can be performed in resource-poor settings, should be evaluated. Different osmotic therapies and management modulating the inflammatory activity in order to decrease the intracranial pressure should be studied.

References

1. Glimaker M, Johansson B, Grindborg O, Bottai M, Lindquist L, Sjolin J. Adult bacterial meningitis: earlier treatment and improved outcome following guideline revision promoting prompt lumbar puncture. Clin Infect Dis. 2015;60(8):1162–9.
2. Koster-Rasmussen R, Korshin A, Meyer CN. Antibiotic treatment delay and outcome in acute bacterial meningitis. J Infect. 2008;57(6):449–54.
3. Thigpen MC, Whitney CG, Messonnier NE, et al. Bacterial meningitis in the United States, 1998-2007. N Engl J Med. 2011;364(21):2016–25.
4. van de Beek D, de Gans J, Spanjaard L, Weisfelt M, Reitsma JB, Vermeulen M. Clinical features and prognostic factors in adults with bacterial meningitis. N Engl J Med. 2004;351(18):1849–59.
5. van Ettekoven CN, van de Beek D, Brouwer MC. Update on community-acquired bacterial meningitis: guidance and challenges. Clin Microbiol Infect. 2017;23(9):601–6.
6. Polkowska A, Toropainen M, Ollgren J, Lyytikainen O, Nuorti JP. Bacterial meningitis in Finland, 1995-2014: a population-based observational study. BMJ Open. 2017;7(5):e015080.
7. De Gaudio M, Chiappini E, Galli L, De Martino M. Therapeutic management of bacterial meningitis in children: a systematic review and comparison of published guidelines from a European perspective. J Chemother. 2010;22(4):226–37.
8. Ouchenir L, Renaud C, Khan S, et al. The epidemiology, management, and outcomes of bacterial meningitis in infants. Pediatrics. 2017;140(1):e20170476.
9. Joubrel C, Tazi A, Six A, et al. Group B streptococcus neonatal invasive infections, France 2007-2012. Clin Microbiol Infect. 2015;21(10):910–6.
10. Weisfelt M, van de Beek D, Spanjaard L, Reitsma JB, de Gans J. Community-acquired bacterial meningitis in older people. J Am Geriatr Soc. 2006;54(10):1500–7.
11. Koopmans MM, Bijlsma MW, Brouwer MC, van de Beek D, van der Ende A. Listeria monocytogenes meningitis in the Netherlands, 1985-2014: a nationwide surveillance study. J Infect. 2017;75(1):12–9.
12. Perera N, Abulhoul L, Green MR, Swann RA. Group A streptococcal meningitis: case report and review of the literature. J Infect. 2005;51(2):E1–4.
13. Aguilar J, Urday-Cornejo V, Donabedian S, Perri M, Tibbetts R, Zervos M. Staphylococcus aureus meningitis: case series and literature review. Medicine (Baltimore). 2010;89(2):117–25.
14. Doran KS, Fulde M, Gratz N, et al. Host-pathogen interactions in bacterial meningitis. Acta Neuropathol. 2016;131(2):185–209.
15. Edberg M, Furebring M, Sjolin J, Enblad P. Neurointensive care of patients with severe community-acquired meningitis. Acta Anaesthesiol Scand. 2011;55(6):732–9.
16. Grände PO, Myhre EB, Nordström CH, Schliamser S. Treatment of intracranial hypertension and aspects on lumbar dural puncture in severe bacterial meningitis. Acta Anaesthesiol Scand. 2002;46(3):264–70.
17. Lindvall P, Ahlm C, Ericsson M, Gothefors L, Naredi S, Koskinen LO. Reducing intracranial pressure may increase survival among patients with bacterial meningitis. Clin Infect Dis. 2004;38(3):384–90.
18. Durand ML, Calderwood SB, Weber DJ, et al. Acute bacterial meningitis in adults. A review of 493 episodes. N Engl J Med. 1993;328(1):21–8.
19. Horwitz SJ, Boxerbaum B, O'Bell J. Cerebral herniation in bacterial meningitis in childhood. Ann Neurol. 1980;7(6):524–8.
20. Kramer AH, Bleck TP. Neurocritical care of patients with central nervous system infections. Curr Treat Options Neurol. 2008;10(3):201–11.
21. Glimaker M, Johansson B, Halldorsdottir H, et al. Neuro-intensive treatment targeting intracranial hypertension improves outcome in severe bacterial meningitis: an intervention-control study. PLoS One. 2014;9(3):e91976.
22. Leib SL, Tauber MG. Pathogenesis of bacterial meningitis. Infect Dis Clin N Am. 1999;13(3):527–48, v–vi.

23. Scheld WM, Koedel U, Nathan B, Pfister HW. Pathophysiology of bacterial meningitis: mechanism(s) of neuronal injury. J Infect Dis. 2002;186(Suppl 2):S225–33.
24. Helweg-Larsen J, Astradsson A, Richhall H, Erdal J, Laursen A, Brennum J. Pyogenic brain abscess, a 15 year survey. BMC Infect Dis. 2012;12:332.
25. Schliamser SE, Bäckman K, Norrby SR. Intracranial abscesses in adults: an analysis of 54 consecutive cases. Scand J Infect Dis. 1988;20(1):1–9.
26. Jaijakul S, Arias CA, Hossain M, Arduino RC, Wootton SH, Hasbun R. Toscana meningoencephalitis: a comparison to other viral central nervous system infections. J Clin Virol. 2012;55(3):204–8.
27. Best J, Hughes S. Evidence behind the WHO Guidelines: hospital care for children – what are the useful clinical features of bacterial meningitis found in infants and children? J Trop Pediatr. 2008;54(2):83–6.
28. McGill F, Heyderman RS, Michael BD, et al. The UK joint specialist societies guideline on the diagnosis and management of acute meningitis and meningococcal sepsis in immunocompetent adults. J Infect. 2016;72(4):405–38.
29. Tunkel AR, Hartman BJ, Kaplan SL, et al. Practice guidelines for the management of bacterial meningitis. Clin Infect Dis. 2004;39(9):1267–84.
30. van de Beek D, Cabellos C, Dzupova O, et al. ESCMID guideline: diagnosis and treatment of acute bacterial meningitis. Clin Microbiol Infect. 2016;22(Suppl 3):S37–62.
31. Khumalo J, Nicol M, Hardie D, Muloiwa R, Mteshana P, Bamford C. Diagnostic accuracy of two multiplex real-time polymerase chain reaction assays for the diagnosis of meningitis in children in a resource-limited setting. PLoS One. 2017;12(3):e0173948.
32. Leber AL, Everhart K, Balada-Llasat JM, et al. Multicenter evaluation of BioFire FilmArray meningitis/encephalitis panel for detection of bacteria, viruses, and yeast in cerebrospinal fluid specimens. J Clin Microbiol. 2016;54(9):2251–61.
33. Brouwer MC, Thwaites GE, Tunkel AR, van de Beek D. Dilemmas in the diagnosis of acute community-acquired bacterial meningitis. Lancet. 2012;380(9854):1684–92.
34. Glimaker M, Johansson B, Bell M, et al. Early lumbar puncture in adult bacterial meningitis-rationale for revised guidelines. Scand J Infect Dis. 2013;45(9):657–63.
35. Joffe AR. Lumbar puncture and brain herniation in acute bacterial meningitis: a review. J Intensive Care Med. 2007;22(4):194–207.
36. Radetsky M. Fulminant bacterial meningitis. Pediatr Infect Dis J. 2014;33(2):204–7.
37. Kastenbauer S, Winkler F, Pfister HW. Cranial CT before lumbar puncture in suspected meningitis. N Engl J Med. 2002;346(16):1248–51. author reply -51.
38. van Crevel H, Hijdra A, de Gans J. Lumbar puncture and the risk of herniation: when should we first perform CT? J Neurol. 2002;249(2):129–37.
39. Costerus JM, Brouwer MC, van der Ende A, van de Beek D. Community-acquired bacterial meningitis in adults with cancer or a history of cancer. Neurology. 2016;86(9):860–6.
40. Salazar L, Hasbun R. Cranial imaging before lumbar puncture in adults with community-acquired meningitis: clinical utility and adherence to the Infectious Diseases Society of America guidelines. Clin Infect Dis. 2017;64(12):1657–62.
41. Costerus JM, Brouwer MC, Bijlsma MW, Tanck MW, van der Ende A, van de Beek D. Impact of an evidence-based guideline on the management of community-acquired bacterial meningitis: a prospective cohort study. Clin Microbiol Infect. 2016;22(11):928–33.
42. Proulx N, Fréchette D, Toye B, Chan J, Kravcik S. Delays in the administration of antibiotics are associated with mortality from adult acute bacterial meningitis. QJM. 2005;98(4):291–8.
43. Aronin SI, Peduzzi P, Quagliarello VJ. Community-acquired bacterial meningitis: risk stratification for adverse clinical outcome and effect of antibiotic timing. Ann Intern Med. 1998;129(11):862–9.
44. Hasbun R, Abrahams J, Jekel J, Quagliarello VJ. Computed tomography of the head before lumbar puncture in adults with suspected meningitis. N Engl J Med. 2001;345(24):1727–33.
45. Kanegaye JT, Soliemanzadeh P, Bradley JS. Lumbar puncture in pediatric bacterial meningitis: defining the time interval for recovery of cerebrospinal fluid pathogens after parenteral antibiotic pretreatment. Pediatrics. 2001;108(5):1169–74.

46. Michael B, Menezes BF, Cunniffe J, et al. Effect of delayed lumbar punctures on the diagnosis of acute bacterial meningitis in adults. Emerg Med J. 2010;27(6):433–8.
47. Prasad K, Singhal T, Jain N, Gupta PK. Third generation cephalosporins versus conventional antibiotics for treating acute bacterial meningitis. Cochrane Database Syst Rev. 2004;(2):Cd001832.
48. Lebel MH, Hoyt MJ, McCracken GH Jr. Comparative efficacy of ceftriaxone and cefuroxime for treatment of bacterial meningitis. J Pediatr. 1989;114(6):1049–54.
49. Peltola H, Anttila M, Renkonen OV. Randomised comparison of chloramphenicol, ampicillin, cefotaxime, and ceftriaxone for childhood bacterial meningitis. Finnish Study Group. Lancet. 1989;1(8650):1281–7.
50. del Rio MA, Chrane D, Shelton S, McCracken GH Jr, Nelson JD. Ceftriaxone versus ampicillin and chloramphenicol for treatment of bacterial meningitis in children. Lancet. 1983;1(8336):1241–4.
51. Odio CM, Faingezicht I, Salas JL, Guevara J, Mohs E, McCracken GH Jr. Cefotaxime vs. conventional therapy for the treatment of bacterial meningitis of infants and children. Pediatr Infect Dis. 1986;5(4):402–7.
52. Schaad UB, Suter S, Gianella-Borradori A, et al. A comparison of ceftriaxone and cefuroxime for the treatment of bacterial meningitis in children. N Engl J Med. 1990;322(3):141–7.
53. Klugman KP, Dagan R. Randomized comparison of meropenem with cefotaxime for treatment of bacterial meningitis. Meropenem Meningitis Study Group. Antimicrob Agents Chemother. 1995;39(5):1140–6.
54. Saez-Llorens X, Castano E, Garcia R, et al. Prospective randomized comparison of cefepime and cefotaxime for treatment of bacterial meningitis in infants and children. Antimicrob Agents Chemother. 1995;39(4):937–40.
55. Schmutzhard E, Williams KJ, Vukmirovits G, Chmelik V, Pfausler B, Featherstone A. A randomised comparison of meropenem with cefotaxime or ceftriaxone for the treatment of bacterial meningitis in adults. Meropenem Meningitis Study Group. J Antimicrob Chemother. 1995;36(Suppl A):85–97.
56. Scholz H, Hofmann T, Noack R, Edwards DJ, Stoeckel K. Prospective comparison of ceftriaxone and cefotaxime for the short-term treatment of bacterial meningitis in children. Chemotherapy. 1998;44(2):142–7.
57. Odio CM, Puig JR, Feris JM, et al. Prospective, randomized, investigator-blinded study of the efficacy and safety of meropenem vs. cefotaxime therapy in bacterial meningitis in children. Meropenem Meningitis Study Group. Pediatr Infect Dis J. 1999;18(7):581–90.
58. Saez-Llorens X, McCoig C, Feris JM, et al. Quinolone treatment for pediatric bacterial meningitis: a comparative study of trovafloxacin and ceftriaxone with or without vancomycin. Pediatr Infect Dis J. 2002;21(1):14–22.
59. Baldwin CM, Lyseng-Williamson KA, Keam SJ. Meropenem: a review of its use in the treatment of serious bacterial infections. Drugs. 2008;68(6):803–38.
60. Ntziora F, Falagas ME. Linezolid for the treatment of patients with central nervous system infection. Ann Pharmacother. 2007;41(2):296–308.
61. Cottagnoud PH, Tauber MG. New therapies for pneumococcal meningitis. Expert Opin Investig Drugs. 2004;13(4):393–401.
62. Nau R, Djukic M, Spreer A, Ribes S, Eiffert H. Bacterial meningitis: an update of new treatment options. Expert Rev Anti-Infect Ther. 2015;13(11):1401–23.
63. Bretonniere C, Jozwiak M, Girault C, et al. Rifampin use in acute community-acquired meningitis in intensive care units: the French retrospective cohort ACAM-ICU study. Crit Care. 2015;19:303.
64. Tauber MG, Khayam-Bashi H, Sande MA. Effects of ampicillin and corticosteroids on brain water content, cerebrospinal fluid pressure, and cerebrospinal fluid lactate levels in experimental pneumococcal meningitis. J Infect Dis. 1985;151(3):528–34.
65. Brouwer MC, McIntyre P, Prasad K, van de Beek D. Corticosteroids for acute bacterial meningitis. Cochrane Database Syst Rev. 2015;(9):CD004405.
66. de Gans J, van de Beek D, European Dexamethasone in Adulthood Bacterial Meningitis Study I. Dexamethasone in adults with bacterial meningitis. N Engl J Med. 2002;347(20):1549–56.

67. Molyneux EM, Walsh AL, Forsyth H, et al. Dexamethasone treatment in childhood bacterial meningitis in Malawi: a randomised controlled trial. Lancet. 2002;360(9328):211–8.
68. Nguyen TH, Tran TH, Thwaites G, et al. Dexamethasone in Vietnamese adolescents and adults with bacterial meningitis. N Engl J Med. 2007;357(24):2431–40.
69. Peltola H, Roine I, Fernandez J, et al. Adjuvant glycerol and/or dexamethasone to improve the outcomes of childhood bacterial meningitis: a prospective, randomized, double-blind, placebo-controlled trial. Clin Infect Dis. 2007;45(10):1277–86.
70. Scarborough M, Gordon SB, Whitty CJ, et al. Corticosteroids for bacterial meningitis in adults in sub-Saharan Africa. N Engl J Med. 2007;357(24):2441–50.
71. McIntyre PB, Berkey CS, King SM, et al. Dexamethasone as adjunctive therapy in bacterial meningitis. A meta-analysis of randomized clinical trials since 1988. JAMA. 1997;278(11):925–31.
72. Glimaker M, Brink M, Naucler P, Sjolin J. Betamethasone and dexamethasone in adult community-acquired bacterial meningitis: a quality registry study from 1995 to 2014. Clin Microbiol Infect. 2016;22(9):814 e1–7.
73. Costerus JM, Brouwer MC, van der Ende A, van de Beek D. Repeat lumbar puncture in adults with bacterial meningitis. Clin Microbiol Infect. 2016;22(5):428–33.
74. Bijlsma MW, Brouwer MC, Kasanmoentalib ES, et al. Community-acquired bacterial meningitis in adults in the Netherlands, 2006-14: a prospective cohort study. Lancet Infect Dis. 2016;16(3):339–47.
75. Heckenberg SG, Brouwer MC, van der Ende A, van de Beek D. Adjunctive dexamethasone in adults with meningococcal meningitis. Neurology. 2012;79(15):1563–9.
76. Ogunlesi TA, Odigwe CC, Oladapo OT. Adjuvant corticosteroids for reducing death in neonatal bacterial meningitis. Cochrane Database Syst Rev. 2015;(11):Cd010435.
77. Syrogiannopoulos GA, Lourida AN, Theodoridou MC, et al. Dexamethasone therapy for bacterial meningitis in children: 2- versus 4-day regimen. J Infect Dis. 1994;169(4):853–8.
78. Schutte CM, van der Meyden CH. A prospective study of Glasgow Coma Scale (GCS), age, CSF-neutrophil count, and CSF-protein and glucose levels as prognostic indicators in 100 adult patients with meningitis. J Infect. 1998;37(2):112–5.
79. Merkelbach S, Rohn S, Konig J, Muller M. Usefulness of clinical scores to predict outcome in bacterial meningitis. Infection. 1999;27(4–5):239–43.
80. van de Beek D, de Gans J, Tunkel AR, Wijdicks EFM. Community-acquired bacterial meningitis in adults. N Engl J Med. 2006;354(1):44–53.
81. van de Beek D, Brouwer MC, Thwaites GE, Tunkel AR. Advances in treatment of bacterial meningitis. Lancet. 2012;380(9854):1693–702.
82. Abulhasan YB, Al-Jehani H, Valiquette MA, et al. Lumbar drainage for the treatment of severe bacterial meningitis. Neurocrit Care. 2013;19(2):199–205.
83. Ajdukiewicz KM, Cartwright KE, Scarborough M, et al. Glycerol adjuvant therapy in adults with bacterial meningitis in a high HIV seroprevalence setting in Malawi: a double-blind, randomised controlled trial. Lancet Infect Dis. 2011;11(4):293–300.
84. Larsen L, Poulsen FR, Nielsen TH, Nordstrom CH, Schulz MK, Andersen AB. Use of intracranial pressure monitoring in bacterial meningitis: a 10-year follow up on outcome and intracranial pressure versus head CT scans. Infect Dis (Lond). 2017;49(5):356–64.
85. Bartek J Jr, Thelin EP, Ghatan PH, Glimaker M, Bellander BM. Neuron-specific enolase is correlated to compromised cerebral metabolism in patients suffering from acute bacterial meningitis; an observational cohort study. PLoS One. 2016;11(3):e0152268.
86. Grande PO, Romner B. Osmotherapy in brain edema: a questionable therapy. J Neurosurg Anesthesiol. 2012;24(4):407–12.
87. Mourvillier B, Tubach F, van de Beek D, et al. Induced hypothermia in severe bacterial meningitis: a randomized clinical trial. JAMA. 2013;310(20):2174–83.
88. Rennick G, Shann F, de Campo J. Cerebral herniation during bacterial meningitis in children. BMJ. 1993;306(6883):953–5.

89. Akpede GO, Ambe JP. Cerebral herniation in pyogenic meningitis: prevalence and related dilemmas in emergency room populations in developing countries. Dev Med Child Neurol. 2000;42(7):462–9.
90. Winkler F, Kastenbauer S, Yousry TA, Maerz U, Pfister H-W. Discrepancies between brain CT imaging and severely raised intracranial pressure proven by ventriculostomy in adults with pneumococcal meningitis. J Neurol. 2002;249(9):1292–7.
91. Baussart B, Cheisson G, Compain M, et al. Multimodal cerebral monitoring and decompressive surgery for the treatment of severe bacterial meningitis with increased intracranial pressure. Acta Anaesthesiol Scand. 2006;50(6):762–5.
92. Perin A, Nascimben E, Longatti P. Decompressive craniectomy in a case of intractable intracranial hypertension due to pneumococcal meningitis. Acta Neurochir. 2008;150(8):837–42. Discussion 42.
93. Bordes J, Boret H, Lacroix G, Prunet B, Meaudre E, Kaiser E. Decompressive craniectomy guided by cerebral microdialysis and brain tissue oxygenation in a patient with meningitis. Acta Anaesthesiol Scand. 2011;55(1):130–3.

Healthcare-Acquired Meningitis and Ventriculitis

3

Tricia Bravo and Adarsh Bhimraj

Introduction

Healthcare-associated meningitis and ventriculitis encompass infections that occur after neurosurgery and spine and otorhinological surgeries where there is dural breach, trauma, and cerebrospinal fluid (CSF) shunt and CSF drain placement and, rarely, infections that occur after lumbar puncture.

CSF shunts are permanent catheters that connect the proximal end (cerebral ventricle or lumbar subarachnoid space) to the distal end located in the peritoneal cavity, the pleural cavity, or the right atrium of the heart. Ventriculoperitoneal (VP) shunts are the most common type of shunt. They require fewer revisions, are easier to implant and revise, and have less serious complications compared to ventriculoatrial (VA) shunts, which terminate in the right atrium [1].

CSF drains, on the other hand, are temporary catheters that act as conduits for external drainage. The proximal end can be located in the cerebral ventricle, the subdural space, an intracranial cyst, or the lumbar subarachnoid space. These drains are connected to a collecting system, which has a drip chamber, ports for intracranial pressure monitoring, sampling and injection ports, and a collection bag. An external ventricular drain, with its proximal end placed in the cerebral ventricle, is used to relieve increased intracranial pressure from acute hydrocephalus caused by intracranial hemorrhage, neoplasms, or trauma. External lumbar drains, which drain the lumbar subarachnoid space, are most often used in the management of operative or post-traumatic CSF leak or in the evaluation of normal pressure hydrocephalus [1].

Both CSF shunts and CSF drains can lead to infection. VP shunt infections can be superficial, involving the skin and subcutaneous tissue surrounding the proximal aspect of the shunt, or can be more invasive, involving the cerebral ventricle or the

T. Bravo · A. Bhimraj (✉)
Section of Neurologic Infectious Diseases, Department of Infectious Diseases,
Cleveland Clinic Foundation, Cleveland, OH, USA
e-mail: bravot@ccf.org; bhimraa@ccf.org

© Springer International Publishing AG, part of Springer Nature 2018
R. Hasbun (ed.), *Meningitis and Encephalitis*,
https://doi.org/10.1007/978-3-319-92678-0_3

peritoneum. CSF drain infections can present as tunnel infections, catheter exit site infections, or ventriculitis. Post-neurosurgical or post-craniotomy infections, based on anatomical involvement, can present as superficial wound infections of the skin, meningitis, empyemas in the epidural or subdural space, parenchymal abscesses, and osteomyelitis of the bone flap.

Epidemiology

The incidence of CSF shunt infections reported in the literature has a wide range (4–17%), but in most studies rates are around 10% [1, 2]. Reported ventricular drain infection rates were also around 10% [3]. In a large meta-analysis of 35 studies which yielded 752 infections from 66,706 catheter days of observation, the overall pooled incidence of external ventricular drain-related CSF infection was 11.4 per 1000 catheter days (95% CI 9.3–13.5); for high-quality studies, the incidence was 10.6 per 1000 catheter days (95% CI 8.3–13) [4]. Infection rates due to lumbar drains are 4.2% [5].

Pathogenesis and Microbiology

The specific causative microorganisms for healthcare-related meningitis or ventriculitis depend on the pathogenesis and the timing of the infection after the predisposing event. During these surgeries, the skull and meninges, which act as natural barriers to pathogens, are breached, making it possible for microorganisms that colonize the scalp and skin of the back, or those that live in the healthcare environment, to enter the subarachnoid space or cerebral ventricles and cause an infection. In patients with ventriculoperitoneal shunts, another less common route by which organisms enter the ventricles is spreading up along the catheter after a peritonitis. On the surface of catheters, these organisms can form biofilms, which are thick sticky polysaccharide layers making them resistant to antimicrobial action [6, 7]. The organisms that usually colonize the skin, especially the scalp, are coagulase-negative *Staphylococcus*, *Staphylococcus aureus*, and *Cutibacterium acnes*, formerly *Propionibacterium acnes*. The organisms that can be present in the healthcare environment *are Staphylococcus aureus* (both methicillin-resistant and methicillin-susceptible strains) and gram-negative bacteria like *Escherichia coli*, *Klebsiella*, *Pseudomonas*, and *Acinetobacter* species (some of the strains can be multidrug resistant).

Staphylococcal species are the most common organisms causing infections, with *Staphylococcus epidermidis* (47–64% of infections) being more common than *Staphylococcus aureus* (12–29% of infections) [1, 3, 8]. Gram-negative bacteria account for 6–20% of the infections [1, 3, 8, 9]. Diphtheroids (especially *Cutibacterium acnes*) account for 1–14% of the infection, but the reason for the low reported rates of *C. acnes* infection in some studies is probably an inadequate culture technique. Anaerobic cultures with prolonged incubation are needed to detect *C. acnes*, but most microbiology labs only perform aerobic cultures and hold CSF cultures for 2–3 days [1–3, 10–12]. Fungi like *Candida*, though reported in the literature, are usually rare [13].

Clinical Presentation

The clinical presentation of healthcare-associated ventriculitis has a wide spectrum from being acute and severe, if caused by virulent organisms like *Staphylococcus aureus* or gram-negative bacteria, to more subtle and chronic, if due to less virulent organisms. Unlike organisms that cause community-acquired bacterial meningitis, those causing CSF catheter-associated ventriculitis, like coagulase-negative *Staphylococci* and *C. acnes*, are indolent, evoke minimal inflammation, and are usually pathogenic in the presence of prosthetic material [6, 7]. Often there may be ventriculitis without meningeal involvement or only mechanical blockage as a result of biofilm formation in or on the catheter, without significant inflammation [14]. In CSF shunt infections, fever can be present only in about half the time (52%) [15]. Headaches (31%) and changes in mental status (29%) can be present less than half the time [15]. Meningismus is rarely found (4%) [15] in these patients, and this is probably because this is mostly a ventriculitis than a meningitis.

Clinical signs and symptoms are even less reliable in ventricular and lumbar drain-related ventriculitis as symptoms like change in mental status, fever, or meningismus could be a manifestation of other neurologic diseases like intracranial hemorrhage or hydrocephalus from other causes. Fever in a patient in the neurocritical care unit can be due to intracranial hemorrhage, central fever, thrombotic episodes, and drug fevers [16] in addition to non-CNS infections like bloodstream infections, hospital-acquired pneumonias, and urinary tract infections.

Blood Tests (WBC Count, C-Reactive Protein, and Procalcitonin)

There are many but suboptimal studies on blood or serum markers like procalcitonin, C-reactive protein (CRP), and peripheral white blood cell counts in patients with healthcare-associated ventriculitis. In a prospective study which recruited consecutive patients with ventricular drains, those with proven bacterial ventriculitis had significantly higher procalcitonin levels (4.7 ± 1.0 vs. 0.2 ± 0.01 ng/mL, $p < 0.0001$), CRP levels (134 ± 29 vs. 51 ± 4 mg/L, $p = 0.0005$), and peripheral white blood cell counts (16.1 ± 1.3 vs. 10.7 ± 0.3 109/L, $p = 0.0008$) [17]. In Martinez et al.'s study, a procalcitonin cutoff value of 1.0 ng/mL or more showed a specificity of 77% and a sensitivity of only 68% for ventriculitis, though it had better diagnostic accuracy in community-acquired bacterial meningitis [18]. In another study in children with suspected CSF shunt infections, the values for serum CRP in infected individuals were higher than in noninfected ones (91.8 ± 70.2 mg/L compared with 16.1 ± 28.3 mg/L, $p < 0.0001$) [19]. Despite the statistically significant p values in some studies, the confidence intervals for calculated sensitivities, based on traditional cutoffs, are wide. Though these markers are easy to obtain and are often presumed to be sensitive indicators of infections, we need further well-designed prospective studies to recommend their routine use in ruling out healthcare-associated ventriculitis, especially in infections with indolent organisms which cause minimal inflammation.

CSF Cell Count and Chemistry (Glucose, Protein, Lactate, and Procalcitonin)

The diagnostic accuracy of CSF markers in healthcare-associated ventriculitis has been evaluated in several studies. Like the blood marker studies, they have design and methodological limitations. One of the major limitations in interpreting these studies is the heterogeneous definition of the reference (gold) standard for the diagnosis of healthcare-associated ventriculitis. To evaluate the diagnostic utility of CSF parameters or any other test, an independent comparison to an acceptable reference standard is required. Often CSF cultures are used as a reference standard in many studies, but diagnosing ventriculitis by a single positive CSF culture will run the risk of a false-positive diagnosis due to colonization or contamination. More specific diagnostic criteria like the presence of multiple CSF cultures with CSF pleocytosis or hypoglycorrhachia with attributable clinical signs and symptoms (fever, headache, photophobia, neck stiffness, decreased level of consciousness) would be clinically meaningful, but using that as a reference standard to calculate diagnostic accuracy like sensitivity and specificity would be erroneous as they are part of the definition of the reference standard and are not statistically independent. There are studies that applied the existing heterogeneous definitions and criteria for ventricular drain-related meningitis and ventriculitis to the same cohort of patients. One of the studies found 16 unique definitions in the published literature. When the definitions were applied to the test cohort, the frequency of infection ranged from 22% to 94% (median 61% with interquartile range (IQR) 56–74%) [20].

In CSF drain-related ventriculitis, the diagnostic utility of CSF WBC count, glucose, and protein is limited, as noninfectious entities like intracranial hemorrhage and neurosurgical procedures can also cause abnormalities in these parameters. Schade et al. [21] performed a prospective study in a cohort of 230 consecutive patients with ventricular drains. Results from analyses of 1516 CSF samples showed no significant differences between the patients with EVD-related ventriculitis and a control group without EVD-related meningitis, with regard to CSF leukocyte count, protein concentration, glucose concentration, and CSF/blood glucose ratio. They evaluated the predictive and diagnostic value of the CSF parameters. For none of the routine CSF parameters could they establish a cutoff value with a sensitivity and specificity of at least 60%. Pfisterer et al. [22] conducted a 3-year prospective study in patients with ventricular drains. Standard laboratory parameters, such as peripheral leukocyte count, CSF glucose, and CSF protein, were not reliable predictors for incipient ventricular catheter infection. The only parameter that significantly correlated with the occurrence of a positive CSF culture was an elevated CSF leukocyte count (unpaired t test, $p < 0.05$). In a prospective study, Pfausler et al. [23] looked at the utility of cell index (CI), which is the ratio of leukocytes to erythrocytes in CSF and leukocytes to erythrocytes in peripheral blood, in predicting ventriculitis. The study was done in patients with intraventricular hemorrhage who had external ventricular drains. Diagnosis of bacterial ventriculitis by CI was possible up to 3 days prior to "conventional diagnosis" which was described as rise of CSF cell count, reduction of CSF/serum glucose, or a positive CSF culture. There are few studies that evaluated the diagnostic utility of CSF lactate in CSF drain-related ventriculitis. In a prospective study of ventricular drain-related ventriculitis, a CSF lactate cutoff value of 4 mmol/L had a sensitivity of 86%, specificity of 86%, positive likelihood ratio of 6.1, and a negative likelihood ratio of 0.16 [24].

There are few studies evaluating the diagnostic accuracy of CSF parameters in CSF shunt infections. In a retrospective study which compared children with VP shunt infection ($n = 10$) to controls ($n = 129$), a CSF leukocyte count over 100/mm^3 had a 96% specificity and 60% sensitivity. The CSF glucose of <40 mg/dL had a 93% specificity and 60% sensitivity. The reference standard (shunt infection) in this study was defined as "clinical signs and symptoms with a positive CSF culture" [25]. Often, less virulent organisms *like Staphylococcus epidermidis* and *C. acnes* might not cause significant inflammation, so a lower cutoff for CSF leukocyte count would have probably increased the sensitivity but that was not addressed in this study. However, CSF shunt infections can present with no CSF pleocytosis at times. In a retrospective analysis of CSF shunt infections in adults, the CSF white blood cell counts and lactate concentrations were normal in approximately 20% of episodes [14]. The CSF parameter values might significantly differ depending on the site from which the CSF is obtained. In one study the leukocyte counts were significantly higher in CSF obtained by the use of lumbar puncture (median leukocyte count, 573 × 10(6) cells/L; $p = 0.001$) and valve puncture (median leukocyte count, 484 × 10(6) cells/L; $p = 0.016$) than in ventricular CSF (median leukocyte count, 8.5 × 10(6) cells/L) [14]. The site of sampling should be considered when interpreting the values as the CSF pleocytosis from ventricular fluid might not be very high even in patients with CSF shunt-related ventriculitis.

There are few studies on the diagnostic accuracy of CSF parameters in post-neurosurgical meningitis and ventriculitis. Often the surgery itself can cause "chemical meningitis" or postoperative meningitis, particularly posterior fossa surgeries. The CSF leukocyte and CSF glucose values can look very similar to infectious meningitis, making it hard to distinguish these entities based on these parameters. In one study only extreme values of CSF leukocyte count >7500/μL (7500 × 10(6)/L) and a glucose level of <10 mg/dL were able to distinguish post-neurosurgical chemical meningitis from bacterial meningitis [26]. Another caveat in post-neurosurgical patients is that the CSF pleocytosis and low CSF glucose might be a result of a bone flap infection, a subgaleal infection, or a deeper infection in the surgical bed-like cerebritis or brain abscess. CSF lactates have shown to perform better in post-neurosurgical meningitis, and CSF procalcitonin have not been well studied. A recent meta-analysis of five studies evaluating CSF lactate in post-neurosurgical meningitis, with a total of 404 patients, showed a pooled sensitivity of 0.92 (95% CI 0.85–0.96) and a pooled specificity of 0.88 (95% CI 0.84–0.92 with significant heterogeneity [27]. In another retrospective study, patients with post-neurosurgical meningitis showed significantly elevated levels of CSF procalcitonin and CSF lactate compared with the non-meningitis group ($p < 0.001$ for both). For CSF procalcitonin, a cutoff value of 0.075 ng/Ml had a sensitivity of 68% and specificity of 73%. For CSF lactate a cutoff value of 3.45 mmol/L had a sensitivity of 90% and specificity of 85% [28].

CSF Microbiology Studies

CSF cultures are traditionally considered the reference standard for the diagnosis of meningitis and ventriculitis. In the context of community-acquired bacterial meningitis, positive CSF cultures for pathogenic organisms like pneumococcus or meningococcus are highly suggestive of meningitis. In the context of healthcare-associated meningitis, the common pathogenic organisms like *S. epidermidis and C. acnes* are skin colonizers, and the possibility of contamination during specimen collection should be considered. Unlike organisms that cause acute community-acquired meningitis, those causing healthcare-associated meningitis are slow to grow on cultures and require anaerobic media. In a study on healthcare-associated ventriculitis and meningitis, a substantial number of positive CSF specimens grew bacteria after >3 days, with some requiring as long as 10 days [29].

The site of specimen collection for microbiology studies is also important, particularly for CSF shunt infections. The site of CSF collection for ventricular catheter infection is generally ventricular fluid, for LP shunts is lumbar subarachnoid fluid, and for post-craniotomy infections is either lumbar subarachnoid fluid or intraoperative ventricular fluid and tissue cultures. For VP shunt infections, the options are CSF by a lumbar puncture, from a "shunt tap" (percutaneous accessing of the shunt reservoir underneath the scalp), or rarely intraoperatively during shunt surgery. In VP shunt infection studies, direct aspiration of the shunt yielded a positive culture in 91–92%, whereas a lumbar puncture CSF culture was positive in only around 45–67% [14, 30]. There is a fear of causing a shunt infection by tapping it, but in a pediatric study with 266 children who underwent 542 shunt taps, there was no evidence of shunt infections. One patient developed an infection after a tap, but there was redness over the shunt tract at the time of the tap, so was not sterile [31].

CSF polymerase chain reaction (PCR) can prove useful to detect organisms that are difficult or slow to grow by culture. In a study that used PCR to detect grampositive bacteria in 86 specimens, 42 were culture negative but PCR positive [32]. There were no positive culture results in patients with a negative CSF PCR, suggesting that a negative PCR result is predictive of the absence of infection. More studies are needed, however, before routine use of PCR can be recommended in this setting.

Diagnostic Approach

Based on the above studies, symptoms, signs, blood tests, and CSF tests have limitations in making the diagnosis of healthcare-associated ventriculitis. There exist many imperfect diagnostic criteria in the literature, especially as cutoffs for CSF parameters to distinguish chemical from infectious ventriculitis are arbitrary. The approach outlined here is based on our clinical experience alone.

CSF Drain-Related Ventriculitis

Lozier et al. [33] proposed a classification system for ventriculitis with a hierarchy based on suspected probability of infection. The diagnostic classification proposed here is a modification of that. In addition to being clinically helpful for deciding when to use antimicrobials, such classification would hopefully establish standard criteria for future research and epidemiological purposes. We have used CSF parameter criteria (the rate of rise or degree of abnormality of inflammatory markers) with microbiologic criteria for the following classification:

Contamination: An isolated positive CSF culture or Gram stain, with expected CSF cell count and glucose with no attributable symptoms or signs

Colonization: Multiple positive CSF cultures or Gram stain, with expected CSF cell count and glucose with no attributable symptoms or signs

Possible ventriculitis: Progressive rise in cell index or progressive decrease in CSF/ blood glucose ratio or an extreme value for CSF WBC count (>1000/μL) or CSF/ blood glucose ratio (<0.2), with attributable symptoms or signs, but negative Gram stain and cultures

Probable ventriculitis: CSF WBC count or CSF/blood glucose ratio more abnormal than expected, but not an extreme value (CSF WBC count > 1000/μL or CSF/ blood glucose ratio < 0.2) and stable (not progressively worsening) with attributable symptoms or signs and positive Gram stain and cultures

Definitive ventriculitis: Progressive rise in cell index or progressive decrease in CSF/blood glucose ratio or an extreme value for CSF WBC count (>1000/μL) or CSF/blood glucose ratio (<0.2), with attributable symptoms or signs and a positive Gram stain and cultures

Contamination and colonization with skin colonizers generally do not need treatment. Antimicrobial treatment of contamination or colonization with virulent organisms is more controversial, but many clinicians might opt to treat positive CSF cultures for *Staphylococcus aureus* or gram-negative rods. Antimicrobial treatment of a possible ventriculitis should also be individualized depending on the circumstances, as at times chemical meningitis from subarachnoid hemorrhage or neurosurgery could cause extreme CSF pleocytosis or hypoglycorrhachia, which a clinician might prefer not to treat. On the other instance, it might be classified as a possible ventriculitis if the CSF cultures are negative due to prior antimicrobial use or if the organism is slow to grow, when one might chose to treat with antimicrobials. Probable and definitive ventriculitis would be treated with antimicrobials by most clinicians.

Post-neurosurgical Meningitis

Post-craniotomy meningitis can also be classified as possible, probable, and definitive meningitis using the above criteria as the confounding comorbidities and organism causing meningitis are similar to CSF drain infections.

CSF Shunt-Related Ventriculitis

A diagnosis of CSF shunt-related ventriculitis should be considered when the WBC count (from a shunt tap) is greater than 10/μL OR CSF/serum glucose ratio < 0.4 with a positive CSF culture and attributable symptoms. The reason for using such a low cutoff for WBC count is because most often indolent organisms evoke minimal inflammation, but the decision to treat based on this should be individualized.

Another instance would be when the WBC count and glucose values are normal, but there are multiple positive CSF cultures (from multiple shunt tap or explanted proximal shunt components) and attributable symptoms. CSF shunt infections can present as shunt blockage due to biofilms formed by organism without significant inflammation.

Approach to Management

Treatment of healthcare-associated ventriculitis is challenging as it is difficult to achieve high CSF antimicrobial levels with intravenous antimicrobials because of the blood-CSF barrier, especially when treating organisms like *Staphylococcus* spp. and gram-negative rods which tend to have high MICs (minimum inhibitory concentrations) for antimicrobials, making it harder to achieve therapeutically effective levels in the CSF. In addition to that these organisms often form biofilms on the catheters, which are mucoid layers into which antimicrobials do not penetrate well. This is especially an issue if the infected catheters are not removed. The below recommendations are based on limited clinical, pharmacokinetic, and pharmacodynamic studies.

Intravenous Antimicrobials

The recommendations for intravenous antimicrobials in patients with a normal renal clearance would be as follows:

Empiric Intravenous Antimicrobial Therapy
If ventriculitis is suspected, first, obtain CSF cultures, and then start empiric treatment with vancomycin (for gram-positive bacteria) as a continuous infusion or divided doses (2–3) of 60 mg/kg/day after a loading dose of 15 mg/kg with intravenous ceftazidime 2 g/8 h or cefepime 2 g/8 h (for gram-negative bacteria).

In a penicillin-allergic patient, start empiric coverage with intravenous vancomycin (same dose as above) and aztreonam 2 g/6 h.

Organism-Specific Intravenous Antimicrobial Therapy
The following antimicrobials can be started for specific organisms pending on antimicrobial susceptibilities, but knowledge of the local antibiogram and susceptibilities at each institution should direct therapy.

MRSA (methicillin-resistant *Staphylococcus aureus*) and MRSE (methicillin-resistant *Staphylococcus epidermidis*) with a vancomycin MIC ≤1 µg/Ml can be treated with vancomycin (same dose as above). If the catheter is retained, rifampin 300 mg IV q 12 h should be added.

MRSA and MRSE with a vancomycin MIC >1 µg/mL or for patient with vancomycin allergy can be treated with linezolid 600 mg IV or PO q 12 h.

Specific treatment for MSSA (methicillin-susceptible *Staphylococcus aureus*) and MSSE (methicillin-susceptible *Staphylococcus epidermidis*) is nafcillin or oxacillin 2 g IV q 4 h.

Specific treatment for *Cutibacterium acnes*, formerly *Propionibacterium acnes*, is penicillin G 2 MU IV q 4 h.

Specific treatment for *Pseudomonas spp.* is ceftazidime 2 g IV q 8 h or cefepime 2 g IV q 8 h or meropenem 2 g IV q 8 h.

Specific treatment for *E. coli* is ceftriaxone 2 g IV q 12 h or meropenem 2 g IV q 8 h; use meropenem if there are epidemiological risk factors for prior colonization or infection with ESBL (extended-spectrum beta-lactamase) producers.

Specific treatment for *Enterobacter spp.* or *Citrobacter spp.* is cefepime 2 g IV q 8 h or meropenem 2 g IV q 8 h.

Intraventricular Antimicrobials

Intraventricular or lumbar intrathecal administration of antimicrobials might be needed when patients do not respond satisfactorily to intravenous treatment or when organisms have high MICs to antimicrobials that do not penetrate the CSF well. This route of administration bypasses the blood-CSF barrier, with controlled delivery directly to the site of infection. CSF pharmacokinetic modeling studies [34–37] show that for most gram-negative bacteria if the MIC for some cephalosporins is greater than 0.5 µg/mL or for meropenem is greater than 0.25 µg/mL and for gram-positive bacteria if the MIC for vancomycin is greater than 1 µg/mL, the target pharmacokinetic-pharmacodynamic (PK-PD) parameters in the CSF with intravenous antimicrobials may not be achieved.

Although no antimicrobial agent has been approved by the US Food and Drug Administration for intraventricular and intrathecal use, there have been several studies on their pharmacokinetics, safety, and efficacy, especially in adults [38–44]. CSF sterility and normalization of CSF parameters were achieved sooner with intraventricular and intravenous use when compared to intravenous use alone. However, the use of intraventricular antimicrobial agents was not recommended in infants based on data in a recent Cochrane review [45]. A clinical trial found a three times higher relative risk of mortality when infants with gram-negative meningitis were treated with intraventricular gentamicin and intravenous antimicrobials, when compared to intravenous therapy alone, although one half of the infants in the intraventricular gentamicin group had received only one dose, raising doubts about the exact cause of death.

Antimicrobial agents administered by the intraventricular or intrathecal route should be preservative-free and should be prepared and given using strict sterile precautions. To avoid increasing the intracranial pressure prior to instilling the drug, a volume of CSF equal to the volume of drug diluent and saline flush should be aspirated and discarded. After administering the drug via a CSF drain, a saline flush can be used to minimize the amount of drug remaining in the draining catheter. When administered through a CSF drain, the drain should be clamped for 15–60 min to allow the antimicrobial solution to equilibrate in the CSF before opening the drain [46]. During and after the procedure, the patient's level of consciousness and ICP should be closely monitored. In treating CSF shunt ventriculitis, administration of the antimicrobials through the shunt reservoir may result in the agent draining distally into the peritoneal cavity; to avoid this issue, antimicrobials can be administered into the cerebral ventricles by placing a ventricular access device separate from the shunt reservoir [47].

Determining the correct dosing regimen is challenging as the CSF concentrations obtained for the same intraventricular dose in pharmacokinetic studies have been highly variable, probably due to the differences among patients in either the volume of distribution depending upon ventricular size or variable CSF clearance as a result of CSF drainage [38–43, 45]. A consensus guideline by the British Society for Antimicrobial Chemotherapy Working Party on Infections in Neurosurgery has recommended that the initial dose of an intraventricular antimicrobial be based on ventricular volume [48]. In adults, the recommended dose of vancomycin is 5 mg in patients with slit ventricles, 10 mg in patients with normal-sized ventricles, and 15–20 mg in patients with enlarged ventricles. Using the same rationale, the initial dosing of an aminoglycoside can also be tailored to ventricular size. The same Working Party recommended that the frequency of dosing be based on the daily volume of CSF drainage: once-daily dosing if CSF drainage is >100 mL/day, every other day if the drainage is 50–100 mL/day, and every third day if drainage is <50 mL/day. The ranges of intraventricular or intrathecal dose/day for other antimicrobials are as follows:

Gentamicin, 4–8 mg
Tobramycin, 5–20 mg
Amikacin, 5–30 mg
Colistimethate sodium, 10 mg, which is 125,000 IU or 3.75 mg CBA (colistin base activity)
Daptomycin, 2–5 mg

Another approach, when drug levels can be monitored, is to base dosing on CSF drug concentrations, after the initial intraventricular dose. However, there are very few studies that have evaluated CSF therapeutic drug monitoring and given the variable CSF clearance of an antimicrobial agent; it is difficult to determine when to obtain CSF to measure peak and trough drug concentrations. A CSF drug concentration can be obtained 24 h after administration of the first dose, which can be presumed to be the trough CSF concentration. The trough CSF concentration divided by the minimal inhibitory concentration of the agent for the isolated organism is termed the inhibitory quotient, which should exceed 10–20 for consistent CSF sterilization [49, 50]. Although not standardized, this approach is reasonable to ensure that adequate CSF concentrations of the antimicrobial are obtained.

Surgical Management

There is a wide range of management approaches to CSF shunt ventriculitis, in the published literature, ranging from conservative treatment with antimicrobials alone to removal of the entire shunt and later reimplanting a shunt after resolution of the ventriculitis [51, 52] There has only been one prospective, randomized trial that evaluated three different approaches to management of infected CSF shunts in 30 children (10 per each arm of the study) [53]. In the study, the arm that received antimicrobial therapy alone with no shunt removal had a 30% cure rate, the arm with the one-stage shunt replacement (removal of the infected CSF shunt with replacement of a new shunt in the same surgery) had a 90% cure rate, and the arm with the two-stage shunt replacement (removal of the infected CSF shunt with replacement of a new shunt in a second surgery after the ventriculitis cleared) had a 100% cure rate. In a decision analysis [51] and a systematic review [52] which synthesized results from many studies, the outcomes were similar to that of the aforementioned trial. They showed that cure rates were better with a two-stage procedure (88–96%) compared to a one-stage procedure (65%), which were better than when treated with antimicrobials alone without removing the infected shunt (34–36%) [51, 52]. In the two-stage approach, there might be a need for a temporary CSF drain, to treat raised ICP or hydrocephalus, while waiting for CSF cultures to clear before reimplanting a new CSF shunt. The optimal timing of shunt reimplantation has not been studied. Early placement may increase the risk of relapse, but a delay in reimplantation may increase the risk of secondary infection of the external ventricular drain. The timing of reimplantation should be individualized based on the isolated organism, severity of ventriculitis, and improvement of CSF parameters and CSF sterilization in response to antimicrobial therapy. Most experts in the field would wait for at least 7–10 days after the CSF cultures become sterile to reimplant a new shunt.

Conservative management without explanting infected prosthetic devices usually has lower cure rates as the organisms adhere to prostheses and form biofilms making them resistant to antimicrobial therapy. However, in one observational study of treatment with systemic and intraventricular antimicrobial agents (instilled via a separate ventricular access device), 84% of 43 patients were cured, with a 92% success rate for infections caused by bacteria other than *S. aureus* [47] suggesting that conservative management may be appropriate for selected patients with CSF shunt infections caused by less virulent microorganisms such as coagulase-negative staphylococci and *P. acnes*. In the treatment of CSF drain infections, removal of the infected drain would be a prudent approach.

Infection Prevention

Systemic Antimicrobial Prophylaxis

In addition to sterile technique and aseptic precautions during neurosurgeries such as craniotomies, the use of periprocedural systemic antimicrobial prophylaxis has been shown to decrease infection rates in most studies [54]. However, there are some studies that show that it does not prevent meningitis [55]. Systemic antimicrobial prophylaxis has also been shown to be effective in reducing CSF shunt infections. In a meta-analysis, the infection rates were found to be decreased with the use of antibiotic prophylaxis for CSF shunt surgery (odds ratio 0.51; 95% confidence interval 0.36–0.73) [56]. The antimicrobials that are generally used are first- or second-generation cephalosporins or vancomycin. Although periprocedural systemic prophylactic antimicrobials are used for CSF drains, the use of prolonged prophylactic systemic antimicrobials for the entire duration of external CSF drainage is more controversial. One study noted that the infection rate was 3.8% in those who received prophylactic antibiotics for the duration of placement of the CSF drain and 4.0% in those who received only periprocedural antibiotics [57], suggesting that prophylactic antibiotics throughout drainage did not significantly decrease the rate of ventriculitis. In contrast, another study demonstrated a lower infection rate with prophylactic antibiotics (2.6% CSF infection rate vs. 10.6% in those who only received periprocedural antibiotics; $p = 0.001$) [58], although the infections in those receiving prophylactic antimicrobials were caused by more drug-resistant, virulent pathogens and had a higher mortality rate (66% vs. 41%). In a systematic review [59] which pooled data from two randomized controlled trials and four observational studies, there was a relative risk reduction of 0.45 with the use of prophylactic prolonged systemic antimicrobials, although there were significant methodological limitations and heterogeneity in the pooled studies, the definitions of ventriculitis were variable, the type and dose of antimicrobials were different, adverse effects were not well studied, and most of the studies were retrospective and prone to bias. Given the availability of a safer efficacious alternative (i.e., antimicrobial-impregnated catheters; see below), it would be prudent to avoid the use of prophylactic prolonged systemic antimicrobials for the prevention of CSF drain infections.

Antimicrobial-Impregnated Catheters

The currently available antimicrobial-impregnated CSF drains and CSF shunts are typically impregnated with either minocycline or clindamycin, combined with rifampin. In a meta-analysis of 12 studies comparing antimicrobial-impregnated to non-antimicrobial-impregnated VP shunts, there was a statistically significant decrease in infections in patients who had received antimicrobial-impregnated shunts (RR 0.37; $p < 0.0001$) [60]. A similar reduction in infection rates has also been shown with the use of antimicrobial-impregnated external ventricular drains. A meta-analysis of five studies showed a statistically significant reduction in infections with antimicrobial-impregnated external ventricular drains (RR of 0.31; $p = 0.009$) [60]. The studies show that antimicrobial-impregnated CSF shunts and CSF drains are effective in preventing infections though larger prospective studies are needed to confirm this.

Combined Interventions (Bundles)

Studies evaluating "bundles" in the prevention of both CSF shunt and CSF drain infections showed that they are effective. In the Hydrocephalus Clinical Research Network Initiative, there was a reduction in infection rates from 8.8% to 5.7% ($p = 0.0028$; RR reduction, 36%), using a 11-step protocol for CSF shunt insertion which included measures to minimize operating room traffic, appropriate and timely prophylactic antimicrobials, hair clipping, chlorhexidine application, proper hand washing, and double gloving [61, 62]. Similarly, in patients requiring placement of an external ventricular drain, following a simple infection control protocol during CSF drain insertion and maintenance reduced ventriculitis rates from 6.3% in the baseline period to 0.8% in the first 3 years of the protocol period [63]. In a 4-year follow-up, the authors reported a further decrease in the ventriculitis rate to 0% [64].

For a more in-depth reading on diagnosis and management, we recommend the IDSA (Infectious Diseases Society of America) guideline on healthcare-associated ventriculitis and meningitis [65].

References

1. Bhimraj A, Drake J, Tunkel A. Cerebrospinal fluid shunt and drain infections. In: Mandell G, Bennett J, Dolin R, editors. Principles and practice of infectious diseases. 8th ed. Philadelphia: Churchill Livingstone; 2014. p. 1186–93.
2. Arnell K, Cesarini K, Lagerqvist-Widh A, Wester T, Sjolin J. Cerebrospinal fluid shunt infections in children over a 13-year period: anaerobic cultures and comparison of clinical signs of infection with Propionibacterium acnes and with other bacteria. J Neurosurg Pediatr. 2008;1(5):366–72.
3. Lozier AP, Sciacca RR, Romagnoli MF, Connolly ES Jr. Ventriculostomy-related infections: a critical review of the literature. Neurosurgery. 2008;62(Suppl 2):688–700.
4. Ramanan M, Lipman J, Shorr A, Shankar A. A meta-analysis of ventriculostomy-associated cerebrospinal fluid infections. BMC Infect Dis. 2015;15:3. https://doi.org/10.1186/s12879-014-0712.
5. Coplin WM, Avellino AM, Kim DK, Winn HR, Grady MS. Bacterial meningitis associated with lumbar drains: a retrospective cohort study. J Neurol Neurosurg Psychiatry. 1999;67(4):468–73.
6. Snowden JN, Beaver M, Smeltzer MS, Kielian T. Biofilm-infected intracerebroventricular shunts elicit inflammation within the central nervous system. Infect Immun. 2012;80(9):3206–14.
7. Braxton EE Jr, Ehrlich GD, Hall-Stoodley L, Stoodley P, Veeh R, Fux C, et al. Role of biofilms in neurosurgical device-related infections. Neurosurg Rev. 2005;28(4):249–55.
8. Wang KW, Chang WN, Shih TY, Huang CR, Tsai NW, Chang CS, et al. Infection of cerebrospinal fluid shunts: causative pathogens, clinical features, and outcomes. Jpn J Infect Dis. 2004;57(2):44–8.

9. Sells CJ, Shurtleff DB, Loeser JD. Gram-negative cerebrospinal fluid shunt-associated infections. Pediatrics. 1977;59(4):614–8.
10. Brook I. Meningitis and shunt infection caused by anaerobic bacteria in children. Pediatr Neurol. 2002;26(2):99–105.
11. Rekate HL, Ruch T, Nulsen FE. Diphtheroid infections of cerebrospinal fluid shunts. The changing pattern of shunt infection in Cleveland. J Neurosurg. 1980;52(4):553–6.
12. Nisbet M, Briggs S, Ellis-Pegler R, Thomas M, Holland D. Propionibacterium acnes: an under-appreciated cause of post-neurosurgical infection. J Antimicrob Chemother. 2007;60(5):1097–103.
13. O'Brien D, Stevens NT, Lim CH, O'Brien DF, Smyth E, Fitzpatrick F, et al. Candida infection of the central nervous system following neurosurgery: a 12-year review. Acta Neurochir. 2011;153(6):1347–50.
14. Conen A, Walti LN, Merlo A, Fluckiger U, Battegay M, Trampuz A. Characteristics and treatment outcome of cerebrospinal fluid shunt-associated infections in adults: a retrospective analysis over an 11-year period. Clin Infect Dis. 2008;47(1):73–82.
15. Moores LE, Ellenbogen RG. Cerebrospinal fluid shunt infections. In: Hall WA, McCutcheon IE, AANS Publications Committee, editors. Infections in neurosurgery. Park Ridge: American Association of Neurological Surgeons; 2000. p. 53.
16. Rabinstein AA, Sandhu K. Non-infectious fever in the neurological intensive care unit: incidence, causes and predictors. J Neurol Neurosurg Psychiatry. 2007;78(11):1278–80.
17. Berger C, Schwarz S, Schaebitz WR, Aschoff A, Schwab S. Serum procalcitonin in cerebral ventriculitis. Crit Care Med. 2002;30(8):1778–81.
18. Martinez R, Gaul C, Buchfelder M, Erbguth F, Tschaikowsky K. Serum procalcitonin monitoring for differential diagnosis of ventriculitis in adult intensive care patients. Intensive Care Med. 2002;28(2):208–10.
19. Schuhmann MU, Ostrowski KR, Draper EJ, Chu JW, Ham SD, Sood S, et al. The value of C-reactive protein in the management of shunt infections. J Neurosurg. 2005;103(3 Suppl):223–30.
20. Lewis A, Wahlster S, Karinja S, Czeisler BM, Kimberly WT, Lord AS. Ventriculostomy-related infections: the performance of different definitions for diagnosing infection. Br J Neurosurg. 2016;30:49–56.
21. Schade RP, Schinkel J, Roelandse FW, Geskus RB, Visser LG, van Dijk JM, et al. Lack of value of routine analysis of cerebrospinal fluid for prediction and diagnosis of external drainage-related bacterial meningitis. J Neurosurg. 2006;104(1):101–8.
22. Pfisterer W, Muhlbauer M, Czech T, Reinprecht A. Early diagnosis of external ventricular drainage infection: results of a prospective study. J Neurol Neurosurg Psychiatry. 2003;74(7):929–32.
23. Pfausler B, Beer R, Engelhardt K, Kemmler G, Mohsenipour I, Schmutzhard E. Cell index – a new parameter for the early diagnosis of ventriculostomy (external ventricular drainage)-related ventriculitis in patients with intraventricular hemorrhage? Acta Neurochir. 2004;146(5):477–81.
24. Grille P, Verga F, Biestro A. Diagnosis of ventriculostomy-related infection: is cerebrospinal fluid lactate measurement a useful tool. J Clin Neurosci. 2017;45:243–7.
25. Lan CC, Wong TT, Chen SJ, Liang ML, Tang RB. Early diagnosis of ventriculoperitoneal shunt infections and malfunctions in children with hydrocephalus. J Microbiol Immunol Infect. 2003;36(1):47–50.
26. Forgacs P, Geyer CA, Freidberg SR. Characterization of chemical meningitis after neurological surgery. Clin Infect Dis. 2001;32(2):179–85.
27. Xiao X, Zhang Y, Kang P, Ji N. The diagnostic value of cerebrospinal fluid lactate for post-neurosurgical bacterial meningitis: a meta-analysis. BMC Infect Dis. 2016;16:483.
28. Li Y, Zhang G, Ma R, Du Y, Zhang L, Li F, Fang F, Lv H, Wang Q, Zhang Y, Kang X. The diagnostic value of cerebrospinal fluids procalcitonin and lactate for the differential diagnosis of post-neurosurgical bacterial meningitis and aseptic meningitis. Clin Biochem. 2015;48(1–2):50–4.

29. Desai A, Lollis SS, Missios S, Radwan T, Zuaro DE, Schwarzman JD, et al. How long should cerebrospinal fluid cultures be held to detect shunt infections? Clinical article. J Neurosurg Pediatr. 2009;4(2):184–9.
30. Noetzel MJ, Baker RP. Shunt fluid examination: risks and benefits in the evaluation of shunt malfunction and infection. J Neurosurg. 1984;61(2):328–32.
31. Spiegelman L, Asija R, Da Silva SL, Krieger MD, McComb JG. What is the risk of infecting a cerebrospinal fluid-diverting shunt with percutaneous tapping? J Neurosurg Pediatr. 2014;14(4):336–9.
32. Banks JT, Bharara S, Tubbs RS, Wolff CL, Gillespie GY, Markert JM, et al. Polymerase chain reaction for the rapid detection of cerebrospinal fluid shunt or ventriculostomy infections. Neurosurgery. 2005;57(6):1237–43. discussion 1237–43.
33. Lozier AP, Sciacca RR, Romagnoli MF, Connolly ES Jr. Ventriculostomy-related infections: a critical review of the literature. Neurosurgery. 2002;51(1):170–81. discussion 181–82.
34. Lodise TP, Nau R, Kinzig M, Drusano GL, Jones RN, Sorgel F. Pharmacodynamics of ceftazidime and meropenem in cerebrospinal fluid: results of population pharmacokinetic modelling and Monte Carlo simulation. J Antimicrob Chemother. 2007;60(5):1038–44.
35. Lodise TP Jr, Rhoney DH, Tam VH, McKinnon PS, Drusano GL. Pharmacodynamic profiling of cefepime in plasma and cerebrospinal fluid of hospitalized patients with external ventriculostomies. Diagn Microbiol Infect Dis. 2006;54(3):223–30.
36. Nau R, Prange HW, Kinzig M, Frank A, Dressel A, Scholz P, et al. Cerebrospinal fluid ceftazidime kinetics in patients with external ventriculostomies. Antimicrob Agents Chemother. 1996;40(3):763–6.
37. Ricard JD, Wolff M, Lacherade JC, Mourvillier B, Hidri N, Barnaud G, et al. Levels of vancomycin in cerebrospinal fluid of adult patients receiving adjunctive corticosteroids to treat pneumococcal meningitis: a prospective multicenter observational study. Clin Infect Dis. 2007;44(2):250–5.
38. Wang JH, Lin PC, Chou CH, Ho CM, Lin KH, Tsai CT, et al. Intraventricular antimicrobial therapy in post neurosurgical Gram-negative bacillary meningitis or ventriculitis: a hospital-based retrospective study. J Microbiol Immunol Infect. 2014;47(3):204–10. https://doi.org/10.1016/j.jmii.2012.08.028.
39. Wilkie MD, Hanson MF, Statham PF, Brennan PM. Infections of cerebrospinal fluid diversion devices in adults: the role of intraventricular antimicrobial therapy. J Infect. 2013;66(3):239–46.
40. Ng K, Mabasa VH, Chow I, Ensom MH. Systematic review of efficacy, pharmacokinetics, and administration of intraventricular vancomycin in adults. Neurocrit Care. 2014;20(1):158–71. https://doi.org/10.1007/s12028-012-9784-z.
41. Tangden T, Enblad P, Ullberg M, Sjolin J. Neurosurgical gram-negative bacillary ventriculitis and meningitis: a retrospective study evaluating the efficacy of intraventricular gentamicin therapy in 31 consecutive cases. Clin Infect Dis. 2011;52(11):1310–6.
42. Imberti R, Cusato M, Accetta G, Marinò V, Procaccio F, Del Gaudio A, et al. Pharmacokinetics of colistin in cerebrospinal fluid after intraventricular administration of colistin methanesulfonate. Antimicrob Agents Chemother. 2012;56(8):4416–21.
43. Ziai WC, Lewin JJ 3rd. Improving the role of intraventricular antimicrobial agents in the management of meningitis. Curr Opin Neurol. 2009;22(3):277–82.
44. Remes F, Tomas R, Jindrak V, Vanis V, Setlik M. Intraventricular and lumbar intrathecal administration of antibiotics in postneurosurgical patients with meningitis and/or ventriculitis in a serious clinical state. J Neurosurg. 2013;119(6):1596–602.
45. Shah SS, Ohlsson A, Shah VS. Intraventricular antibiotics for bacterial meningitis in neonates. Cochrane Database Syst Rev. 2012;7:CD004496.
46. Cook AM, Mieure KD, Owen RD, Pesaturo AB, Hatton J. Intracerebroventricular administration of drugs. Pharmacotherapy. 2009;29(7):832–45.
47. Brown EM, Edwards RJ, Pople IK. Conservative management of patients with cerebrospinal fluid shunt infections. Neurosurgery. 2006;58(4):657–65. discussion 657–65.

48. The management of neurosurgical patients with postoperative bacterial or aseptic meningitis or external ventricular drain-associated ventriculitis. Infection in Neurosurgery Working Party of the British Society for Antimicrobial Chemotherapy. Br J Neurosurg. 2000;14(1):7–12.
49. Ellner PD, Neu HC. The inhibitory quotient. A method for interpreting minimum inhibitory concentration data. JAMA. 1981;246(14):1575–8.
50. Tunkel AR, Hartman BJ, Kaplan SL, Kaufman BA, Roos KL, Scheld WM, et al. Practice guidelines for the management of bacterial meningitis. Clin Infect Dis. 2004;39(9):1267–84.
51. Schreffler RT, Schreffler AJ, Wittler RR. Treatment of cerebrospinal fluid shunt infections: a decision analysis. Pediatr Infect Dis J. 2002;21(7):632–6.
52. Yogev R. Cerebrospinal fluid shunt infections: a personal view. Pediatr Infect Dis. 1985;4(2):113–8.
53. James HE, Walsh JW, Wilson HD, Connor JD, Bean JR, Tibbs PA. Prospective randomized study of therapy in cerebrospinal fluid shunt infection. Neurosurgery. 1980;7(5):459–63.
54. Barker FG 2nd. Efficacy of prophylactic antibiotics against meningitis after craniotomy: a meta-analysis. Neurosurgery. 2007;60(5):887–94. discussion 887–94.
55. Korinek AM, Baugnon T, Golmard JL, van Effenterre R, Coriat P, Puybasset L. Risk factors for adult nosocomial meningitis after craniotomy: role of antibiotic prophylaxis. Neurosurgery. 2006;59(1):126–33. discussion 126–33.
56. Ratilal B, Costa J, Sampaio C. Antibiotic prophylaxis for surgical introduction of intracranial ventricular shunts: a systematic review. J Neurosurg Pediatr. 2008;1(1):48–56.
57. Alleyne CH Jr, Hassan M, Zabramski JM. The efficacy and cost of prophylactic and periproce-dural antibiotics in patients with external ventricular drains. Neurosurgery. 2000;47(5):1124–7. discussion 1127–9.
58. Poon WS, Ng S, Wai S. CSF antibiotic prophylaxis for neurosurgical patients with ventriculos-tomy: a randomised study. Acta Neurochir Suppl. 1998;71:146–8.
59. Sonabend AM, Korenfeld Y, Crisman C, Badjatia N, Mayer SA, Connolly ES Jr. Prevention of ventriculostomy-related infections with prophylactic antibiotics and antibiotic-coated external ventricular drains: a systematic review. Neurosurgery. 2011;68(4):996–1005.
60. Thomas R, Lee S, Patole S, Rao S. Antibiotic-impregnated catheters for the prevention of CSF shunt infections: a systematic review and meta-analysis. Br J Neurosurg. 2012;26(2):175–84.
61. Kestle JRW, Riva-Cambrin J, Wellons JC 3rd, et al. A standardized protocol to reduce cere-brospinal fluid shunt infection: the Hydrocephalus Clinical Research Network Quality Improvement Initiative. J Neurosurg Pediatr. 2011;8:22–9.
62. Kestle JR, Holubkov R, Douglas Cochrane D. A new Hydrocephalus Clinical Research Network protocol to reduce cerebrospinal fluid shunt infection. J Neurosurg Pediatr. 2016;17:391–6.
63. Flint AC, Rao VA, Renda NC, Faigeles BS, Lasman TE, Sheridan W. A simple protocol to prevent external ventricular drain infections. Neurosurgery. 2013;72:993–9.
64. Flint AC, Toossi S, Chan SL, Rao VA, Sheridan W. A simple infection control protocol durably reduces external ventricular drain infections to near-zero levels. World Neurosurg. 2017;99:518 523.
65. Tunkel AR, Hasbun R, Bhimraj A, et al. 2017 Infectious Diseases Society of America's clini-cal practice guidelines for healthcare-associated ventriculitis and meningitis. Clin Infect Dis. 2017;64:e34–65.

Acute Aseptic Meningitis Syndrome

4

Rodrigo Hasbun

Wallgren initially described the aseptic meningitis syndrome in 1925 as an acute community-acquired syndrome with cerebrospinal fluid (CSF) pleocytosis in the absence of a positive Gram stain and culture, without a parameningeal focus or a systemic illness and with a good clinical outcome [1]. It was not until the 1950s when advances in diagnostic virology identified seasonal patterns and a major role for viruses. Since then this clinical syndrome has been used more broadly and includes more than 100 infectious and noninfectious etiologies with some of them being treatable (see Table 4.1). The most common etiologies of aseptic meningitis in the United States (USA) are viruses such as *Enterovirus*, herpes simplex type 2, and West Nile virus although up to 81% of adults remain with unknown etiologies, especially when PCR testing is not routinely done [2]. Acute meningitis is defined as duration of symptoms of less than 5 days and accounts for 75% of all community-acquired meningitis cases [3]. In this chapter, we will review the diagnostic and management challenges to some of the most common causes of acute aseptic meningitis syndrome. We will briefly discuss herpes viruses, arboviruses, dengue, Zika, chikungunya, syphilis, partially treated bacterial meningitis, human immunodeficiency virus, and Lyme disease as other chapters in this book cover these etiologies extensively.

R. Hasbun
UT Health-McGovern Medical School, Houston, TX, USA
e-mail: Rodrigo.Hasbun@uth.tmc.edu

© Springer International Publishing AG, part of Springer Nature 2018
R. Hasbun (ed.), *Meningitis and Encephalitis*,
https://doi.org/10.1007/978-3-319-92678-0_4

Table 4.1 Differential diagnosis of acute aseptic meningitis syndrome

Infectious etiologies
Viruses
Enteroviruses[a]; arboviruses[b]; herpes viruses[c]; mumps virus; polio viruses
Lymphocytic choriomeningitis virus; human immunodeficiency virus[d]
Adenovirus; parainfluenza virus; influenza A and B; measles; rubella
Bacteria
Bacterial meningitis; parameningeal focus[e]; *Rickettsia* species; endocarditis
Ehrlichia; *Anaplasma* spp.; *Brucella* species; *Bartonella henselae*;
Nocardia spp.; *Mycoplasma* spp.; *Mycobacterium tuberculosis*
Spirochetes
Treponema pallidum (syphilis); *Borrelia burgdorferi* (Lyme disease); *Leptospira* spp.;
Protozoa and helminths
Naegleria fowleri; Angiostrongylus cantonensis; Baylisascaris procyonis
Taenia solium; Toxocara spp.; *Strongyloides stercoralis* (hyperinfection syndrome)
Noninfectious etiologies
Intracranial tumors and cysts
Craniopharyngioma; teratoma[f]; dermoid/epidermoid cyst
Medications
Antimicrobial agents[g]; nonsteroidal anti-inflammatory agents[h]; muromonab-CD3 (OKT3)
Azathioprine; cytarabine; carbamazepine[h]; immune intravenous globulin; ranitidine
Systemic illnesses
Systemic lupus erythematosus; Behçet's disease; sarcoidosis; Vogt-Koyanagi-Harada
Procedure related
After neurosurgery ("chemical meningitis"); spinal anesthesia; intrathecal injections[i]
Miscellaneous
Seizures; migraine or migraine-like syndromes; postvaccination; meningeal carcinomatosis
Multiple sclerosis; heavy metal (lead and mercury) poisoning; vein of Galen aneurysm

[a]Primarily echoviruses and coxsackieviruses

[b]In the USA, the major etiologic agents are the mosquito-borne West Nile virus, California, St. Louis, and Eastern equine encephalitis and the tick-borne Colorado tick fever

[c]Primarily herpes simplex virus type 2 but also herpes simplex virus type 1, varicella-zoster virus, cytomegalovirus, Epstein-Barr virus, and human herpesvirus 6

[d]During the acute HIV seroconversion syndrome

[e]Brain abscess, sinusitis, otitis, mastoiditis, subdural empyema, epidural abscess, venous sinus thrombophlebitis, pituitary abscess, cranial osteomyelitis

[f]Main association of the anti-NMDA receptor encephalitis in young women

[g]Trimethoprim, sulfamethoxazole, trimethoprim-sulfamethoxazole, ciprofloxacin, penicillin, isoniazid, metronidazole, cephalosporins, pyrazinamid, Ibuprofen, sulindac, naproxen, tolmetin, diclofenac, ketoprofene

[h]In patients with connective tissue diseases

[i]Air, isotopes, antimicrobial agents, antineoplastic agents, corticosteroids, radiographic contrast media

Infectious Causes

Viral Meningitis

Enteroviruses

Enteroviruses (EV) are the leading recognizable cause of aseptic meningitis syndrome [1, 2]. As the surveillance of EV infections to the Centers for Disease Control and Prevention (CDC) is passive [4] and because enteroviral infections are underdiagnosed as only 15% of adults with aseptic meningitis get a CSF EV polymerase chain reaction (PCR) done [2], the true prevalence of this infection is unknown. A total of 118 types of enteroviruses and 16 types of human parechoviruses (HPeV) have been described as causes of viral meningitis in the USA [4, 5]. EV can sometimes also cause acute flaccid paralysis, encephalitis, myocarditis, and sepsis with worse clinical presentations most commonly seen in neonates or infants [5, 6]. Enterovirus D68 has been implicated as a possible cause of acute flaccid paralysis (AFP) in the USA as 43% of cases have had the virus isolated from respiratory specimens by PCR [6]. Enteroviruses have a worldwide distribution, and in temperate climates they have a summer/fall seasonality [1, 2, 5]. Transmission is via the fecal-oral route and less likely by respiratory droplets [5]. A report from the National Enterovirus Surveillance System from the CDC from 2009 to 2013 documented the seasonal pattern (April to November) with the two most common viruses identified as coxsackievirus A6 and human parechovirus type 3 [4].

Infants and young children most commonly suffer from enteroviral meningitis because they are the most susceptible host population within the community. Risk factors for severe disease in children are absence of oral lesions, seizures, and lethargy [7]. In adults, enteroviruses more commonly present with aseptic meningitis with good clinical outcomes [2]. Rarely, patients can present with an enteroviral meningoencephalitis after receiving chimeric anti-CD20 monoclonal antibody rituximab [8]. Additionally, neonates can present with a severe form of meningoencephalitis with symptoms and signs developing at birth after transplacental transmission of the virus. With disease progression, a sepsis-like syndrome characterized by multiorgan involvement, disseminated intravascular coagulation, seizures, focal neurological signs, and cardiovascular collapse may develop [5]. A recent small clinical trial showed that pleconaril improved clearance of the virus and mortality in neonates with enteroviral sepsis, but the Federal Drug Administration (FDA) [9] has not approved the drug.

Severe disease and poor outcome are rare in infants, children, and adults [2, 10]. Infants usually present with fever, irritability, feeding difficulties, and rash with the majority of them having a good clinical outcome [5, 10]. Approximately one-third of patients have stiff neck with less than 2% of patients presenting with altered mental status. Headache is nearly always present in adults, but photophobia is seen in ~ one-third of patients [11]. Patients may also present with nonspecific symptoms and signs such as vomiting, anorexia, rash, diarrhea, cough, upper respiratory tract findings, and myalgias. The duration of illness in enteroviral meningitis is usually less than 1 week, with many patients reporting improvement after lumbar puncture, presumably from reduction in intracranial pressure [1, 5].

Herpes Viruses

Herpes viruses include herpes simplex virus (HSV) types 1 and 2, varicella-zoster virus, cytomegalovirus, Epstein-Barr virus, and human herpes viruses 6, 7, and 8 [1]. Although neurologic complications are known to occur with some of these viruses, complications associated with HSV are of the most significance. In a recent study of 404 adults with aseptic meningitis, HSV was the most common identified viral pathogen even though only 39% of patients had a CSF HSV PCR performed [2]. In patients beyond the neonatal period, it is critical to differentiate between HSV encephalitis (usually HSV type 1), a potentially fatal infection, and HSV meningitis (most commonly by HSV type 2), a self-limited syndrome. The syndrome of HSV-2 aseptic meningitis is most commonly associated with primary genital infection and has a benign clinical outcome that does not appear to be impacted by antiviral therapy [12]. HSV-2 is also the most common cause Mollaret's meningitis (now termed *recurrent benign lymphocytic meningitis*), although a few cases have been associated with HSV-1 and Epstein-Barr virus have been reported [13]. The majority of patients are female, have no history of genital HSV and have no active lesions on presentation [13]. A recent double blind, randomized clinical trial of valacyclovir suppression showed no impact on decreasing recurrent rates in patients with HSV-2 meningitis [14]. Acute aseptic meningitis has also been associated with varicella-zoster virus (VZV) in patients with or without typical skin lesions, [12] the latter known as *zoster sine herpete*. VZV is most likely an underdiagnosed treatable etiology as only 1.2% of patients with aseptic meningitis undergo a CSF VZV PCR [2]. A recent study using a multiplex PCR documented that human herpes virus 6 (HHV-6) was more commonly detected than HSV-1 or HSV-2 in adults and children with meningitis and encephalitis [15]. The proportion that these HHV-6 cases represent a true infection versus reactivation or chromosomal integration remains to be determined [16]. Cytomegalovirus and Epstein-Barr virus may cause aseptic meningitis in association with a mononucleosis syndrome, particularly in an immunocompetent host [1].

Arboviruses

Arboviruses (arthropod-borne virus) include several families of viruses that are transmitted by either mosquitos, ticks, or sandflies [17]. The most common arthropod-transmitted cause of aseptic meningitis in the USA is West Nile virus (WNV), a flavivirus. WNV infection is most commonly asymptomatic with approximately 20% having a febrile illness and 1% presenting with neuroinvasive disease [18]. Neuroinvasive disease may present with an aseptic meningitis, with encephalitis, or with an acute flaccid paralysis/myelitis but may be underdiagnosed as only approximately one-third of adults and children with meningitis or encephalitis get tested [19]. There is no vaccine or therapy for WNV.

Neuroinvasive disease develops in approximately 1% of patients with West Nile virus infections during the summer months in the USA [19]. Patients can present with meningitis, encephalitis, or acute flaccid paralysis with up to 50% of patients with encephalitis having concomitant chorioretinitis [20]. Patients with meningitis typically presents with fever, headache, nausea, vomiting, stiff neck, photophobia, and occasionally with a maculopapular rash [17]. In addition, patients may have persistent headaches, memory impairment, and chronic fatigue years after infection [21].

Other less common arboviruses in the USA that can cause aseptic meningitis are the two mosquito-borne illnesses, St. Louis encephalitis (a flavivirus) and the California encephalitis group of viruses (e.g., La Crosse, Jamestown Canyon, and snowshoe hare viruses, which are bunyaviruses), and two tick-borne illnesses, Powassan virus in northern central and eastern USA and coltivirus (agent of Colorado tick fever) in the mountainous and western regions of the USA and Canada [17]. In 2015, the CDC reported a total incidence of 2175 cases of WNV followed by La Crosse (55), St. Louis (23), Jamestown canyon (11), Powassan (7), and Eastern equine encephalitis (6) [22]. In Europe, tick-borne encephalitis can be associated with a complex syndrome of meningoencephaloradiculitis (MER), which is associated with a relatively high risk of severe disease (requirement for intensive care and mechanical ventilation). Age, male sex, and preexisting diabetes mellitus were predictive of the more severe MER [23]. Toscana virus has emerged as one of the most common causes of meningitis or encephalitis during the summer in the Mediterranean countries [11]. It is transmitted by sandflies and is caused by a bunyavirus.

Other Viruses

Lymphocytic choriomeningitis virus (LCMV) can cause aseptic meningitis; this virus is now rarely reported as an etiologic agent [1]. A seroprevalence of 5% for LCMV was seen in 400 patients with neurological infections in Finland [24]. LCMV is transmitted to humans by contact with rodents (e.g., hamsters, rats, mice) or their excreta [1, 24]; the greatest risk for infection is in laboratory workers, pet owners, and persons living in impoverished and unhygienic situations. Recent outbreaks have been reported in rodent breeding factories or infected households [25, 26]. No evidence of human-to-human transmission has been reported.

In an unimmunized population, mumps can cause aseptic meningitis [1]. With the introduction of the measles-mumps-rubella (MMR) vaccine, the incidence of mump-associated meningitis has dramatically decreased with now only accounting for <1% of all cases of meningitis and encephalitis in the UK and US [27, 28].

Human immunodeficiency virus (HIV) can cause aseptic meningitis during HIV seroconversion presenting clinically with a mononucleosis-like picture [1]. HIV may also cause an encephalitis presentation in those with acquired immunodeficiency syndrome (AIDS) who are not receiving antiretroviral therapy (ART) (known as AIDS encephalopathy or HIV encephalitis) or in those patients on ART with CSF viral escape (detectable viral load in the CSF with undetectable or low-level viremia) [29]. This latter form is referred to as CD8 encephalitis and can be treated with steroids and by optimizing ART.

Japanese encephalitis is a vaccine preventable infection that continues to cause both meningitis and encephalitis in countries where routine vaccination is not available [30]. Dengue, chikungunya, and Zika virus are emerging causes of meningitis or encephalitis in several parts of the world [31, 32]. The epidemic of Ebola disease in West Africa has revealed unusual characteristics of the disease not previously described, including viral relapse with acute meningitis, with high levels of virus in the cerebrospinal fluid. Antiviral therapy with an experimental agent and adjuvant corticosteroids led to resolution of the disease [33].

Bacterial Etiologies

Patients with bacterial meningitis may present with a negative Gram stain [34]. Patients with bacterial meningitis classically present with fever, headache, meningismus, and signs of cerebral dysfunction; however, clinical presentation may vary based on age and underlying disease status and as a result of infection by specific bacterial pathogens. Even though the CSF typically shows a >1000 WBC per mm^3 with a neutrophilic predominance, a CSF protein >100 mg/dl and a glucose <40 mg/dl, a neutrophilic pleocytosis, and hypoglycorrhachia may be seen in viral meningitis as well [35, 36]. Patients with infective endocarditis due to *Staphylococcus aureus* and *Streptococcus pneumoniae* can sometimes present with meningitis [1]. Additionally, patients with parameningeal focus of infections may sometimes present with meningitis. Epidural or subdural empyemas may sometimes occur to contiguous osteomyelitis complicating sinusitis, otitis, or mastoiditis [1].

Spirochetal Meningitis

Treponema pallidum disseminates to the CNS during early infection [37]. The organism can be isolated from the CSF of patients with primary syphilis, and CSF laboratory abnormalities are detected in 5–9% of patients with seronegative primary syphilis. The actual rate of invasion of the CNS during these early stages is likely to be considerably higher, however. Clinical neurosyphilis can be divided into four distinct syndromes [37]: syphilitic meningitis, meningovascular syphilis, parenchymatous neurosyphilis, and gummatous neurosyphilis.

Lyme disease, most commonly caused by *Borrelia burgdorferi*, can cause an aseptic meningitis in the secondary phase typically 2–10 weeks after the erythema migrans rash [38]. Because viral meningitis is an important differential diagnosis, a clinical prediction rule has been used to help clinicians differentiate these two conditions. The "Rule of 7's" classifies children at low risk for Lyme meningitis when each of the following 3 criteria are met: <7 days of headache, <70% cerebrospinal fluid (CSF) mononuclear cells, and absence of seventh or other cranial nerve palsy [39]. The best currently available laboratory test for the diagnosis of Lyme disease is demonstration of specific serum antibody to *B. burgdorferi,* and this positive test in a patient with a compatible neurologic abnormality is strong evidence for the diagnosis [38].

Leptospirosis can cause aseptic meningitis during the second (immune) phase of the illness and is typically associated with uveitis, rash, conjunctival suffusion, adenopathy, and hepatosplenomegaly [40]. The CSF profile resembles viral meningitis with the diagnosis being established by CSF or urine culture using Fletcher's medium or by serology. The treatment is doxycycline.

Protozoal and Helminthic Meningitis

Amebas

Despite the hundreds of species of free-living amebas that are known, only a few have been reported to infect humans [41]. The most important are in the genera *Naegleria, Acanthamoeba,* and *Balamuthia. Naegleria fowleri,* the main protozoan causing primary amebic meningoencephalitis in humans, has been recovered from lakes, puddles, pools, ponds, rivers, sewage sludge, tap water, air conditioner drains, and soil [41, 42]. Sporadic cases of primary amebic meningoencephalitis occur when persons, usually children and young adults, swim or play in water containing the amebas or when swimming pools or water supplies have become contaminated, often through failure of chlorination. In the largest review of 142 cases reported in the USA from 1937 to 2013, cases were reported in most southern states and occurred primarily in previously healthy young males exposed to warm recreational waters, especially lakes and ponds, in warm weather locations during summer months [42]. Clinical presentation and CSF formula resembles bacterial meningitis with a mortality of 98%. Recently, miltefosine has resulted in survival in a few cases with *Naegleria fowleri* and *Acanthamoeba* [43, 44].

Eosinophilic Meningitis

Infection of humans by larvae of the nematode *Angiostrongylus cantonensis* is the most common cause of eosinophilic meningitis [45]. Humans become infected by eating infected intermediate hosts (i.e., mollusks, such as snails and slugs) or paratenic (i.e., freshwater prawns, crabs, frogs, and planaria) hosts or by eating food such as leafy green vegetables contaminated by these hosts. The larvae invade the brain either directly from the bloodstream or after migrating through other organs before reaching the spinal cord and brain. Once in the CNS, the larvae mature into adult worms that migrate through the brain. *A. cantonensis* is widespread, and human infection is fairly common and reported from many parts of the world. Other infectious causes of eosinophilic meningitis include *Gnathostoma* species, *Baylisascaris procyonis, Toxocara* species, and *Taenia solium* [45].

Diagnosis

The empirical management of patients is challenging as approximately 93% of patients with community-acquired meningitis present with a negative Gram stain [3]. Furthermore, as the differential diagnosis is broad and available CSF is limited, the majority of patients do not undergo comprehensive diagnostic evaluations, and several pathogens go undiagnosed [2, 3, 19]. Rapid multiplex PCR testing of the CSF may offer a solution to this dilemma. The BioFire FilmArray Meningitis/ Encephalitis (FA ME) (BioFire Diagnostics, Salt Lake City, UT) is the first FDA-approved multiplex PCR panel which detects six bacteria (*S. pneumoniae, N. meningitidis, S. agalactiae, H. influenzae, L. monocytogenes,* and *E. coli* K1), seven viruses (HSV types 1 and 2 [HSV-1 and -2], human herpesvirus 6 [HHV-6], cytomegalovirus [CMV], enterovirus, parechovirus, varicella-zoster virus [VZV]), and two fungi (*Cryptococcus gattii/neoformans*) using 0.2 ml of CSF in 1 h. A strategy that uses the panel in meningitis with a negative Gram stain found an increase of 22.9% in diagnoses rendered, mostly commonly viral pathogens, but also two cases with *S. pneumoniae* and a case of *C. gattii/neoformans*. However, 15.2% (5/33) of FA ME-negative isolates were positive by standard assays (four cases of West Nile virus and a case of *Histoplasma capsulatum*, pathogens not included in the panel) [46]. In a retrospective analysis of CSF from HIV patients with cryptococcosis in Uganda, the test was considered useful in distinguishing culture-positive relapse from culture-negative immune reconstitution syndrome [47]. A multicenter prospective study of 1560 patients tested with the panel showed a high sensitivity and specificity for the 14 pathogens in the panel [15]. Other multiplex PCRs that are currently being studied are the Fasttrack, Seegene, and the TaqMan array card assays [48]. Of all these assays, the most comprehensive one is the TaqMan array card that includes 21 pathogens: 2 parasites (*Balamuthia mandrillaris* and *Acanthamoeba*), 6 bacteria (*Streptococcus pneumoniae, Haemophilus influenzae, Neisseria meningitidis, Mycoplasma pneumoniae, Mycobacterium tuberculosis, and Bartonella*), and 13 viruses (*parechovirus, dengue virus, Nipah virus, varicella-zoster virus, mumps virus, measles virus, lyssavirus, herpes simplex viruses 1 and 2, Epstein-Barr virus, enterovirus, cytomegalovirus, and chikungunya virus*).

Viral Meningitis

Cerebrospinal Fluid Examination
CSF pleocytosis is almost always present in patients with enteroviral meningitis, although some enteroviruses have been isolated from young infants with clinical evidence of meningitis but no CSF white blood cells [5]. A study of 390 patients with enteroviral meningitis showed that 16–18% of children and 68–77% of neonates had no CSF pleocytosis with younger age, lower serum white blood cell count, and shorter duration of symptoms prior to the lumbar puncture being predictors for lack of CSF pleocytosis [49]. The cell count is usually 100–1000/mm^3, although counts in the several thousands have also been reported [5]. Enterovirus can present with a neutrophilic pleocytosis in 39% of patients [35]. If a repeat lumbar puncture is done more than 8 h later, this may switch to a lymphocytic pleocytosis [50], but this practice is done currently in only 0.5% of patients with viral CNS infections [35]. Additionally, a retrospective study of 158 cases of meningitis (138 aseptic and 20 bacterial) showed that 51% of the 53 patients with aseptic meningitis and

duration of symptoms of less than 24 h had a neutrophil predominance in CSF, suggesting that a CSF neutrophil predominance is not useful as a sole criterion in distinguishing between aseptic and bacterial meningitis [51].

Patients with HSV-2 meningitis also present most commonly with a lymphocytic meningitis (<500/mm^3) and a normal glucose content but occasionally can present with a mild hypoglycorrhachia (30–45 mg/dl) or with a neutrophilic pleocytosis [35, 36]. PCR has also become the standard method for diagnosis for all herpes viruses (HSV1, HSV 2, HHSV 6, CMV, EBV, VZV). VZV PCR assay has also confirmed several cases of herpes zoster meningitis even without the typical vesicular rash (zoster sine herpete) [12, 51]. The CSF formula for West Nile virus resembles enteroviral meningitis, and the diagnosis is made by a positive West Nile IgM [19].

Differentiation of Bacterial from Viral Meningitis

Even though the most common causes of meningitis and encephalitis are viral, the majority of patients are admitted and receive empirical antibiotic therapy [28, 34]. In order to aid clinicians, several clinical models have been developed. In one study of 422 immunocompetent patients older than 1 month of age with acute bacterial or viral meningitis, a CSF glucose concentration less than 34 mg/dl, a CSF-to-blood glucose ratio less than 0.23, a CSF protein concentration greater than 220 mg/dl, more than 2000 leukocytes/mm^3 of CSF, and more than 1180 neutrophils/mm^3 of CSF were found to be individual predictors of bacterial rather than viral meningitis, with 99% certainty or better [52]. The Bacterial Meningitis Score has been derived and validated in a total of 4896 patients which identifies children with CSF pleocytosis who were at very low risk for bacterial meningitis (low-risk features were negative CSF Gram stain, CSF absolute neutrophil count <1000 cell/mm^3, CSF protein <80 mg/dl, and peripheral absolute neutrophil count <10,000 cells/mm^3) [53]. Not surprisingly, one of the most important predictors for bacterial meningitis in this scoring system is a positive Gram stain where the diagnosis is not a dilemma to clinicians. A recent study of 960 adults derived and validated a risk score in patients with meningitis and a negative Gram stain that identified a "zero risk" subgroup for any urgent treatable etiology (e.g., bacterial meningitis, herpes simplex encephalitis, fungal encephalitis, etc.) with 100% sensitivity [34]. Even though these clinical models are available, physicians are still treating empirically for bacterial meningitis in the majority of patients [28].

Biomarkers may also aid in the differentiation of viral versus bacterial meningitis. Elevated CSF lactate concentrations may also be useful in differentiating bacterial from nonbacterial meningitis in patients who have not received prior antimicrobial therapy [54, 55]. Two meta-analyses, one including 25 studies with 1692 patients (adults and children) [54] and the other including 31 studies with 1885 patients [55], concluded that the diagnostic accuracy of CSF lactate is better than that of the CSF white blood cell count, glucose concentration, and protein level in the differentiation of bacterial from aseptic meningitis; sensitivities of 93% and 97% and specificities of 96% and 94%, respectively, were seen. C-reactive protein (CRP), detected either in serum or CSF, and serum procalcitonin concentrations have been elevated in patients with acute bacterial meningitis and may be useful in discriminating between bacterial and viral meningitis. In one study, serum CRP was capable of distinguishing Gram stain-negative bacterial meningitis from viral meningitis on admission with a sensitivity of 96%, a specificity of 93%, and a negative predictive value of 99% [56]. In another study, a serum procalcitonin concentration of more than 0.2 ng/ml had a sensitivity and specificity of up to 100% in the diagnosis of bacterial meningitis, [57] although false-negative results have been reported [58].

Cranial Imaging

Due to the fear of herniation in patients with a possible brain mass, the Infectious Diseases Society of America recommends a head CT before the lumbar puncture with the following criteria: new-onset seizures, an immunocompromised state, signs that are suggestive of space-occupying lesions (papilledema or focal neurologic signs, not including cranial nerve palsy), or moderate to severe impairment of consciousness [59]. Despite these recommendations, the majority of patients with community-acquired meningitis undergo CT scanning with no indications [60]. In a large study of adults and children with aseptic meningitis, all head CT scans that were done were normal [2]. This practice increases costs and delays the diagnosis and therapy of patients with meningitis [61].

Summary of Challenges

- The etiologies of the aseptic meningitis syndrome remain unknown for a large proportion of cases fostering costly admissions, unnecessary antibiotic therapy, and exposure to nosocomial hazards for the majority of patients.
- Utilization of clinical models, biomarkers, and rapid multiplex PCR tests could help identify patients that do not require hospital admission or empiric antibiotic therapy. This could reduce costs and nosocomial complications.
- Cranial imaging is of no diagnostic value in aseptic meningitis and should not be done in patients without indications.

References

1. Hasbun R. The acute aseptic meningitis syndrome. Curr Infect Dis Rep. 2000;2(4):345–51.
2. Shukla B, Aguilera EA, Salazar L, et al. Aseptic meningitis in adults and children: diagnostic and management challenges. J Clin Virol. 2017;94:110–4.
3. Sulaiman T, Salazar L, Hasbun R. Acute versus subacute community-acquired meningitis in adults: an analysis of 611 patients. Medicine. 2017;96(36):e7984.
4. Centers for Disease Control and Prevention. Enterovirus and human parechovirus surveillance—United States, 2009–2013. MMWR Morb Mortal Wkly Rep. 2015;64:940–3.

5. Rudolph H, Schroten H, Tenenbaum T. Enterovirus infections of the central nervous system in children: an update. Pediatr Infect Dis J. 2016;35(5):567–9.
6. Messacar K, Schreiner TL, Van Haren K, et al. Acute flaccid paralysis: a clinical review of US cases 2012–2015. Ann Neurol. 2016;80:326–38.
7. Owatanapanich S, Wutthanarungsan R, Jaksupa W, Thisyakorn U. Risk factors for severe enteroviral infections in children. J Med Assoc Thai. 2016;99(3):322–30.
8. Grisariu S, Vaxman I, Gatt M, et al. Enteroviral infections in patients treated with rituximbab for non-Hodgkin lymphoma: a case series and review of the literature. Hematol Oncol. 2017;35(4):591–8.
9. Abzug MJ, Michaels MG, Wald E, et al. A randomized, double-blind, placebo-controlled trial of pleconaril for the treatment of neonates with enterovirus sepsis. J Pediatric Infect Dis Soc. 2016;5(1):53–62.
10. March B, Eastwood K, Wright IM, Tilbrook L, Durrheim DN. Epidemiology of enteroviral meningoencephalitis in neonates and young infants. J Paediatr Child Health. 2014;50(3):216–20.
11. Jaijakul S, Arias CA, Hossain M, et al. Toscana meningoencephalitis: a comparison to other viral central nervous system infections. J Clin Virol. 2012;55(3):204–8.
12. Kaewpoowat Q, Salazar L, Aguilera E, Wootton SH, Hasbun R. Herpes simplex and varicella zoster CNS infections: clinical presentations, treatment and outcomes. Infection. 2016;44(3):337–45.
13. Rosenberg J, Galen BT. Recurrent meningitis. Curr Pain Headache Rep. 2017;21(7):33.
14. Aurelius E, Franzen-Rohl E, Glimaker M, et al. Long-term valacyclovir suppressive treatment after herpes simplex virus type 2 meningitis: a double-blind, randomized controlled trial. Clin Infect Dis. 2012;54(9):1304–13.
15. Leber AL, Everhart K, Ballada-Llasat JM, et al. Multicenter evaluation of the BioFire film array meningitis encephalitis panel for detection of bacteria, viruses, and yeast in cerebrospinal fluid specimens. J Clin Microbiol. 2016;54(9):2251–61.
16. Pantry SN, Medveckzky PG. Latency, integration and reactivation of Human Herpes simplex type 6. Viruses. 2017;9(7):194.
17. Beckham JD, Tyler KL. Arbovirus infections. Continuum (Minneap Minn). 2015;21(6):1599–611.
18. Athar P, Hasbun R, Garcia MN, et al. Long-term neuromuscular outcomes of West Nile virus infection: a clinical and electromyograph evaluation of patients with a history of infection. Muscle Nerve. 2017;57(1):77–82.
19. Vanichanan J, Salazar L, Wootton SH, et al. Use of testing for West Nile virus and other arboviruses. Emerg Infect Dis. 2016;22(9). https://doi.org/10.3201/eid2209.152050.
20. Hasbun R, Garcia MN, Kellaway J, Baker L, Salazar L, Woods SP, Murray KM. West Nile virus retinopathy and associations with long term neurological and neurocognitive sequelae. PLoS One. 2016;11(3):e0148898.
21. Garcia MN, Hause AM, Walker CM, Orange JS, Hasbun R, Murray KO. Evaluation of prolonged fatigue post-West Nile virus infection and association of fatigue with elevated antiviral and pro-inflammatory cytokines. Viral Immunol. 2014;27(7):327–33.
22. Krow-Lucal E, Lindsey NP, Lehman J, Fischer M, Staples JE. West Nile virus and other nationally notifiable arboviral diseases — United States, 2015. MMWR Morb Mortal Wkly Rep. 2017;66:51–5.
23. Lenhard T, Ott D, Jakob NJ, et al. Predictors, neuroimaging characteristics and long-term outcome of severe European tick-borne encephalitis: a prospective cohort study. PLoS One. 2016;11:e0154143.
24. Fevola C, Kuivanen S, Smura T, et al. Seroprevalence of lymphocytic choriomeningitis virus and Ljungan virus in Finnish patients with suspected neurological infections. J Med Virol. 2018;90(3):429–35.
25. Centers for Disease Control and Prevention. Lymphocytic choriomeningitis virus infection in employees of a rodent breeding facility—Indiana, May–June 2012. MMWR Morb Mortal Wkly Rep. 2012;61:622–3.

26. Talley P, Holzbauer S, Smith K, et al. Notes from the field: lymphocytic choriomeningitis virus meningoencephalitis from a household rodent infestation—Minnesota, 2015. MMWR Morb Mortal Wkly Rep. 2016;65:248–9.
27. Martin NG, Iro MA, Sadarangani M, et al. Hospital admissions for viral meningitis in children in England over five decades: a population-based observational study. Lancet Infect Dis. 2016;16:2279–87.
28. Hasbun R, Rosenthal N, Balada-Llasat JM, et al. Epidemiology of meningitis and encephalitis in adults in the United States from 2011–2014. Clin Infect Dis. 2017;65(3):359–63.
29. Lescure FX, Moulignier A, Savatovsky J, et al. CD8 encephalitis in HIV-infected patients receiving cART: a treatable entity. Clin Infect Dis. 2013;57(1):101–8.
30. Dubot Peres A, Sengvilaipaseuth O, Changthonthip A, Newton PN, Lamballerie X. How many patients with anti-JEV IgM in cerebrospinal fluid really have Japanese encephalitis? Lancet Infect Dis. 2015;15(12):1376–7.
31. Puccioni-Sohler M, Roveroni N, Rosadas C, et al. Dengue infection in the nervous system: lessons learned for Zika and Chikungunya. Arq Neuropsiquiatr. 2017;75(2):123–6.
32. Waterman SH, Margolis HS, Sejvar JJ. Surveillance for dengue and dengue-associated neurologic syndromes in the United States. Am J Trop Med Hyg. 2015;92:996–8.
33. Jacobs M, Rodger A, Bell DJ, et al. Late Ebola virus relapse causing meningoencephalitis: a case report. Lancet. 2016;388(10043):498–503.
34. Hasbun R, Bijlsma M, Brouwer MC, et al. Risk score for identifying adults with CSF pleocytosis and negative CSF Gram stain at low risk for an urgent treatable cause. J Infect. 2013;67(2):102–10.
35. Jaijakul S, Salazar L, Wooton SH, Aguilera EA, Hasbun R. The clinical significance of neutrophilic pleocytosis in viral central nervous system infections. Int J Infect Dis. 2017;59:77–81.
36. Shrikanth V, Salazar L, Khoury N, Wootton S, Hasbun R. Hypoglycorrhachia in adults with community-acquired meningitis: etiologies and prognostic significance. Int J Infect Dis. 2015;39:39–43.
37. Marra CM. Chapter 38. Neurosyphilis. In:Scheld WM, Whitley RJ, Marra CM, editors. Infections of the central nervous system. 4th edition. Philadelphia:Lippincott Williamsn & Walkins. 2014:659–673.
38. Halperin JJ. Neurologic manifestations of Lyme disease. Curr Infect Dis Rep. 2011;13:360–6.
39. Cohn KA, Thompson AD, Shah SS, et al. Validation of a clinical prediction rule to distinguish Lyme meningitis from aseptic meningitis. Pediatrics. 2012;129(1):e46–53.
40. Jimenez JIS, Marroquin JLH, Richards GA, Amin P. Leptospirosis: report from the task force on tropical diseases by the World Federation of Societies of Intensive and Critical Care Medicine. J Crit Care. 2018;43:361–5.
41. Cope JR, Ali IK. Primary amebic meningoencephalitis: what have we learned in the last 5 years? Curr Infect Dis Rep. 2016;18:31.
42. Capewell LG, Harris AM, Yoder JS, et al. Diagnosis, clinical course, and treatment of primary amoebic meningoencephalitis in the United States, 1937–2013. J Pediatric Infect Dis Soc. 2015;4(4):e68–75.
43. Linam WM, Ahmed M, Cope JR, et al. Successful treatment of an adolescent with *Naegleria fowleri* primary amebic meningoencephalitis. Pediatrics. 2015;135(3):e744–8.
44. El Sahly H, Udayamurthy M, Parkerson G, Hasbun R. Survival of an AIDS patient after infection with Acanthamoeba sp of the central nervous system. Infection. 2017;45(5):715–8.
45. Morassutti AL, Thiengo SC, Fernandez M, et al. Eosinophilic meningitis caused by *Angiostrongylus cantonensis*: an emergent disease in Brazil. Mem Inst Oswaldo Cruz. 2014;109:399–407.
46. Wootton SH, Aguilera E, Salazar L, et al. Enhancing pathogen identification in patients with meningitis and a negative Gram stain using the BioFire FilmArray Meningitis/Encephalitis panel. Ann Clin Microbiol Antimicrob. 2016;15:26.
47. Rhein J, Bahr NC, Hemmert AC, et al. Diagnostic performance of a multiplex PCR assay for meningitis in an HIV-infected population in Uganda. Diagn Microbiol Infect Dis. 2016;84:268–73.

48. Onyango CO, Loparev V, Lidechi S, et al. Evaluation of a TaqMan Array card for detection of a central nervous system infection. J Clin Microbiol. 2017;55(7):2035–44.
49. Yun KW, Choi EH, Cheon DS, et al. Enteroviral meningitis without pleocytosis in children. Arch Dis Child. 2012;97(10):874–8.
50. Feigin RD, Shackelford PG. Value of repeat lumbar puncture in the differential diagnosis of meningitis. N Engl J Med. 1973;289(11):571–4.
51. Jarrin I, Sellier P, Lopes A, et al. Etiologies and management of aseptic meningitis in patients admitted to an internal medicine department. Medicine. 2016;95(2):e2372.
52. Spanos A, Harreli FE, Durack DT. Differential diagnosis of acute meningitis. An analysis of the predictive value of initial observations. JAMA. 1989;262:2700–7.
53. Nigrovic LE, Malley R, Kuppermann N. Meta-analysis of bacterial meningitis score validation studies. Arch Dis Child. 2012;97:799–805.
54. Huy NT, Thao NTH, Diep DTN, et al. Cerebrospinal fluid lactate concentration to distinguish bacterial from aseptic meningitis: a systemic review and meta-analysis. Crit Care. 2010;14:R240.
55. Sakushima K, Hayashino Y, Kawaguchi T, et al. Diagnostic accuracy of cerebrospinal fluid lactate for differentiating bacterial meningitis from aseptic meningitis: a meta-analysis. J Infect. 2011;62:255–62.
56. Sormunen P, Kallio MJ, Kilpi T, et al. C-reactive protein is useful in distinguishing Gram stain-negative bacterial meningitis from viral meningitis in children. J Pediatr. 1999;134:725–9.
57. Viallon A, Zeni F, Lambert C, et al. High sensitivity and specificity of serum procalcitonin levels in adults with bacterial meningitis. Clin Infect Dis. 1999;28:1313–6.
58. Schwarz S, Bertram M, Schwab S, et al. Serum procalcitonin levels in bacterial and abacterial meningitis. Crit Care Med. 2000;28:1828–32.
59. Tunkel AR, Hartman BJ, Kaplan SL, et al. Practice guidelines for the management of bacterial meningitis. Clin Infect Dis. 2004;39:1267–84.
60. Salazar L, Hasbun R. Cranial imaging before lumbar puncture in adults with community-acquired meningitis: clinical utility and adherence to the Infectious Diseases Society of America guidelines. Clin Infect Dis. 2017;64(12):1657–62.
61. Glimåker M, Johansson B, Grindborg Ö, et al. Adult bacterial meningitis: earlier treatment and improved outcome following guideline revision promoting prompt lumbar puncture. Clin Infect Dis. 2015;60:1162–9.

Cryptococcal Meningitis

5

Ahmed Al Hammadi and Luis Ostrosky-Zeichner

Abbreviations

5-FC	Flucytosine, 5-fluorocytosine
ABLC	Amphotericin B lipid complex
AIDS	Acquired immune deficiency syndrome
AmB	Amphotericin B
ART	Antiretroviral therapy
CM	Cryptococcal meningitis
CMV	Cytomegalovirus
CNS	Central nervous system
CrAg	Cryptococcal antigen
CSF	Cerebrospinal fluid
CT	Computed tomography
CYP51	Cytochrome P51
ELISA	Enzyme-linked immunosorbent assay
GM-CSF	Granulocyte macrophage colony-stimulating factor
HIV	Human immunodeficiency virus
Hsp90	Heat shock protein 90
IDSA	Infectious Disease Society of America
IFN-γ	Interferon-γ
IL	Interleukin
IRIS	Immune reconstitution inflammatory syndrome
LA	Latex agglutination
LFA	Lateral flow assay
LFAmB	Lipid formulations of AmB

A. Al Hammadi · L. Ostrosky-Zeichner (✉)
UT Health-McGovern Medical School, Houston, TX, USA
e-mail: Ahmed.Alhammadi@uth.tmc.edu; Luis.Ostrosky-Zeichner@uth.tmc.edu

MALDI-TOF-MS	Matrix-assisted laser desorption/ionization time-of-flight mass spectrometry
MIC	Minimal inhibitory concentrations
MRI	Magnetic resonance imaging
PIIRS	Post-infectious inflammatory response syndrome
SOT	Solid organ transplantation
Th-1	T-helper type 1 response
TNF-α	Tumor necrosis factor-α
VP	Ventriculoperitoneal
WCC	White cell count
WHO	World Health Organization

Introduction

Ecology and Mycology of *Cryptococcus*

First identified in 1894, the genus of *Cryptococcus* comprises more than 30 known species, of which human infections are almost always caused by *Cryptococcus neoformans* and *Cryptococcus gattii* [1, 2]. Based on antigenic determinants on the polysaccharide capsule, the two varieties of *C. neoformans* are identified as *var. grubii* [serotype A] and *var. neoformans* [serotype D], while *C. gattii* includes serotypes B and C [3]. Recent genetic studies propose to redivide the two species into seven separate species and genotypes [4].

   C. neoformans and *C. gattii* are encapsulated, heterobasidiomycetous fungi that exist in asexual or sexual stages [1]. *C. neoformans* was isolated from soil, avian excreta especially pigeons, and many other environmental sources, while *C. gattii* is restricted to red gum trees (*Eucalyptus*) [5–9]. The filaments that result from the mating of the two opposite types "*alpha*" and "*a*" have basidia that produce 1–2 micron basidiospores, thought to be the infectious propagules [10]. Most environmental and clinical isolates of *C. neoformans* only have the *alpha* mating locus shown to be more virulent in mice [11, 12]. This predominance can be explained by the yeast's ability under certain conditions to produce haploid fruiting without mating and sexual reproduction within the same mating type which may have explained the emergence of the Vancouver Island *C. gattii* outbreak [11–14].

Epidemiology and Risk Factors of Cryptococcal Meningitis (CM)

Cryptococcus is not considered a part of the human normal flora [15]. Prior to the era of acquired immune deficiency syndrome (AIDS), data analyzed from 725 isolates revealed that 100% of the isolates from Europe and Japan and more than 85% of the isolates from Canada, the UK, and the USA (except Southern California and Hawaii) were *C. neoformans* (serotypes A, D, or AD), while 35–100% of the isolates from tropical and subtropical areas were *C. gattii* (serotypes B and C). Overall,

C. neoformans serotypes were 86% of the isolates, and *C. gattii* serotypes were 13%, and 1% was not typeable [16].

Cryptococcosis remains a rare infection in normal hosts [15]. In fact, most adults and children in New York City were found to have antibodies to *C. neoformans* antigens, indicating that most of these infections are asymptomatic [17, 18]. In patients with AIDS, most infections are caused by *C. neoformans* serotype A [19], and *C. gattii* is much less common even in tropical and subtropical areas [20]. *C. gattii* is thought to cause disease predominantly in immunocompetent hosts, whereas *C. neoformans* mostly affects immunosuppressed patients [21], although *C. neoformans* (serotype A) in Vietnam has been associated with high prevalence of CM in human immunodeficiency virus (HIV)-negative, immunocompetent patients [22].

CM is the most common cause of adult meningitis in HIV patients in areas with high prevalence of HIV [23, 24]. The lower the CD4+ count in HIV patients, the higher the incidence of cryptococcosis, and that skyrockets with CD4+ count <100 cells/μL [25, 26]. The incidence of CM has declined significantly in Europe and the USA following the wide availability of antiretroviral therapy (ART) since 1997. Similarly, the rate of hospitalization in the USA declined from 16.6 million in 1997 to 7.7 million total population in 2009 [27, 28]. This was not seen in Africa as many patients present with a history of ART use and low CD4+ count due to nonadherence and loss of follow-up [29]. The updated analysis of the global burden of HIV-associated CM in 2014 estimated the global annual rate of CM as 223,100 cases and global deaths of 181,100, of which 73% and 75%, respectively, were in sub-Saharan Africa [30]. This is, however, a remarkable reduction from 957,000 annual CM cases and 600,000 deaths estimated in 2009 [31].

In HIV-negative patients, most patients with disseminated cryptococcosis have an identifiable underlying disease. For example, these infections are seen in patients with hematologic malignancies, treatment with corticosteroids, sarcoidosis with or without corticosteroids, and solid organ transplantation (SOT) but not in bone marrow transplantation likely due to the routine use of azole antifungal prophylaxis in these patients. Other populations at risk are patients with abnormalities in cell-mediated immunity [32, 33].

Of note, 51% of HIV-negative patients with cryptococcosis had central nervous system (CNS) involvement, and of that 30% had no apparent predisposing conditions [34]. The "normal host" may actually have subtle or uncommon immune abnormalities [2]. Furthermore, smoking and outdoor occupations was associated with increased risk of cryptococcal infections in HIV-infected patients [35]. Table 5.1 shows common predisposing conditions for CM [34, 36–44].

Clinical Manifestations of Cryptococcosis

Pathogenesis, Immune Responses, and Neurotropism

After inhaling the aerosolized basidiospores from the environment, the immune system of a normal host can efficiently kill the yeast [1]. Alternatively, the initial possibly asymptomatic infection is contained in a primary complex in the hilar lymph

Table 5.1 Predisposing conditions to cryptococcal meningitis

Autoimmune disorders
  • Sarcoidosis
  • Systemic lupus erythematosus

Comorbidities
  • Cirrhosis
  • Diabetes mellitus
  • Hepatic disease
  • Lymphoproliferative diseases
  • Peritoneal dialysis

Drugs
  • Corticosteroids
  • Monoclonal antibodies (adalimumab, alemtuzumab, infliximab)

Immunodeficiencies
  • Chronic granulomatous disease
  • FCg receptor II polymorphism
  • GATA2 mutations
  • Hyperimmunoglobulin E (Job syndrome)
  • Hyper-IgM syndrome

Infections
  • HIV infection

Syndromes and autoantibodies
  • Autoantibodies to IFN-γ
  • Autoantibodies to GM-CSF
  • Idiopathic CD4$^+$ lymphopenia
  • Pulmonary alveolar proteinosis

Transplantation
  • Solid organ transplantation

nodes similar to primary tuberculosis [45]. This process involves CD4$^+$ T cells, interleukin-2 (IL-2), and tumor necrosis factor-α (TNF-α) [1, 46]. On the hand, the infection may disseminate outside the lungs in immunocompromised hosts and sometimes in normal hosts following a primary infection or a reactivation in dormant hosts after a decline of the CD4$^+$ count or the use of corticosteroids [1, 47].

C. *neoformans* has many virulence factors, of which the capsule is the most defined [48]. The polysaccharide capsule helps to evade phagocytosis by macrophages [49], activates the alternative complement pathway leading to depletion of complements [50], inhibits T-cell activation and pro-inflammatory cytokines such as TNF-α [51, 52], downregulates the antigen-presentation capacity of monocytes [53], and decreases the production of interferon-γ (IFN-γ) which suppresses the IL-12 production leading to inhibition of the protective T-helper type 1 response (Th-1) against C. *neoformans* [54, 55]. It also enhances HIV replication and resists oxidative stress [1, 48].

Other important virulence factors in C. *neoformans* which can explain the yeast neurotropism are (A) a laccase enzyme that converts CNS catecholamines to melanin that protects against oxidative stress and exerts multiple cell-wall functions [56], (B) thermotolerance of C. *neoformans* to high temperatures up to 43 °C compared to C. *gattii* and serotype D that do not tolerate heat above 40° [57], (C) a urease and metalloprotease Mpr1 enzymes in C. *neoformans* that facilitate its transcellular migration into the mouse brain [58, 59], and (D) mechanisms in *C. neoformans* that allow it to survive nutrient starvation in the brain [60].

Pulmonary, Disseminated Disease and Atypical Sites of Infections

Cryptococcus causes a wide spectrum of infections with two major sites: the lungs and the CNS [15]. In immunocompetent hosts, pulmonary infections may be asymptomatic or may present with fever, chills, cough, chest pain, productive cough, hemoptysis, weight loss, and night sweats [61]. *C. neoformans* may colonize the respiratory tract of patients with chronic lung disease without underlying immune dysfunction. Infection may only involve the lungs associated with negative serum cryptococcal antigen (CrAg), but serum CrAg positivity should prompt ruling out an extrapulmonary focus of infection [62].

Most immunosuppressed patients present symptomatically, and pneumonia may progress faster and cause acute respiratory distress syndrome [63]. These patients may present with meningeal rather than pneumonia symptoms despite having both infections. Other coinfections have to be considered in AIDS patients with CD4+ count <100 cells/µL especially cytomegalovirus (CMV), *Nocardia*, *Pneumocystis*, and typical and atypical mycobacteria [1, 64].

Cryptococcus can infect any organ system of the body. Noteworthy, skin involvement is almost exclusively associated with disseminated disease, and lesions can be of any type. Lesions may mimic bacterial cellulitis or abscess, acne vulgaris, molluscum contagiosum, and squamous or basal carcinoma and may originate deeper from the underlying bone or subcutaneous tissue [1, 65, 66]. Of note, SOT recipients on tacrolimus were found to have more skin and soft tissue infections than CNS infections. This may be explained by the antifungal activity of tacrolimus at 37–39 °C and the lower skin temperatures [67]. Another site of the infection is the prostate which is usually asymptomatic, and the isolation of *Cryptococcus* in the urine indicates disseminated disease [1]. Of note, the prostate may be a reservoir for the yeast which may grow in the urine even after the successful treatment of CM in AIDS patients [68].

CNS and Ocular Disease

CM may present with fever, headache, altered mental status, cranial nerve palsies, lethargy, coma, and memory loss [1, 15]. HIV patients with CM usually present after 2 weeks of the onset of symptoms and have a more disseminated disease, while non-HIV patients with CM may present after 6–12 weeks of the onset, a diagnosis often delayed by the absence of fever in non-HIV patients [2]. HIV patients with CM have more yeast burden, higher CSF CrAg titers, and higher rates of increased cerebrospinal fluid (CSF) pressure [1, 69]. In fact, 51% of HIV patients with CM have an opening pressure of >250 mm H_2O [70]. Also, HIV patients are also more likely to have other infections such as *Toxoplasma gondii* or CNS lymphomas [1]. Interestingly, *C. gattii* is associated with more cryptococcomas and hydrocephalus than *C. neoformans* [71].

Ocular disease is frequently seen in patients with CM. The most common findings are papilledema, cranial nerve palsies, and decreased visual acuity due to raised intracranial pressure [72, 73]. Visual loss may occur secondary to optic neuritis or endophthalmitis [74]. Furthermore, ocular coinfection may be seen with CMV and HIV [75]. In addition, compression of the ophthalmic artery may occur during the antifungal therapy due to raised intracranial pressure [1].

Outcomes and Prognostic Factors of CM

A study in Botswana showed no significant difference between the presentation and outcome in HIV-associated CM due to *C. neoformans* or *C. gattii* [76]. The updated analysis of the global burden of HIV-associated CM in 2014 estimated the 1-year mortality in patients in care to be 70% in low-income countries, 40% in middle-income countries, 20% in North America, and 30% in Europe, with 1.5 times higher mortality in patients not in care in these regions [30]. Risk factors that influence mortality in HIV-associated CM are CSF fungal burden, decreased sensorium, and the rate of clearance of infection [70]. In addition, HIV infection and cryptococcemia were associated with higher mortality rates, whereas hematologic malignancy and organ failure were not associated with mortality [77]. Also, low CSF white cell count (WCC) (<20 cell/µL) and high CSF CrAg titers >1:1024 were associated with worse outcomes [78].

In the USA, the mortality of HIV-negative patients was higher than HIV-positive patients (35% vs 26%) [77]. This may be attributed to the late presentation, delayed diagnosis, and possibly subtle immune dysfunction [77, 79]. Furthermore, the predictors of mortality of cryptococcosis in HIV-negative patients were shown to be age ≥60 years, hematologic neoplasm and organ dysfunction [34]. Also, a study of *C. gattii* CM in Australia showed that a CSF CrAg titer of ≥256 was associated with worse neurological consequences and death [80].

Cryptococcal Immune Reconstitution Inflammatory Syndrome (IRIS) in Patients with CM

Although the association between IRIS and CM in HIV patients is well established [81], IRIS has been described also in normal hosts, solid and bone marrow transplant recipients, and hematological malignancy patients on chemotherapy [1, 2, 82] after the immunosuppressive or antirejection regimens have been reduced to strengthen the immune system [83]. In apparently immunocompetent hosts, post-infectious inflammatory response syndrome (PIIRS) happens when cerebral edema and neurological damage are exacerbated by the immune response [79]. Two forms of IRIS identified in HIV patients are paradoxical IRIS in CM patients responding to antifungal therapy who relapse after initiating ART and unmasking IRIS in patients developing CM after starting ART [84].

IRIS may present with relapsing aseptic meningitis, abscess development, increased intracranial pressure, new focal findings, cryptococcomas, or other CNS findings [85, 86]. Risk factors for CM-IRIS include high fungal burden which inhibits leukocyte migration into the CNS [87]; low initial CSF WCC and CSF protein levels as well as lower CSF IFN-γ, TNF-α, IL-2, IL-6, IL-8, and IL-17 cytokines; and higher CSF chemokines of macrocyte chemotactic protein-1, macrophage inflammatory protein-1α, and granulocyte macrophage colony-stimulating factor (GM-CSF). In addition, a rapid improvement of low CD4+ cell count after starting ART is another major risk factor [88–91]. Predictors of IRIS in transplant patients include host immune responses and discontinuation of calcineurin inhibitors which causes a five times increased risk for IRIS [83]. The optimal time of starting ART and management options of IRIS will be discussed below in the management of CM section.

Diagnosis of CM

CSF Findings

HIV-negative patients with CM have increased CSF protein levels and WCC, while HIV patients have lower CSF protein levels and CSF WCC (median 15×10^6 cells/L) [70]. Low glucose levels and lymphocytic predominance are seen in both groups [2, 92]. India ink staining is a rapid tool for the diagnosis of CM and has a sensitivity of 50–70% in HIV-negative patients [93, 94] and a sensitivity/specificity of 84%/53% in HIV patients [95]. The performance of this test is highly operator-dependent.

CSF Cultures

Most bacterial and fungal media cultures of the CSF can detect the yeast in 3–7 days, with a sensitivity of 50–80% [93]. Biochemical reactions and DNA-based methods can help to identify isolates and distinguish between *C. neoformans* and *C. gattii* [96, 97]. Quantitative fungal cultures have been used to assess the rate of clearance and the fungicidal activity of various antifungal drugs [98]. Recently, matrix-assisted laser desorption/ionization time-of-flight mass spectrometry (MALDI-TOF-MS) has been studied and can rapidly identify species and genotypes of *Cryptococcus* [99].

Serum and CSF CrAg

Detection of cryptococcal capsular polysaccharide (glucuronoxylomannan, GXM) Ag in serum and CSF by latex agglutination (LA) and enzyme-linked immunosorbent assay (ELISA) has a sensitivity of 100% for disseminated disease and 94% for meningeal disease [100]. Specificity for CSF and serum CrAg was at least 90% for both LA and ELISA regardless of HIV status [101, 102]. In addition, cross-reactive serum CrAg has been seen in infections with *Trichosporon beigelii* [103] and *Stomatococcus mucilaginosus* [104].

A simple, quick, and cheap point-of-care test for the detection of CSF and serum CrAg has been developed; this new bedside lateral flow assay (LFA) has a sensitivity and specificity of 99% [105]. It has a preemptive role in resource-limited settings in the early diagnosis of asymptomatic CM and prevention of IRIS after starting ART [106] and in ART-naïve patients [107]. In addition, LFA's improved sensitivity offers an advantage over LA and cultures in diagnosing HIV-negative *C. gattii* meningitis [108].

Radiographic Findings

Brain magnetic resonance imaging (MRI) is more sensitive than computed tomography (CT) in CM, but there are no pathognomonic findings. Findings include lesions in the basal ganglia and midbrain that hyperenhance with T2-weighted images but do not enhance with T1-weighted postcontrast images [1]. Also, findings include hydrocephalus, single or multiple nodules with or without enhancement, dilated Virchow-Robin spaces, pseudocysts, masses, gyral enhancement, cryptococcomas, and lacunar and cortical infarcts [109, 110]. Even with the initiation of ART, these lesions may not resolve in months or years after successful treatment [111]; thus, cultures, symptoms, and clinical findings have to be considered before declaring treatment failure, and in the case of CNS parenchymal lesions, CNS lymphoma and coinfections with *Nocardia* or *Toxoplasma* should be ruled out [1]. Chest radiographs (chest X-ray, CT) can show single to multiple, well-defined noncalcified nodules in normal hosts diagnosed by lung biopsy. Other findings include lobar and mass-like infiltrates, hilar lymphadenopathy, lung cavities, and pleural effusions [112]. Disease may progress more rapidly in immunosuppressed patients such as AIDS patients or those receiving high-dose corticosteroids [63].

Management and Complications of CM

Antifungal Therapy

If untreated, CM can progress to altered sensorium, seizures, coma, and even death [2]. The rate of progression of the disease depends on host factors and fungal burden of *Cryptococcus*. The management of CM according to the practice guidelines of the Infectious Disease Society of America (IDSA) is based on three risk groups: HIV-infected individuals, organ transplant recipients, and non-HIV-infected nontransplant hosts [113]. The course is divided into three steps: induction, consolidation, and maintenance.

The use of Amphotericin B (AmB) has been imperative in the management of CM [114], and its combination with flucytosine (5-Fluorocytosine, 5-FC) was shown to be more fungicidal than AmB alone in sterilizing CSF [115]. The combination of AmB/5-FC was also associated with improved survival [116], reduced nephrotoxicity, shorter hospitalization [117], and prevention of relapse [118].

Patients with or predisposed to renal dysfunction or organ transplant recipients should not receive AmB deoxycholate (AmBd) but should be placed on lipid formulations of AmB (LFAmB) either with liposomal AmB (L-AmB) or AmB lipid complex (ABLC). Monitoring the kidney function is important during therapy with AmBd or LFAmB, and the dose of 5-FC has to be adjusted accordingly [113].

HIV-infected individual should receive induction with AmB/5-FC for at least 2 weeks until clinical response is seen, followed by consolidation with 400–800 mg fluconazole daily for 8–10 weeks and maintenance with 200 mg fluconazole daily for at least 1 year which can be stopped when CD4 count is ≥100 cells/μL, viral load is low or undetectable for ≥3 months, and serum CrAg is negative or low [113]. This requires the successful introduction of ART with the possibility of inducing paradoxical IRIS [113]. Current IDSA 2010 practice guidelines for CM recommend to start ART in 2–10 weeks after initiating induction, although more recent studies suggested 4–6 weeks as the most optimal time to start ART and prevent IRIS [70, 119]. Please see Table 5.2 for detailed recommendations of treatment of CM in HIV patients, SOT recipients, and HIV-negative patients.

5-FC is used in combination with one of AmB formulations for induction for at least 2 weeks (a dose of 100 mg/kg/day or renally adjusted) and should not be used alone as monotherapy can lead to resistance [120]. Monitoring of complete blood counts for bone marrow suppression is important, but it is not necessary to monitor serum drug levels [116, 121]. Also, monitoring of hypokalemia, hypomagnesemia, and acute kidney injury is essential in patients on AmB, and routine intravenous hydration and preemptive electrolyte replacement reduced the rates of hypokalemia and renal toxicity [122].

Azoles such as fluconazole have been used in the management of CM due to its safe profile and excellent penetration into the brain [123, 124]. However, due to its fungistatic properties, fluconazole should not be used in the induction phase when there is a high fungal burden in the CSF [1]. Itraconazole, although has less CSF penetration, was shown to successfully treat CM [125]. When 5-FC is not available, AmB plus fluconazole (800 mg/day superior to 400 mg/day) can be used [126]. Furthermore, fluconazole 1200 mg daily was shown to be more fungicidal than 800 mg daily in HIV-associated CM [127], and its combination with 5-FC (100 mg/kd/day) had early fungicidal activity close to that of AmB alone [128]. Also, voriconazole, posaconazole, and isavuconazole were used as salvage therapy in refractory cases with 38–60% response rates [129–131]. Echinocandins are not effective against *Cryptococcus* [132]. CNS cryptococcomas are treated similarly to CM but may require longer duration and surgical resection is rarely needed [133].

Persistence of CM Infection

Studies showed that in patients with AIDS and CM, at 10 weeks of therapy with AmB or fluconazole alone, 60–65% did not have a successful outcome compared to 35–45% failure rate in those who received a combination of AmB/5-FC or fluconazole/5-FC [134–137].

Table 5.2 Treatment recommendation of CM per IDSA 2010 guidelines

Stage	Regimen	Duration	Alternatives
Induction			
HIV patients	AmBd (0.7–1.0 mg/kg per day) plus 5-FC (100 mg/kg per day)	2 weeks	AmBd plus fluconazole, fluconazole plus 5-FC, fluconazole, itraconazole
	L-AmB (3–4 mg/kg per day) or ABLC (5 mg/kg per day) plus 5-FC (100 mg/kg per day)	2 weeks	–
	AmBd (0.7–1.0 mg/kg per day), L-AmB (3–4 mg/kg per day) or ABLC (5 mg/kg per day) alone in patient intolerant to 5-FC	4 weeks	–
Transplant recipients	L-AmB (3–4 mg/kg per day) or ABLC (5 mg/kg per day) plus 5-FC (100 mg/kg per day)	2 weeks	L-AmB (6 mg/kg per day), ABLC (5 mg/kg per day) or AmBd (0.7 mg/kg per day) all for 4–6 weeks
Non-HIV, nontransplant patients	AmBd (0.7–1.0 mg/kg per day) plus 5-FC (100 mg/kg per day)	≥4 weeks	–
	AmBd (0.7–1.0 mg/kg per day) alone in patient intolerant to 5-FC	≥6 weeks	–
	L-AmB (3–4 mg/kg per day) or ABLC (5 mg/kg per day) plus 5-FC (100 mg/kg per day) for AmBd-intolerant patients	≥4 weeks	–
Consolidation			
HIV patients	Fluconazole 400 mg daily	8 weeks	–
Transplant recipients	Fluconazole 400–800 mg daily	8 weeks	–
Non-HIV, nontransplant patients	Fluconazole 400–800 mg daily	8 weeks	–
Maintenance			
HIV patients	Fluconazole 200 mg daily	≥1 year	Itraconazole 400 mg daily (for ≥1 year)
			AmBd (1 mg/kg per week for ≥1 year)
Transplant recipients	Fluconazole 200–400 mg daily	6–12 months	–
Non-HIV, nontransplant patients	Fluconazole 200 mg daily	6–12 months	–

Persistence or relapse of infection may be difficult to identify but should be considered after at least 4 weeks of therapy with new signs or symptoms or repeat positive cultures and should not be based only on the persistence of positive India ink staining or CSF CrAg titers [1]. Also, a diagnosis of unmasking IRIS has to be considered in these settings. Most initial isolates of *C. neoformans* and *C. gattii* have low minimal inhibitory concentrations (MICs) to AmB, 5-FC, and azoles by in vitro susceptibility testing [138]. Mechanisms of drug resistance in *C. neoformans* were described [139], and in fact, the clinical response may correlate with MIC levels [140]. Of note, molecular testing confirmed that most recurrent infections represented relapse of the initial strain rather than a new strain [141].

Management of IRIS in Patients with CM

The percentage of patients who develop IRIS (including paradoxical and unmasking) was shown to be 30% by 30 days of starting ART [142]. For patients who are worsening despite a sterile CSF, the IDSA guidelines recommend continuing antifungal therapy and using corticosteroids (0.5–1 mg/kg/day of prednisone equivalent) or dexamethasone at higher doses for severe CNS signs and symptoms [113]. Doses are to be tapered over the next 2–6 weeks. Nonsteroidal anti-inflammatory drugs and thalidomide were used but data is limited [113]. Also, recent cases suggest using TNF-α blockade with adalimumab in patients with severe CM-associated IRIS [143, 144]. Of note, chloroquine was used successfully to treat IRIS that resulted from withdrawal of corticosteroids due to its antifungal effects on *Cryptococcus* [145].

Management of Increased Intracranial Pressures in Patients with CM

Elevated intracranial pressure plays a critical role in the initial management of HIV-associated CM and improvement clinically and microbiologically [146]. Patients with severe CM often have CSF opening pressure >250 mm, acutely worsening brain edema, and possible development of CSF outflow obstruction [147]. Increased intracranial pressure may cause uncal herniation, tonsillar-cerebellar herniation, or compression of the midbrain [1]. During the early phase of treatment, controlling the increased intracranial pressure may be critical with external drainage by repeat lumbar punctures and ventricular or lumbar drains [148]. Hydrocephalus in patients with CM can be managed safely with placement of ventriculoperitoneal (VP) shunt even with positive CSF cultures [149]. Corticosteroids should only be used in patients with concomitant increased intracranial pressure and IRIS and not without IRIS [150].

Salvage and Adjunctive Immunomodulating Therapy

The use of adjunctive corticosteroids during initial combination antifungal treatment of CM was associated with increased disability, adverse side effects, and decreased rates of fungal clearance of CSF [150]. Stopping corticosteroids in SOT recipients is recommended to optimize immunity [83]; however, discontinuing calcineurin agents was associated with IRIS owing to the synergistic activity of calcineurin inhibitors with antifungals against *Cryptococcus* [151]. The HIV-negative, apparently immunocompetent host may develop CM due to virulent strains; however, ruling our subtle immunodeficiencies (as outlined in Table 5.1) or idiopathic lymphopenia is recommended [152].

Adding sertraline to AmB and fluconazole has been associated with increased rates of CSF fungal clearance and less IRIS incidence and relapse [153]. Mycograb® which is a humanized Ab against heat shock protein 90 (hsp90) was shown to synergistically render AmB fungicidal and mirror the effects of 5-FC on the killing of *C. neoformans* [154]. Cytokine therapy with IFN-γ improved the fungal CSF clearance of *Cryptococcus* without increased adverse events [155]. Also, GM-CSF may enhance the anti-cryptococcal activity of monocytes and neutrophils in HIV patients [156, 157]. In addition, a new oral tetrazole, cytochrome P51 (CYP51) inhibitor Viamet 1129 showed potent in vitro activity against *C. neoformans* and *C. gattii* in animal models and may be used for fluconazole-resistant isolates [158, 159].

Screening and Prevention of CM

The goal of this approach is early diagnosis of HIV patients at high risk of developing CM through early detection of CrAg in the blood [106], detectable at median of 22 days before CNS symptoms [160]. The 100% negative predictive value supports its use in screening and preemptive fluconazole in CrAg-positive patients [2, 161]. In fact, the World Health Organization (WHO) supports its use in screening ART-naïve HIV patients with CD4+ count <100 cells/μL and high prevalence of cryptococcal antigenemia (≥3%) [106, 162].

Research Gaps

Despite the use of combination therapy with AmB and 5-FC, CM mortality remains significantly high [30]. Many agents with potential antifungal properties remain under investigation [152]. A vaccine against cryptococcal GXM-tetanus toxoid conjugate was developed and elicited protective antibodies in mice [163]; however, human trials are yet to be conducted. The use of monoclonal antibodies could be promising but is to be further investigated and may require repeated injections [164]. Viamet 1129 is a new oral azole-like agent and may be promising but needs to be evaluated clinically. Further investigations of subtle immune deficiencies that predispose apparently immunocompetent hosts to cryptococcal infections may lead to the discovery of new agents and new mechanisms to better target and treat *Cryptococcus*.

References

1. Perfect JR. Cryptococcosis (Cryptococcus neoformans and Cryptococcus gattii). In: Bennett JE, Dolin R, Blaser MJ, editors. Mandell, Douglas, and Bennett's principles and practice of infectious diseases. 8th ed. Philadelphia: Elsevier; 2015. p. 2934–48.

2. Williamson PR, Jarvis JN, Panackal AA, Fisher MC, Molloy SF, Loyse A, et al. Cryptococcal meningitis: epidemiology, immunology, diagnosis and therapy. Nat Rev Neurol. 2017;13(1):13–24.
3. Kwon-Chung K, Boekhout T, Fell J, Diaz M. Proposal to conserve the name Cryptococcus gattii against C. hondurianus and C. bacillisporus (Basidiomycota, Hymenomycetes, Tremellomycetidae). Taxon. 2002;51(4):804–6.
4. Hagen F, Khayhan K, Theelen B, Kolecka A, Polacheck I, Sionov E, et al. Recognition of seven species in the Cryptococcus gattii/Cryptococcus neoformans species complex. Fungal Genet Biol. 2015;78:16–48.
5. Emmons CW. Isolation of Cryptococcus neoformans from soil. J Bacteriol. 1951;62(6):685–90.
6. Emmons CW. Saprophytic sources of Cryptococcus neoformans associated with the pigeon (Columba livia). Am J Hyg. 1955;62(3):227–32.
7. Muchmore HG, Rhoades ER, Nix GE, Felton FG, Carpenter RE. Occurrence of Cryptococcus neoformans in the environment of three geographically associated cases of Cryptococcal meningitis. N Engl J Med. 1963;268(20):1112–4.
8. Bauwens L, Swinne D, De Vroey C, De Meurichy W. Isolation of Cryptococcus neoformans var. neoformans in the aviaries of the Antwerp zoological gardens. Mykosen. 1986;29(7):291.
9. Levitz SM. The ecology of Cryptococcus neoformans and the epidemiology of cryptococcosis. Rev Infect Dis. 1991;13(6):1163–9.
10. Botts MR, Giles SS, Gates MA, Kozel TR, Hull CM. Isolation and characterization of Cryptococcus neoformans spores reveal a critical role for capsule biosynthesis genes in spore biogenesis. Eukaryot Cell. 2009;8(4):595–605.
11. Kwon-Chung KJ, Bennett JE. Distribution of alpha and alpha mating types of Cryptococcus neoformans among natural and clinical isolates. Am J Epidemiol. 1978;108(4):337–40.
12. Kwon-Chung KJ, Edman JC, Wickes BL. Genetic association of mating types and virulence in Cryptococcus neoformans. Infect Immun. 1992;60(2):602–5.
13. Wickes BL, Mayorga ME, Edman U, Edman JC. Dimorphism and haploid fruiting in Cryptococcus neoformans: association with the alpha-mating type. Proc Natl Acad Sci U S A. 1996;93(14):7327–31.
14. Fraser JA, Giles SS, Wenink EC, Geunes-Boyer SG, Wright JR, Diezmann S, et al. Same-sex mating and the origin of the Vancouver Island Cryptococcus gattii outbreak. Nature. 2005;437(7063):1360–4.
15. Perfect JR, Casadevall A. Cryptococcosis. Infect Dis Clin N Am. 2002;16(4):837–74, v–vi.
16. Kwon-Chung KJ, Bennett JE. Epidemiologic differences between the two varieties of Cryptococcus neoformans. Am J Epidemiol. 1984;120(1):123–30.
17. Chen LC, Goldman DL, Doering TL, Pirofski L, Casadevall A. Antibody response to Cryptococcus neoformans proteins in rodents and humans. Infect Immun. 1999;67(5):2218–24.
18. Goldman DL, Khine H, Abadi J, Lindenberg DJ, Pirofski L, Niang R, et al. Serologic evidence for Cryptococcus neoformans infection in early childhood. Pediatrics. 2001;107(5):E66.
19. Steenbergen JN, Casadevall A. Prevalence of Cryptococcus neoformans var. neoformans (serotype D) and Cryptococcus neoformans var. grubii (serotype A) isolates in New York City. J Clin Microbiol. 2000;38(5):1974–6.
20. Morgan J, McCarthy KM, Gould S, Fan K, Arthington-Skaggs B, Iqbal N, et al. Cryptococcus gattii infection: characteristics and epidemiology of cases identified in a South African province with high HIV seroprevalence, 2002–2004. Clin Infect Dis. 2006;43(8):1077–80.
21. Speed B, Dunt D. Clinical and host differences between infections with the two varieties of Cryptococcus neoformans. Clin Infect Dis. 1995;21(1):28–34; discussion 5–6.
22. Chau TT, Mai NH, Phu NH, Nghia HD, Chuong LV, Sinh DX, et al. A prospective descriptive study of cryptococcal meningitis in HIV uninfected patients in Vietnam—high prevalence of Cryptococcus neoformans var grubii in the absence of underlying disease. BMC Infect Dis. 2010;10:199.

23. Rajasingham R, Rhein J, Klammer K, Musubire A, Nabeta H, Akampurira A, et al. Epidemiology of meningitis in an HIV-infected Ugandan cohort. Am J Trop Med Hyg. 2015;92(2):274–9.
24. Jarvis JN, Meintjes G, Williams A, Brown Y, Crede T, Harrison TS. Adult meningitis in a setting of high HIV and TB prevalence: findings from 4961 suspected cases. BMC Infect Dis. 2010;10:67.
25. Crowe SM, Carlin JB, Stewart KI, Lucas CR, Hoy JF. Predictive value of CD4 lymphocyte numbers for the development of opportunistic infections and malignancies in HIV-infected persons. J Acquir Immune Defic Syndr. 1991;4(8):770–6.
26. Sorvillo F, Beall G, Turner PA, Beer VL, Kovacs AA, Kerndt PR. Incidence and factors associated with extrapulmonary cryptococcosis among persons with HIV infection in Los Angeles County. AIDS. 1997;11(5):673–9.
27. Dromer F, Mathoulin-Pelissier S, Fontanet A, Ronin O, Dupont B, Lortholary O. Epidemiology of HIV-associated cryptococcosis in France (1985–2001): comparison of the pre- and post-HAART eras. AIDS. 2004;18(3):555–62.
28. Pyrgos V, Seitz AE, Steiner CA, Prevots DR, Williamson PR. Epidemiology of cryptococcal meningitis in the US: 1997–2009. PLoS One. 2013;8(2):e56269.
29. Wall EC, Everett DB, Mukaka M, Bar-Zeev N, Feasey N, Jahn A, et al. Bacterial meningitis in Malawian adults, adolescents, and children during the era of antiretroviral scale-up and Haemophilus influenzae type b vaccination, 2000–2012. Clin Infect Dis. 2014;58(10):e137–45.
30. Rajasingham R, Smith RM, Park BJ, Jarvis JN, Govender NP, Chiller TM, et al. Global burden of disease of HIV-associated cryptococcal meningitis: an updated analysis. Lancet Infect Dis. 2017;17(8):873–81.
31. Park BJ, Wannemuehler KA, Marston BJ, Govender N, Pappas PG, Chiller TM. Estimation of the current global burden of cryptococcal meningitis among persons living with HIV/AIDS. AIDS. 2009;23(4):525–30.
32. Diamond RD, Bennett JE. Disseminated cryptococcosis in man: decreased lymphocyte transformation in response to Cryptococcus neoformans. J Infect Dis. 1973;127(6):694–7.
33. Graybill JR, Alford RH. Cell-mediated immunity in Cryptococcosis. Cell Immunol. 1974;14(1):12–21.
34. Pappas PG, Perfect JR, Cloud GA, Larsen RA, Pankey GA, Lancaster DJ, et al. Cryptococcosis in human immunodeficiency virus-negative patients in the era of effective azole therapy. Clin Infect Dis. 2001;33(5):690–9.
35. Hajjeh RA, Conn LA, Stephens DS, Baughman W, Hamill R, Graviss E, et al. Cryptococcosis: population-based multistate active surveillance and risk factors in human immunodeficiency virus-infected persons. Cryptococcal Active Surveillance Group. J Infect Dis. 1999;179(2):449–54.
36. Zonios DI, Falloon J, Huang CY, Chaitt D, Bennett JE. Cryptococcosis and idiopathic CD4 lymphocytopenia. Medicine (Baltimore). 2007;86(2):78–92.
37. Nath DS, Kandaswamy R, Gruessner R, Sutherland DE, Dunn DL, Humar A. Fungal infections in transplant recipients receiving alemtuzumab. Transplant Proc. 2005;37(2):934–6.
38. Tsiodras S, Samonis G, Boumpas DT, Kontoyiannis DP. Fungal infections complicating tumor necrosis factor alpha blockade therapy. Mayo Clin Proc. 2008;83(2):181–94.
39. Rosen LB, Freeman AF, Yang LM, Jutivorakool K, Olivier KN, Angkasekwinai N, et al. Anti-GM-CSF autoantibodies in patients with cryptococcal meningitis. J Immunol. 2013;190(8):3959–66.
40. Saijo T, Chen J, Chen SC, Rosen LB, Yi J, Sorrell TC, et al. Anti-granulocyte-macrophage colony-stimulating factor autoantibodies are a risk factor for central nervous system infection by Cryptococcus gattii in otherwise immunocompetent patients. MBio. 2014;5(2):e00912–4.
41. Lee YC, Chew GT, Robinson BW. Pulmonary and meningeal cryptococcosis in pulmonary alveolar proteinosis. Aust NZ J Med. 1999;29(6):843–4.

42. Browne SK, Burbelo PD, Chetchotisakd P, Suputtamongkol Y, Kiertiburanakul S, Shaw PA, et al. Adult-onset immunodeficiency in Thailand and Taiwan. N Engl J Med. 2012;367(8):725–34.
43. Vinh DC, Patel SY, Uzel G, Anderson VL, Freeman AF, Olivier KN, et al. Autosomal dominant and sporadic monocytopenia with susceptibility to mycobacteria, fungi, papillomaviruses, and myelodysplasia. Blood. 2010;115(8):1519–29.
44. Hu XP, Wu JQ, Zhu LP, Wang X, Xu B, Wang RY, et al. Association of Fcgamma receptor IIB polymorphism with cryptococcal meningitis in HIV-uninfected Chinese patients. PLoS One. 2012;7(8):e42439.
45. Salyer WR, Salyer DC, Baker RD. Primary complex of Cryptococcus and pulmonary lymph nodes. J Infect Dis. 1974;130(1):74–7.
46. Hill JO. CD4+ T cells cause multinucleated giant cells to form around Cryptococcus neoformans and confine the yeast within the primary site of infection in the respiratory tract. J Exp Med. 1992;175(6):1685–95.
47. Garcia-Hermoso D, Janbon G, Dromer F. Epidemiological evidence for dormant Cryptococcus neoformans infection. J Clin Microbiol. 1999;37(10):3204–9.
48. Zaragoza O, Chrisman CJ, Castelli MV, Frases S, Cuenca-Estrella M, Rodriguez-Tudela JL, et al. Capsule enlargement in Cryptococcus neoformans confers resistance to oxidative stress suggesting a mechanism for intracellular survival. Cell Microbiol. 2008;10(10):2043–57.
49. Kozel TR, Gotschlich EC. The capsule of Cryptococcus neoformans passively inhibits phagocytosis of the yeast by macrophages. J Immunol. 1982;129(4):1675–80.
50. Levitz SM. Overview of host defenses in fungal infections. Clin Infect Dis. 1992;14(Suppl 1):S37–42.
51. Mody CH, Syme RM. Effect of polysaccharide capsule and methods of preparation on human lymphocyte proliferation in response to Cryptococcus neoformans. Infect Immun. 1993;61(2):464–9.
52. Vecchiarelli A, Retini C, Pietrella D, Monari C, Tascini C, Beccari T, et al. Downregulation by cryptococcal polysaccharide of tumor necrosis factor alpha and interleukin-1 beta secretion from human monocytes. Infect Immun. 1995;63(8):2919–23.
53. Retini C, Vecchiarelli A, Monari C, Bistoni F, Kozel TR. Encapsulation of Cryptococcus neoformans with glucuronoxylomannan inhibits the antigen-presenting capacity of monocytes. Infect Immun. 1998;66(2):664–9.
54. Pietrella D, Monari C, Retini C, Palazzetti B, Kozel TR, Vecchiarelli A. HIV type 1 envelope glycoprotein gp120 induces development of a T helper type 2 response to Cryptococcus neoformans. AIDS. 1999;13(16):2197–207.
55. Decken K, Kohler G, Palmer-Lehmann K, Wunderlin A, Mattner F, Magram J, et al. Interleukin-12 is essential for a protective Th1 response in mice infected with Cryptococcus neoformans. Infect Immun. 1998;66(10):4994–5000.
56. Salas SD, Bennett JE, Kwon-Chung KJ, Perfect JR, Williamson PR. Effect of the laccase gene CNLAC1, on virulence of Cryptococcus neoformans. J Exp Med. 1996;184(2):377–86.
57. Martinez LR, Garcia-Rivera J, Casadevall A. Cryptococcus neoformans var. neoformans (serotype D) strains are more susceptible to heat than C. neoformans var. grubii (serotype A) strains. J Clin Microbiol. 2001;39(9):3365–7.
58. Shi M, Li SS, Zheng C, Jones GJ, Kim KS, Zhou H, et al. Real-time imaging of trapping and urease-dependent transmigration of Cryptococcus neoformans in mouse brain. J Clin Invest. 2010;120(5):1683–93.
59. Vu K, Tham R, Uhrig JP, Thompson GR 3rd, Na Pombejra S, Jamklang M, et al. Invasion of the central nervous system by Cryptococcus neoformans requires a secreted fungal metalloprotease. MBio. 2014;5(3):e01101–14.
60. Coelho C, Bocca AL, Casadevall A. The tools for virulence of Cryptococcus neoformans. Adv Appl Microbiol. 2014;87:1–41.
61. Warr W, Bates JH, Stone A. The spectrum of pulmonary cryptococcosis. Ann Intern Med. 1968;69(6):1109–16.

62. Randhawa HS, Pal M. Occurrence and significance of Cryptococcus neoformans in the respiratory tract of patients with bronchopulmonary disorders. J Clin Microbiol. 1977;5(1):5–8.
63. Henson DJ, Hill AR. Cryptococcal pneumonia: a fulminant presentation. Am J Med Sci. 1984;288(5):221–2.
64. Riley E, Cahan WG. Pulmonary cryptococccis followed by pulmonary tuberculosis. A case report. Am Rev Respir Dis. 1972;106(4):594–9.
65. Schupbach CW, Wheeler CE Jr, Briggaman RA, Warner NA, Kanof EP. Cutaneous manifestations of disseminated cryptococcosis. Arch Dermatol. 1976;112(12):1734–40.
66. Pema K, Diaz J, Guerra LG, Nabhan D, Verghese A. Disseminated cutaneous cryptococcosis. Comparison of clinical manifestations in the pre-AIDS and AIDS eras. Arch Intern Med. 1994;154(9):1032–4.
67. Odom A, Del Poeta M, Perfect J, Heitman J. The immunosuppressant FK506 and its nonimmunosuppressive analog L-685,818 are toxic to Cryptococcus neoformans by inhibition of a common target protein. Antimicrob Agents Chemother. 1997;41(1):156–61.
68. Larsen RA, Bozzette S, McCutchan JA, Chiu J, Leal MA, Richman DD. Persistent Cryptococcus neoformans infection of the prostate after successful treatment of meningitis. California Collaborative Treatment Group. Ann Intern Med. 1989;111(2):125–8.
69. Jongwutiwes U, Sungkanuparph S, Kiertiburanakul S. Comparison of clinical features and survival between cryptococcosis in human immunodeficiency virus (HIV)-positive and HIV-negative patients. Jpn J Infect Dis. 2008;61(2):111–5.
70. Jarvis JN, Bicanic T, Loyse A, Namarika D, Jackson A, Nussbaum JC, et al. Determinants of mortality in a combined cohort of 501 patients with HIV-associated Cryptococcal meningitis: implications for improving outcomes. Clin Infect Dis. 2014;58(5):736–45.
71. Chen S, Sorrell T, Nimmo G, Speed B, Currie B, Ellis D, et al. Epidemiology and host- and variety-dependent characteristics of infection due to Cryptococcus neoformans in Australia and New Zealand. Australasian Cryptococcal Study Group. Clin Infect Dis. 2000;31(2):499–508.
72. Okun E, Butler WT. Ophthalmologic complications of cryptococcal meningitis. Arch Ophthalmol. 1964;71:52–7.
73. Johnston SR, Corbett EL, Foster O, Ash S, Cohen J. Raised intracranial pressure and visual complications in AIDS patients with cryptococcal meningitis. J Infect. 1992;24(2):185–9.
74. Rex JH, Larsen RA, Dismukes WE, Cloud GA, Bennett JE. Catastrophic visual loss due to Cryptococcus neoformans meningitis. Medicine. 1993;72(4):207–24.
75. Doft BH, Curtin VT. Combined ocular infection with cytomegalovirus and cryptococcosis. Arch Ophthalmol. 1982;100(11):1800–3.
76. Steele KT, Thakur R, Nthobatsang R, Steenhoff AP, Bisson GP. In-hospital mortality of HIV-infected cryptococcal meningitis patients with C. gattii and C. neoformans infection in Gaborone, Botswana. Med Mycol. 2010;48(8):1112–5.
77. Brizendine KD, Baddley JW, Pappas PG. Predictors of mortality and differences in clinical features among patients with Cryptococcosis according to immune status. PLoS One. 2013;8(3):e60431.
78. Anekthananon T, Manosuthi W, Chetchotisakd P, Kiertiburanakul S, Supparatpinyo K, Ratanasuwan W, et al. Predictors of poor clinical outcome of cryptococcal meningitis in HIV-infected patients. Int J STD AIDS. 2011;22(11):665–70.
79. Panackal AA, Williamson KC, van de Beek D, Boulware DR, Williamson PR. Fighting the monster: applying the host damage framework to human central nervous system infections. MBio. 2016;7(1):e01906–15.
80. Chen SC, Slavin MA, Heath CH, Playford EG, Byth K, Marriott D, et al. Clinical manifestations of Cryptococcus gattii infection: determinants of neurological sequelae and death. Clin Infect Dis. 2012;55(6):789–98.
81. Sungkanuparph S, Filler SG, Chetchotisakd P, Pappas PG, Nolen TL, Manosuthi W, et al. Cryptococcal immune reconstitution inflammatory syndrome after antiretroviral therapy in

AIDS patients with cryptococcal meningitis: a prospective multicenter study. Clin Infect Dis. 2009;49(6):931–4.

82. Singh N, Lortholary O, Alexander BD, Gupta KL, John GT, Pursell K, et al. An immune reconstitution syndrome-like illness associated with Cryptococcus neoformans infection in organ transplant recipients. Clin Infect Dis. 2005;40(12):1756–61.

83. Sun HY, Alexander BD, Huprikar S, Forrest GN, Bruno D, Lyon GM, et al. Predictors of immune reconstitution syndrome in organ transplant recipients with cryptococcosis: implications for the management of immunosuppression. Clin Infect Dis. 2015;60(1):36–44.

84. Haddow LJ, Colebunders R, Meintjes G, Lawn SD, Elliott JH, Manabe YC, et al. Cryptococcal immune reconstitution inflammatory syndrome in HIV-1-infected individuals: proposed clinical case definitions. Lancet Infect Dis. 2010;10(11):791–802.

85. Meya DB, Okurut S, Zziwa G, Rolfes MA, Kelsey M, Cose S, et al. Cellular immune activation in cerebrospinal fluid from Ugandans with cryptococcal meningitis and immune reconstitution inflammatory syndrome. J Infect Dis. 2015;211(10):1597–606.

86. Boulware DR, Meya DB, Bergemann TL, Wiesner DL, Rhein J, Musubire A, et al. Clinical features and serum biomarkers in HIV immune reconstitution inflammatory syndrome after cryptococcal meningitis: a prospective cohort study. PLoS Med. 2010;7(12):e1000384.

87. Dong ZM, Murphy JW. Intravascular cryptococcal culture filtrate (CneF) and its major component, glucuronoxylomannan, are potent inhibitors of leukocyte accumulation. Infect Immun. 1995;63(3):770–8.

88. Longley N, Harrison TS, Jarvis JN. Cryptococcal immune reconstitution inflammatory syndrome. Curr Opin Infect Dis. 2013;26(1):26–34.

89. Boulware DR, Bonham SC, Meya DB, Wiesner DL, Park GS, Kambugu A, et al. Paucity of initial cerebrospinal fluid inflammation in cryptococcal meningitis is associated with subsequent immune reconstitution inflammatory syndrome. J Infect Dis. 2010;202(6):962–70.

90. Chang CC, Lim A, Omarjee S, Levitz SM, Gosnell BI, Spelman T, et al. Cryptococcosis-IRIS is associated with lower cryptococcus-specific IFN-gamma responses before antiretroviral therapy but not higher T-cell responses during therapy. J Infect Dis. 2013;208(6):898–906.

91. Jarvis JN, Meintjes G, Bicanic T, Buffa V, Hogan L, Mo S, et al. Cerebrospinal fluid cytokine profiles predict risk of early mortality and immune reconstitution inflammatory syndrome in HIV-associated cryptococcal meningitis. PLoS Pathog. 2015;11(4):e1004754.

92. Liu Y, Kang M, Wu SY, Ma Y, Chen ZX, Xie Y, et al. Different characteristics of cryptococcal meningitis between HIV-infected and HIV-uninfected patients in the southwest of China. Med Mycol. 2017;55(3):255–61.

93. Saha DC, Xess I, Jain N. Evaluation of conventional & serological methods for rapid diagnosis of cryptococcosis. Indian J Med Res. 2008;127(5):483–8.

94. Chen M, Zhou J, Li J, Li M, Sun J, Fang WJ, et al. Evaluation of five conventional and molecular approaches for diagnosis of cryptococcal meningitis in non-HIV-infected patients. Mycoses. 2016;59(8):494–502.

95. Gal AA, Evans S, Meyer PR. The clinical laboratory evaluation of cryptococcal infections in the acquired immunodeficiency syndrome. Diagn Microbiol Infect Dis. 1987;7(4):249–54.

96. el-Zaatari M, Pasarell L, McGinnis MR, Buckner J, Land GA, Salkin IF. Evaluation of the updated Vitek yeast identification data base. J Clin Microbiol. 1990;28(9):1938–41.

97. Mitchell TG, Freedman EZ, White TJ, Taylor JW. Unique oligonucleotide primers in PCR for identification of Cryptococcus neoformans. J Clin Microbiol. 1994;32(1):253–5.

98. Bicanic T, Muzoora C, Brouwer AE, Meintjes G, Longley N, Taseera K, et al. Independent association between rate of clearance of infection and clinical outcome of HIV-associated cryptococcal meningitis: analysis of a combined cohort of 262 patients. Clin Infect Dis. 2009;49(5):702–9.

99. Firacative C, Trilles L, Meyer W. MALDI-TOF MS enables the rapid identification of the major molecular types within the Cryptococcus neoformans/C. gattii species complex. PLoS One. 2012;7(5):e37566.

100. Kauffman CA, Bergman AG, Severance PJ, McClatchey KD. Detection of cryptococcal antigen. Comparison of two latex agglutination tests. Am J Clin Pathol. 1981;75(1):106–9.

101. Panackal AA, Dekker JP, Proschan M, Beri A, Williamson PR. Enzyme immunoassay versus latex agglutination cryptococcal antigen assays in adults with non-HIV-related cryptococcosis. J Clin Microbiol. 2014;52(12):4356–8.
102. Feldmesser M, Harris C, Reichberg S, Khan S, Casadevall A. Serum cryptococcal antigen in patients with AIDS. Clin Infect Dis. 1996;23(4):827–30.
103. McManus EJ, Jones JM. Detection of a Trichosporon beigelii antigen cross-reactive with Cryptococcus neoformans capsular polysaccharide in serum from a patient with disseminated Trichosporon infection. J Clin Microbiol. 1985;21(5):681–5.
104. Chanock SJ, Toltzis P, Wilson C. Cross-reactivity between Stomatococcus mucilaginosus and latex agglutination for cryptococcal antigen. Lancet. 1993;342(8879):1119–20.
105. Boulware DR, Rolfes MA, Rajasingham R, von Hohenberg M, Qin Z, Taseera K, et al. Multisite validation of cryptococcal antigen lateral flow assay and quantification by laser thermal contrast. Emerg Infect Dis. 2014;20(1):45–53.
106. Meya DB, Manabe YC, Castelnuovo B, Cook BA, Elbireer AM, Kambugu A, et al. Cost-effectiveness of serum cryptococcal antigen screening to prevent deaths among HIV-infected persons with a CD4+ cell count < or = 100 cells/microL who start HIV therapy in resource-limited settings. Clin Infect Dis. 2010;51(4):448–55.
107. Letang E, Muller MC, Ntamatungiro AJ, Kimera N, Faini D, Furrer H, et al. Cryptococcal antigenemia in immunocompromised human immunodeficiency virus patients in rural Tanzania: a preventable cause of early mortality. Open Forum Infect Dis. 2015;2(2):ofv046.
108. Jitmuang A, Panackal AA, Williamson PR, Bennett JE, Dekker JP, Zelazny AM. Performance of the cryptococcal antigen lateral flow assay in non-HIV-related cryptococcosis. J Clin Microbiol. 2016;54(2):460–3.
109. Loyse A, Moodley A, Rich P, Molloy SF, Bicanic T, Bishop L, et al. Neurological, visual, and MRI brain scan findings in 87 South African patients with HIV-associated cryptococcal meningoencephalitis. J Infect. 2015;70(6):668–75.
110. Zhong Y, Zhou Z, Fang X, Peng F, Zhang W. Magnetic resonance imaging study of cryptococcal neuroradiological lesions in HIV-negative cryptococcal meningitis. Eur J Clin Microbiol Infect Dis. 2017;36(8):1367–72.
111. Hospenthal DR, Bennett JE. Persistence of cryptococcomas on neuroimaging. Clin Infect Dis. 2000;31(5):1303–6.
112. Feigin DS. Pulmonary cryptococcosis: radiologic-pathologic correlates of its three forms. AJR Am J Roentgenol. 1983;141(6):1262–72.
113. Perfect JR, Dismukes WE, Dromer F, Goldman DL, Graybill JR, Hamill RJ, et al. Clinical practice guidelines for the management of cryptococcal disease: 2010 update by the infectious diseases society of America. Clin Infect Dis. 2010;50(3):291–322.
114. Sarosi GA, Parker JD, Doto IL, Tosh FE. Amphotericin B in cryptococcal meningitis. Long-term results of treatment. Ann Intern Med. 1969;71(6):1079–87.
115. Brouwer AE, Rajanuwong A, Chierakul W, Griffin GE, Larsen RA, White NJ, et al. Combination antifungal therapies for HIV-associated cryptococcal meningitis: a randomised trial. Lancet. 2004;363(9423):1764–7.
116. Day JN, Chau TT, Wolbers M, Mai PP, Dung NT, Mai NH, et al. Combination antifungal therapy for cryptococcal meningitis. N Engl J Med. 2013;368(14):1291–302.
117. Utz JP, Garriques IL, Sande MA, Warner JF, Mandell GL, McGehee RF, et al. Therapy of cryptococcosis with a combination of flucytosine and amphotericin B. J Infect Dis. 1975;132(4):368–73.
118. van der Horst CM, Saag MS, Cloud GA, Hamill RJ, Graybill JR, Sobel JD, et al. Treatment of cryptococcal meningitis associated with the acquired immunodeficiency syndrome. National Institute of Allergy and Infectious Diseases Mycoses Study Group and AIDS Clinical Trials Group. N Engl J Med. 1997;337(1):15–21.
119. Boulware DR, Meya DB, Muzoora C, Rolfes MA, Huppler Hullsiek K, Musubire A, et al. Timing of antiretroviral therapy after diagnosis of cryptococcal meningitis. N Engl J Med. 2014;370(26):2487–98.

120. Utz JP. Flucytosine. N Engl J Med. 1972;286(14):777–8.
121. Loyse A, Dromer F, Day J, Lortholary O, Harrison TS. Flucytosine and cryptococcosis: time to urgently address the worldwide accessibility of a 50-year-old antifungal. J Antimicrob Chemother. 2013;68(11):2435–44.
122. Bicanic T, Bottomley C, Loyse A, Brouwer AE, Muzoora C, Taseera K, et al. Toxicity of amphotericin B deoxycholate-based induction therapy in patients with HIV-associated cryptococcal meningitis. Antimicrob Agents Chemother. 2015;59(12):7224–31.
123. Stern JJ, Hartman BJ, Sharkey P, Rowland V, Squires KE, Murray HW, et al. Oral fluconazole therapy for patients with acquired immunodeficiency syndrome and cryptococcosis: experience with 22 patients. Am J Med. 1988;85(4):477–80.
124. Yamaguchi H, Ikemoto H, Watanabe K, Ito A, Hara K, Kohno S. Fluconazole monotherapy for cryptococcosis in non-AIDS patients. Eur J Clin Microbiol Infect Dis. 1996;15(10):787–92.
125. Denning DW, Tucker RM, Hanson LH, Hamilton JR, Stevens DA. Itraconazole therapy for cryptococcal meningitis and cryptococcosis. Arch Intern Med. 1989;149(10):2301–8.
126. Pappas PG, Chetchotisakd P, Larsen RA, Manosuthi W, Morris MI, Anekthananon T, et al. A phase II randomized trial of amphotericin B alone or combined with fluconazole in the treatment of HIV-associated cryptococcal meningitis. Clin Infect Dis. 2009;48(12):1775–83.
127. Longley N, Muzoora C, Taseera K, Mwesigye J, Rwebembera J, Chakera A, et al. Dose response effect of high-dose fluconazole for HIV-associated cryptococcal meningitis in southwestern Uganda. Clin Infect Dis. 2008;47(12):1556–61.
128. Nussbaum JC, Jackson A, Namarika D, Phulusa J, Kenala J, Kanyemba C, et al. Combination flucytosine and high-dose fluconazole compared with fluconazole monotherapy for the treatment of cryptococcal meningitis: a randomized trial in Malawi. Clin Infect Dis. 2010;50(3):338–44.
129. Perfect JR, Marr KA, Walsh TJ, Greenberg RN, DuPont B, de la Torre-Cisneros J, et al. Voriconazole treatment for less-common, emerging, or refractory fungal infections. Clin Infect Dis. 2003;36(9):1122–31.
130. Pitisuttithum P, Negroni R, Graybill JR, Bustamante B, Pappas P, Chapman S, et al. Activity of posaconazole in the treatment of central nervous system fungal infections. J Antimicrob Chemother. 2005;56(4):745–55.
131. Thompson GR 3rd, Rendon A, Ribeiro Dos Santos R, Queiroz-Telles F, Ostrosky-Zeichner L, Azie N, et al. Isavuconazole treatment of cryptococcosis and dimorphic mycoses. Clin Infect Dis. 2016;63(3):356–62.
132. Feldmesser M, Kress Y, Mednick A, Casadevall A. The effect of the echinocandin analogue caspofungin on cell wall glucan synthesis by Cryptococcus neoformans. J Infect Dis. 2000;182(6):1791–5.
133. Fujita NK, Reynard M, Sapico FL, Guze LB, Edwards JE Jr. Cryptococcal intracerebral mass lesions: the role of computed tomography and nonsurgical management. Ann Intern Med. 1981;94(3):382–8.
134. Bennett JE, Dismukes WE, Duma RJ, Medoff G, Sande MA, Gallis H, et al. A comparison of amphotericin B alone and combined with flucytosine in the treatment of cryptoccal meningitis. N Engl J Med. 1979;301(3):126–31.
135. Larsen RA, Bozzette SA, Jones BE, Haghighat D, Leal MA, Forthal D, et al. Fluconazole combined with flucytosine for treatment of cryptococcal meningitis in patients with AIDS. Clin Infect Dis. 1994;19(4):741–5.
136. Larsen RA, Leal MA, Chan LS. Fluconazole compared with amphotericin B plus flucytosine for cryptococcal meningitis in AIDS. A randomized trial. Ann Intern Med. 1990;113(3):183–7.
137. Robinson PA, Bauer M, Leal MA, Evans SG, Holtom PD, Diamond DA, et al. Early mycological treatment failure in AIDS-associated cryptococcal meningitis. Clin Infect Dis. 1999;28(1):82–92.
138. Espinel-Ingroff A, Aller AI, Canton E, Castanon-Olivares LR, Chowdhary A, Cordoba S, et al. Cryptococcus neoformans-Cryptococcus gattii species complex: an international study of wild-type susceptibility endpoint distributions and epidemiological cutoff values for

fluconazole, itraconazole, posaconazole, and voriconazole. Antimicrob Agents Chemother. 2012;56(11):5898–906.
139. Perfect JR, Cox GM. Drug resistance in Cryptococcus neoformans. Drug Resist Updat. 1999;2(4):259–69.
140. Aller AI, Martin-Mazuelos E, Lozano F, Gomez-Mateos J, Steele-Moore L, Holloway WJ, et al. Correlation of fluconazole MICs with clinical outcome in cryptococcal infection. Antimicrob Agents Chemother. 2000;44(6):1544–8.
141. Spitzer ED, Spitzer SG, Freundlich LF, Casadevall A. Persistence of initial infection in recurrent Cryptococcus neoformans meningitis. Lancet. 1993;341(8845):595–6.
142. Shelburne SA 3rd, Darcourt J, White AC Jr, Greenberg SB, Hamill RJ, Atmar RL, et al. The role of immune reconstitution inflammatory syndrome in AIDS-related Cryptococcus neoformans disease in the era of highly active antiretroviral therapy. Clin Infect Dis. 2005;40(7):1049–52.
143. Gaube G, De Castro N, Gueguen A, Lascoux C, Zagdanski AM, Alanio A, et al. Treatment with adalimumab for severe immune reconstitution inflammatory syndrome in an HIV-infected patient presenting with cryptococcal meningitis. Med Mal Infect. 2016;46(3):154–6.
144. Scemla A, Gerber S, Duquesne A, Parize P, Martinez F, Anglicheau D, et al. Dramatic improvement of severe cryptococcosis-induced immune reconstitution syndrome with adalimumab in a renal transplant recipient. Am J Transplant. 2015;15(2):560–4.
145. Narayanan S, Banerjee C, Holt PA. Cryptococcal immune reconstitution syndrome during steroid withdrawal treated with hydroxychloroquine. Int J Infect Dis. 2011;15(1):e70–3.
146. Graybill JR, Sobel J, Saag M, van Der Horst C, Powderly W, Cloud G, et al. Diagnosis and management of increased intracranial pressure in patients with AIDS and cryptococcal meningitis. The NIAID Mycoses Study Group and AIDS Cooperative Treatment Groups. Clin Infect Dis. 2000;30(1):47–54.
147. Denning DW, Armstrong RW, Lewis BH, Stevens DA. Elevated cerebrospinal fluid pressures in patients with cryptococcal meningitis and acquired immunodeficiency syndrome. Am J Med. 1991;91(3):267–72.
148. Rolfes MA, Hullsiek KH, Rhein J, Nabeta HW, Taseera K, Schutz C, et al. The effect of therapeutic lumbar punctures on acute mortality from cryptococcal meningitis. Clin Infect Dis. 2014;59(11):1607–14.
149. Park MK, Hospenthal DR, Bennett JE. Treatment of hydrocephalus secondary to cryptococcal meningitis by use of shunting. Clin Infect Dis. 1999;28(3):629–33.
150. Beardsley J, Wolbers M, Kibengo FM, Ggayi AB, Kamali A, Cuc NT, et al. Adjunctive dexamethasone in HIV-associated cryptococcal meningitis. N Engl J Med. 2016;374(6):542–54.
151. Kontoyiannis DP, Lewis RE, Alexander BD, Lortholary O, Dromer F, Gupta KL, et al. Calcineurin inhibitor agents interact synergistically with antifungal agents in vitro against Cryptococcus neoformans isolates: correlation with outcome in solid organ transplant recipients with cryptococcosis. Antimicrob Agents Chemother. 2008;52(2):735–8.
152. Coelho C, Casadevall A. Cryptococcal therapies and drug targets: the old, the new and the promising. Cell Microbiol. 2016;18(6):792–9.
153. Rhein J, Morawski BM, Hullsiek KH, Nabeta HW, Kiggundu R, Tugume L, et al. Efficacy of adjunctive sertraline for the treatment of HIV-associated cryptococcal meningitis: an open-label dose-ranging study. Lancet Infect Dis. 2016;16(7):809–18.
154. Nooney L, Matthews RC, Burnie JP. Evaluation of mycograb, amphotericin B, caspofungin, and fluconazole in combination against Cryptococcus neoformans by checkerboard and time-kill methodologies. Diagn Microbiol Infect Dis. 2005;51(1):19–29.
155. Jarvis JN, Meintjes G, Rebe K, Williams GN, Bicanic T, Williams A, et al. Adjunctive interferon-gamma immunotherapy for the treatment of HIV-associated cryptococcal meningitis: a randomized controlled trial. AIDS. 2012;26(9):1105–13.
156. Tascini C, Vecchiarelli A, Preziosi R, Francisci D, Bistoni F, Baldelli F. Granulocyte-macrophage colony-stimulating factor and fluconazole enhance anti-cryptococcal activity of monocytes from AIDS patients. AIDS. 1999;13(1):49–55.

157. Coffey MJ, Phare SM, George S, Peters-Golden M, Kazanjian PH. Granulocyte colony-stimulating factor administration to HIV-infected subjects augments reduced leukotriene synthesis and anticryptococcal activity in neutrophils. J Clin Invest. 1998;102(4):663–70.
158. Lockhart SR, Fothergill AW, Iqbal N, Bolden CB, Grossman NT, Garvey EP, et al. The investigational fungal Cyp51 inhibitor VT-1129 demonstrates potent in vitro activity against Cryptococcus neoformans and Cryptococcus gattii. Antimicrob Agents Chemother. 2016;60(4):2528–31.
159. Nielsen K, Vedula P, Smith KD, Meya DB, Garvey EP, Hoekstra WJ, et al. Activity of VT-1129 against Cryptococcus neoformans clinical isolates with high fluconazole MICs. Med Mycol. 2017;55(4):453–6.
160. French N, Gray K, Watera C, Nakiyingi J, Lugada E, Moore M, et al. Cryptococcal infection in a cohort of HIV-1-infected Ugandan adults. AIDS. 2002;16(7):1031–8.
161. Jarvis JN, Lawn SD, Vogt M, Bangani N, Wood R, Harrison TS. Screening for cryptococcal antigenemia in patients accessing an antiretroviral treatment program in South Africa. Clin Infect Dis. 2009;48(7):856–62.
162. WHO Guidelines Approved by the Guidelines Review Committee. Rapid advice: diagnosis, prevention and management of cryptococcal disease in HIV-infected adults, adolescents and children. Geneva: World Health Organization; 2011. http://www.who.int/hiv/pub/cryptococcal_disease2011/en/. Accessed 19 Dec 2017.
163. Devi SJ, Schneerson R, Egan W, Ulrich TJ, Bryla D, Robbins JB, et al. Cryptococcus neoformans serotype A glucuronoxylomannan-protein conjugate vaccines: synthesis, characterization, and immunogenicity. Infect Immun. 1991;59(10):3700–7.
164. Mukherjee J, Zuckier LS, Scharff MD, Casadevall A. Therapeutic efficacy of monoclonal antibodies to Cryptococcus neoformans glucuronoxylomannan alone and in combination with amphotericin B. Antimicrob Agents Chemother. 1994;38(3):580–7.

Challenges in Tuberculous Meningitis

6

Jeffrey R. Starke and Andrea T. Cruz

Tuberculosis continues to be one of the most important infectious diseases in the world. Although 85% of tuberculosis cases occur in the lungs, 15% of cases occur outside of the respiratory system, with the central nervous system (CNS) being the second most common site of extrathoracic involvement. Children are more prone to extrapulmonary tuberculosis in general and to CNS tuberculosis because of their relative inability to contain the infection. Although tuberculous meningitis is uniformly fatal if untreated, early detection, combined with appropriate medical and surgical intervention, can lead to greatly improved outcomes for many patients. Tuberculous meningitis is the most common form of CNS tuberculosis, but tuberculoma, an inflammatory mass in the brain, is common in certain areas of the world [1]. In some developing countries, tuberculomas are the most common cause of mass-occupying CNS lesions, and *Mycobacterium tuberculosis* is the most common cause of bacterial meningitis [2].

Epidemiology

It is estimated that in 2016 10.4 million people developed tuberculosis disease in the world, with approximately 1.8 million associated deaths [3]. Tuberculosis cases in children are grossly underestimated because of the difficulty in obtaining microbiologic confirmation from young children. Many children with CNS tuberculosis are misdiagnosed as having a "bacterial meningitis." It is not known how many cases of

J. R. Starke (✉) · A. T. Cruz
Department of Pediatrics, Baylor College of Medicine, Texas Children's Hospital, Houston, TX, USA
e-mail: jrstarke@texaschildrens.org

© Springer International Publishing AG, part of Springer Nature 2018
R. Hasbun (ed.), *Meningitis and Encephalitis*,
https://doi.org/10.1007/978-3-319-92678-0_6

CNS tuberculosis actually occur, but 10–15% of children <2 years of age with untreated tuberculosis infection develop tuberculous meningitis.

There are two separate risk factors for developing tuberculosis disease. The first is the risk of becoming infected with *M. tuberculosis*, which depends on the person's chance of coming into contact with a person with contagious tuberculosis. In many developing countries, infection rates of 3–5% per year are common so that the majority of young adults carry infection with *M. tuberculosis*. It is estimated that one third of the world's population is infected, serving as reservoirs for future disease cases. For children, the likelihood of becoming infected with *M. tuberculosis* depends on the risk factors of the adults in their environment, because children rarely are contagious. Most children are infected in the home, but outbreaks of childhood tuberculosis centered in elementary and high schools, nursery schools, day care homes, churches, school buses, and stores still occur [4].

The second risk factor is the likelihood of developing disease after infection has occurred. A variety of medical conditions increase an infected person's chance of developing disease, especially conditions that suppress the immune system. Corticosteroids and tumor necrosis factor-α antibodies are the major classes of drugs that increase the risk of infection progressing to disease. For adults with tuberculosis infection, the most important risk factor for the development of tuberculosis, including CNS tuberculosis, is coinfection with HIV. Adults who are infected with both HIV and *M. tuberculosis* have a 5–10% annual chance of developing tuberculosis disease, and adults with immune systems that have been damaged by HIV are more likely to develop CNS tuberculosis. The HIV epidemic has had a profound effect on the epidemiology of tuberculosis among children by two major mechanisms. First, HIV- infected adults with pulmonary tuberculosis may transmit *M. tuberculosis* to children, some of whom will develop tuberculosis disease, including meningitis. Second, children with HIV infection are at increased risk of experiencing progression from tuberculosis infection to disease and developing CNS tuberculomas as a complication of immune reconstitution inflammatory syndrome (IRIS). Unfortunately, both pulmonary and CNS tuberculosis in HIV-infected adults and children can be similar in clinical presentation to many other opportunistic infections that are common in this population. In general, adults and children living with HIV infection in an area endemic for tuberculosis who develop severe acute CNS disease should be given empiric antituberculosis chemotherapy until a definite diagnosis can be established.

Pathophysiology

The portal of entry for *M. tuberculosis* is the lung in more than 95% of cases. During the development of the lesion in the lung, bacilli escape via the bloodstream and lymphatic systems to infect many other parts of the body, most commonly the apices of the lungs, liver, spleen, lymph nodes, and meninges. This dissemination can involve either large numbers of bacilli, which leads to disseminated tuberculosis disease, or small numbers of bacilli that cause asymptomatic microscopic tuberculous foci scattered in tissues, including the meninges, which can be the origin of CNS tuberculosis that occurs years to decades later.

It was initially thought that tuberculous meningitis was a direct result of infection of the meninges from organisms spread through the blood [5]. Patients with HIV infection and tuberculosis have a higher incidence of tuberculous meningitis, including occult meningeal disease. This observation may be a result, at least in part, of the finding that up to 40% of patients with HIV infection and severe immune suppression have detectable mycobacteremia associated with their tuberculosis disease, increasing the likelihood of meningeal seeding. On the other hand, pathologic studies performed in the 1930s showed that tuberculous meningitis can occur without disease in other parts of the body; meningitis may be absent in the most extreme cases of disseminated bloodstream tuberculosis; and introduction of large numbers of bacilli into the bloodstream of susceptible laboratory animals invariably produces bloodstream tuberculosis but fails to cause tuberculous meningitis [6]. From these observations, investigators postulated that tuberculous meningitis usually arises in two stages. First, tuberculous lesions form in the brain or in the meninges from the blood-borne dissemination of bacilli early in the infection. Meningitis develops by discharge of bacilli from a subjacent focus directly into the subarachnoid space. This may explain why tuberculous meningitis is extremely rare in infants younger than 6 months of age: it takes at least 6 months for the lesion to develop. Rarely, a tuberculous lesion develops in the spinal cord or arises from a site of tuberculous spondylitis or a skull lesion. Second, proteins and other chemicals from the organisms leak into the cerebrospinal fluid (CSF), producing an intense immune reaction not unlike the reaction to a tuberculin skin test. As a result, inflammation occurs around the brain and meninges. This inflammatory reaction may damage nerves, block the circulation of CSF, and thrombose small blood vessels producing multiple cerebral infarcts. The type and extent of CNS lesions that follow this discharge of organisms and proteins into the CSF depend on the number of bacilli, their virulence, and the inflammation caused by the immune response of the host.

Several basic pathological mechanisms are responsible for the damage and symptoms caused by tuberculous meningitis. Initially, a thick exudate fills the cisterns. This exudate surrounds the base of the brain, affecting the cranial nerves and the major blood vessels at the base. The brain tissue underlying this exudate develops a variable degree of edema. As the exudate enlarges, circulation of CSF is blocked, and some degree of hydrocephalus is usually present in patients with tuberculous meningitis who have survived more than several weeks. The blockage occurs most frequently in the basal cisterns or around the outflow foramina of the fourth ventricle; it rarely occurs between the third and fourth ventricle causing aqueductal stenosis. At the same time, the inflammation causes vasculitis involving large, medium, and small arteries as well as veins emanating from the circle of Willis. Partial or complete occlusion of the arteries—most often the middle and anterior cerebral arteries—may be seen, and the venous sinuses may become thrombosed. These vascular changes result in ischemic damage or infarction that occasionally is hemorrhagic. These infarctions may be superficial but often include the basal ganglia or hypothalamus and watershed areas. In children, infarction of the brainstem also has been observed.

The pathogenesis of tuberculomas is incompletely described. They may originate from a small area of necrosis surrounded by some very large cells that form in or just below the cortex of the brain. These lesions continue to enlarge and aggregate, producing a nodule. The bacilli stimulate a local immune reaction, with resulting edema and continued inflammation in the surrounding brain. Occasionally, these lesions may stimulate extensive necrosis, causing a tuberculous brain abscess. Patients with tuberculous brain abscess become ill very rapidly and usually require immediate surgical intervention for survival.

Clinical Manifestations

Prior to the development of treatment for tuberculosis, tuberculous meningitis had a progressive course that inevitably resulted in death. However, during the past four decades, the clinical presentation has become increasingly varied, and atypical cases are now more common, particularly in developed countries [7, 8]. The clinical manifestations in an individual depend on the degree of severity of the basic pathological processes: the thick basilar exudates (resulting in cranial nerve palsies and hydrocephalus), vasculitis (resulting in infarct and focal neurological deficits), allergic reaction to antigens of the organism, cerebral edema (causing impaired consciousness and seizures), and the presence of tuberculomas. It is interesting to note that the organism genotype, drug resistance pattern, coinfection with HIV, and BCG immunization status do not consistently change the clinical manifestations.

Early diagnosis of tuberculous meningitis is notoriously difficult and delayed because the clinical onset is often gradual, occurring over 1–3 weeks [9, 10]. As a result, the presentation is subacute, and neck stiffness, the classic sign of acute meningitis, is usually lacking during the early stages. Unfortunately, early diagnosis and rapid initiation of treatment are the most important factors for determining the clinical outcome. Rarely, the onset is abrupt and marked by convulsions or rapid progression of neurological deficits.

The natural history of TB meningitis was described in the prechemotherapy era and was divided into three stages. The first stage is characterized by personality change, irritability, anorexia, weight loss, listlessness, fever, and general ill health, but no focal neurological findings on examination. Infants and toddlers in this stage often lose developmental milestones. These nonspecific signs and symptoms are differentiated from more common and less serious illnesses by their persistence and usually can be recognized as caused by tuberculous meningitis only in retrospect. After 1–2 weeks, the second stage begins with drowsiness, stiff neck, cranial nerve palsies (especially of cranial nerves III, VI, and VII), papillary abnormalities, vomiting, and convulsions. In some patients, headache and vomiting are the major complaints until a devastating neurological event occurs. In many cases, children present to medical attention repeatedly and may be misdiagnosed as having more common acute conditions [4, 7]. The second stage of tuberculous meningitis may be heralded by a sudden onset of focal neurological deficits and stroke. Hemiplegia may occur at the onset of disease or at a later stage but usually correlates with ischemic infarction in the territory of the middle cerebral artery. Quadriplegia occurs only in advanced cases after bilateral infarctions or severe generalized edema has occurred. Monoplegia is uncommon and is caused by a small vascular lesion that occurs at an early stage of disease. Rare cases of tuberculous meningitis are dominated early by abnormal movements such as choreiform or hemiballistic movements, athetosis, tremors, myoclonic jerks, or ataxia due to infarcts in the basal ganglia or thalamus. In addition, a variety of neurological and psychiatric syndromes have been described in association with tuberculous meningitis in older children and adults: acute-onset somnolence, transient amnesia, psychosis, and agoraphobia. Tuberculous encephalopathy is restricted to children and characterized by convulsions, stupor, or coma without signs of meningitis. The third stage of tuberculous meningitis is characterized by coma or stupor, irregular pulse and respirations, rising fever, and, eventually, death. Papilledema may be seen but is not a universal finding. Once the classic signs and symptoms of tuberculous meningitis have appeared, the diagnosis is easier to establish but the outcomes are far worse [11].

A tuberculoma usually presents with the symptoms and signs that occur with any intracranial space-occupying lesion. The clinical picture depends on the size and location of the tuberculoma(s), the amount of associated inflammation and edema, and the pressure they produce on adjacent structures. Headache, seizures, paralysis, personality changes, and focal neurological problems occur frequently. Children are more prone to developing infratentorial lesions, so ataxia and sudden onset of severe neurological dysfunction are more common. Children also are more likely to develop a single tuberculoma, whereas multiple and supratentorial tuberculomas are more common in adults. Small tuberculomas can be clinically silent, discovered only by neuroimaging, especially if the inflammatory reaction is minimal or suppressed.

Tuberculosis-related IRIS of the CNS is often a life-threatening complication caused by the interactions of HIV and *M. tuberculosis* and their respective therapies [12–15]. "Unmasking" IRIS occurs when previously unrecognized tuberculosis infection suddenly arises after starting antiretroviral therapy (ART), while "paradoxical" IRIS occurs when new or worsening signs and symptoms of CNS tuberculosis develop in a patient already under treatment for tuberculosis in whom ART was recently started. The most common manifestations are neck stiffness, symptoms caused by new intracranial and/or spinal mass lesions, radiculomyelitis, new onset or worsening of hydrocephalus, visual impairment, and seizures, which can be focal or generalized. Tuberculosis-related IRIS appears to be more common in adults than children, and associated mortality is up to 30% in adults [16]. The optimal time to initiate ART in a patient with HIV-associated CNS tuberculosis is unknown; however, it appears that the timing of the start of ART makes little difference in mortality.

Diagnosis: Some General Principles (Box 6.1)

Box 6.1 Major Challenges and Research Needs in Diagnosis

- The initial signs and symptoms are nonspecific and mimic common less severe conditions, making early diagnosis difficult. Their persistence is characteristic of tuberculous meningitis.
- In children, tuberculous meningitis often arises within weeks to a few months after infection. The source case often has not yet been diagnosed so the exposure history is "negative."
- The tests of tuberculosis infection, acid-fast stain, and PCR of the CSF are often negative, and the correct diagnosis is not considered.
- CSF cultures for *M. tuberculosis* are positive in fewer than 50% of cases in most series, meaning diagnosis cannot be confirmed microbiologically and drug susceptibility results are not available.
- All of these difficulties are greater when patients also have immune compromise, especially poorly controlled HIV infection.
- There currently are no biomarkers or patterns of biomarkers that improve the diagnosis of CNS tuberculosis.
- Neuroradiology is essential to support the diagnosis of tuberculous meningitis in most cases but is often unavailable in high-burden settings. The key to early diagnosis is often clinical presentation and suggestive neuroradiology findings (basilar enhancement, hydrocephalus, evidence of ischemia, or stroke).
- Standardized methods of diagnosis should be utilized across studies to enhance the quality and comparability of tuberculous meningitis studies [17–19].

Diagnosis is often delayed in industrialized nations, as the lower incidence of tuberculosis results in clinicians having a low index of suspicion for the disease. *As a general rule, any child or adult who presents with basilar meningitis without an obvious cause and one or a combination of stroke, cranial nerve abnormalities, or hydrocephalus should be considered to have tuberculous meningitis until proven otherwise; antituberculosis chemotherapy should be started immediately while the workup is in progress.*

Establishing the diagnosis of CNS tuberculosis is often difficult because detecting the organism is not easy. One key to establishing the diagnosis is often finding another focus of tuberculosis disease, such as pulmonary tuberculosis. Many adults with CNS tuberculosis have a normal chest radiograph, but over 90% of children with meningeal tuberculosis have an abnormal chest radiograph showing adenopathy, pulmonary infiltrates, or atelectasis caused by the bronchial obstruction that is a classic sign of childhood tuberculosis. Differences in the utility of chest radiographs between children and adults may be explained at least partly by the incubation period. In children, there is a very short time between infection and the development of tuberculosis meningitis, and insufficient time has passed to heal the lung parenchyma or for adenopathy to have resolved. In adults, tuberculous meningitis may be caused by reactivation of a remote infection, and the chest radiograph is more likely to be normal. *At any age, the combination of meningitis and an abnormal chest X-ray should suggest the diagnosis of tuberculous meningitis.* Because tuberculous meningitis tends to be an early complication of tuberculosis infection in children, the infected patient may have had recent contact with an adult with contagious tuberculosis. However, because of the short incubation time of tuberculous meningitis in children, the contagious person may not yet have been diagnosed. Whenever tuberculous meningitis is suspected, it is critical to evaluate the adolescent and adult contacts of the patient immediately to determine if any of them have evidence of contagious pulmonary tuberculosis. Some hospitals routinely screen adults accompanying children with suspected tuberculosis by chest radiograph. This strategy prevents potentially contagious adults from nosocomial transmission of the bacteria and allows for rapid referral for medical evaluation; it also may help assist in the diagnosis of the ill child.

General Laboratory Evaluation

Most patients with tuberculous meningitis have a normal complete blood count and differential. Basic blood chemistries are often normal, although hyponatremia can be seen secondary to either the syndrome of inappropriate antidiuretic hormone secretion or salt wasting. Serum chloride and bicarbonate may be altered due to dehydration from decreased intake and emesis. The erythrocyte sedimentation rate is elevated in up to 80% of cases of tuberculous meningitis, but this is a nonspecific abnormality.

Tests of Tuberculosis Infection

The tuberculin skin test is used to determine if a patient has been infected with *M. tuberculosis*. A small amount of purified protein derivative is injected into the upper layer of the skin. A positive result is induration (firmness) or blistering that occurs 48–72 h after placement of the test; erythema alone should not be considered positive. Reactions of various sizes may occur, but the larger the reaction, the more likely it is caused by infection with *M. tuberculosis*. However, when evaluating a child for possible tuberculous meningitis, any induration in response to a tuberculin skin test should be considered significant. Unfortunately, up to 50% of adults and children with tuberculous meningitis have a negative tuberculin skin test at the time of diagnosis. Therefore, a positive tuberculin skin test can be very helpful in diagnosing tuberculous meningitis, but a negative tuberculin skin test never eliminates tuberculosis as a cause of disease.

Interferon-γ release assays (IGRAs) are also tests of infection that measure the immunological response to *M. tuberculosis* antigens [20]. In contrast to the tuberculin skin test, IGRAs contain only two or three proteins found primarily in *M. tuberculosis* and only a few nontuberculous species, increasing the specificity of the test; there is no cross-reaction with the BCG vaccine. The sensitivity of IGRAs is similar to that of the tuberculin skin test for most forms of tuberculosis disease. However, when evaluating a patient for tuberculous meningitis, optimizing sensitivity is critical, and any test (tuberculin skin test or IGRA) being positive should be considered. Often, a positive IGRA or tuberculin skin test may be the first specific evidence that a patient has tuberculosis. To maximize sensitivity, we routinely obtain a tuberculin skin test and send both commercially available IGRAs licensed in the United States (QuantiFERON [Qiagen, Inc., Hilden, Germany] and T-SPOT.*TB* [Oxford Immunotec, Abingdon, United Kingdom]) in patients in whom we suspect tuberculosis disease, particularly CNS disease.

Cerebrospinal Fluid Examination

Lumbar puncture reveals an elevated opening pressure in most cases of tuberculous meningitis. The CSF is usually clear and colorless but may show a pellicle or clot on standing. There is usually a moderate degree of pleocytosis not exceeding 500–1000 cells/mm^3. Although polymorphonuclear cells may predominate early in the course, a change to a predominance of lymphocytes develops fairly quickly. However, an abundance of neutrophils may predict a poorer outcome and increased tendency for IRIS to occur. The lumbar CSF protein concentration is usually in the range of 100–500 mg/dl, but can be much higher. Simultaneously obtained ventricular CSF may have a normal cell count and protein because the fluid is obtained proximal to the inflammation. The protein concentration may increase as the disease progresses and may increase suddenly—to several gm/dl—if spinal block occurs because of obstruction of the outflow of CSF. Initial protein concentrations higher than 300 mg/dl correlate with a poor prognosis in adults. The CSF glucose concentration initially is in the low-normal range but declines steadily as illness progresses. One study of adults with tuberculous meningitis demonstrated that low levels of CSF glucose and high levels of lactate were associated with mortality. The measurement of adenosine deaminase levels in the CNS might be a useful adjunctive test to suggest the diagnosis of tuberculous meningitis; the reported sensitivities have ranged from 50% to 70% and the specificities from 60% to 90%, but inconsistencies in study methodology have made the results difficult to interpret [21].

Microbiology, Biomarkers, and Genetics

Microscopic examination of the spinal fluid for *M. tuberculosis* organisms, using an acid-fast stain, is the most important procedure for the early diagnosis of tuberculous meningitis. The frequency with which organisms are seen varies widely but depends on the amount of CSF that is sampled and the time devoted to searching for the organisms. The auramine-rhodamine (Truant) fluorescent stain is the most sensitive. Some studies have demonstrated organisms in more than 90% of consecutive cases of tuberculous meningitis in adults, but most studies have shown a far lower percentage, particularly in children. The gold standard for the diagnosis of tuberculous meningitis is to isolate *M. tuberculosis* in culture from the CSF. In most series of tuberculous meningitis, the organism has been isolated from the CSF in 10–50% of patients depending on the quantity of fluid cultured and the laboratory facilities. *A negative CSF culture never rules out tuberculous meningitis.* Gastric aspirate cultures are positive in up to 20% of children with CNS tuberculosis. Polymerase chain reaction (PCR) and other nucleic acid amplification tests performed on CSF, including GeneXpert MTB-RIF (Cepheid, Sunnyvale, California), have sensitivities of 50–85% and specificities of 88–100%, respectively, when compared with CSF stain and cultures [22, 23]. As with most tests, a positive result is valuable, but a negative result never excludes tuberculous meningitis [24].

Because of the difficulties in directly detecting *M. tuberculosis*, there is increasing interest in developing biomarkers both for diagnosis and to detect or monitor the degree of inflammation. While there are many specific proteins and transcriptional patterns in the CSF, no specific diagnostic biosignature of tuberculous meningitis has yet emerged. However, some patterns of biomarkers have been associated with intensity and type of inflammation and neuron cell damage; these markers may ultimately help predict and monitor anti-inflammatory therapy and establish prognosis for neurologic function [25]. There is also growing interest in host genotypes [26]. As one example, a single nucleotide polymorphism in the leukotriene A4 hydrolase (*LTA4H*) promoter influences the balance between proinflammatory leukotriene B4 and immunosuppressive A4; in tuberculous meningitis, this polymorphism is associated with bacterial load, inflammatory cell recruitment, patient survival, and response to anti-inflammatory therapy.

Neuroradiology

The findings on neuroimaging mirror the pathology described previously [27, 28]. Although a computed tomography (CT) scan cannot definitely establish the diagnosis of tuberculous meningitis, it is useful to rule out other diseases in patients who have an obscure illness, or evidence of increased intracranial pressure or generalized or focal neurological deficits, and to identify patients in need of prompt neurosurgical or enhanced medical intervention [29]. The most common imaging feature seen in CNS tuberculosis is hydrocephalus, noted in 80–100% of patients. The most sensitive radiologic feature (89%) is basal enhancement on a contrast-enhanced CT, with thickened meninges in the basilar areas of the brain. The most specific feature (almost 100%) is the presence of high density within the basal cisterns on a noncontrast CT. Additional findings suggestive of tuberculosis include vasculitis and thromboses causing ischemia, often visible as areas of radiolucency, particularly when located in the basal ganglia or near the Sylvian fissure. The hydrocephalus that occurs with tuberculous meningitis may increase as the patient improves; this is not a poor prognostic sign but may need to be treated with a CSF shunt or acetazolamide [30]. Magnetic resonance imaging has some advantages over CT in the evaluation of tuberculous meningitis because it allows better visualization of the exudate in the basilar cisterns and smaller infarcts in strategic locations such as the brainstem [31]. It also is better for identifying miliary leptomeningeal tubercles present in most patients with tuberculous meningitis [32].

Neuroimaging is important in monitoring the appearance and evolution of tuberculomas which usually present as one or several mass lesions surrounded by edema. The lesions are relatively avascular. The neuroradiological images of tuberculoma are nonspecific; diagnosis is usually established by biopsy or strong epidemiological or other clinic evidence of tuberculosis. These lesions can develop in patients with tuberculous meningitis who are being adequately treated [33]. With increased use of MRI, more patients have been recognized as having tuberculomas; in some case series, almost two thirds of adults with tuberculous meningitis have tuberculomas on presentation, and up to three quarters have them when imaged 2–3 months after starting therapy [34]. These so-called paradoxical tuberculomas develop after chemotherapy is started. It is thought that the development of these lesions represents an immunological phenomenon caused by inflammation as organisms are killed and proteins are released into the surrounding tissues, and is one form of IRIS.

Additional imaging should include chest radiographs, which are abnormal in >80% of children with CNS tuberculosis. The most common findings include hilar adenopathy (33%), infiltrates (33%), and miliary disease (20%).

Differential Diagnosis

While the diagnosis of tuberculous meningitis is often difficult in previously normal hosts, the difficulties are increased in patients with immune compromise, especially HIV infection, as other opportunistic infections can mimic tuberculosis [35–37]. The differential diagnosis of tuberculous meningitis includes fungal (e.g., cryptococcal) meningitis, viral meningoencephalitis (e.g., cytomegalovirus), and noninfectious processes such as CNS lymphoma, meningeal metastases, and sarcoidosis. Rare infectious diseases that may present a clinical picture similar to that of tuberculous meningitis include leptospirosis, brucellosis, cat-scratch encephalitis (bartonellosis), toxoplasmosis, and infection due to *Naegleria*. Additional considerations are focal parameningeal infections such as brain abscess, cancer, sarcoidosis, and meningitis or encephalitis that result from embolic complications of infective endocarditis. CNS vasculitis can mimic tuberculous meningitis. The differential diagnosis of tuberculomas includes infectious (abscesses, septic emboli, fungal balls) and noninfectious (primary and metastatic malignancies) causes of mass-occupying lesions.

Management and Treatment (Box 6.2)

Box 6.2 Major Challenges and Research Needs in Management and Treatment

- As cultures are positive in only about 50% of cases, drug susceptibility results also are unknown for half the cases, meaning significant drug resistance is often missed in locales with a high prevalence of drug-resistant tuberculosis.
- Although ethambutol is part of the WHO-recommended regimen for initial treatment of tuberculous meningitis, it penetrates into the CSF poorly. Most experts prefer a different fourth drug, classically ethionamide or amikacin, and more recently a fluoroquinolone.
- Rifampin also penetrates poorly into the CSF. Emerging evidence has demonstrated improved outcomes using larger doses of rifampin, 20–30 mg/kg/day, with no increase in adverse drug effects.
- Outcomes are generally poor with traditional management. Clinical trials in adults have suggested that when a fluoroquinolone, usually moxifloxacin, is included in the initial regimen, the outcomes are improved.
- Management of acute hydrocephalus is critical. While ventriculostomy and ventriculoperitoneal shunts provide immediate relief, medical management using acetazolamide and furosemide also can be effective.
- There is increasing emphasis on the management of the inflammation of CNS tuberculosis. Corticosteroids sometimes have limited effectiveness and a large number of potential adverse effects. More specific therapies aimed at specific cytokines or other mediators of inflammation are needed. Thalidomide has shown great potential to decrease inflammation and even restore vision in some children.
- The prognosis of tuberculous meningitis is extremely variable and difficult to predict. Recent work on neurologic biomarkers and specific genetic alleles has demonstrated some predictive associations, but much more work is needed.
- Management of multidrug-resistant tuberculous (MDR-TB) meningitis is extremely challenging as many second-line drugs do not penetrate well into the CSF. In addition to fluoroquinolones, linezolid has been identified as a very useful drug for MDR-TB meningitis.

Despite the use of effective antituberculosis drugs, morbidity and mortality rates from tuberculous meningitis remain high throughout the world [38]. Early death and poor clinical response are usually due to failure to recognize the disease and begin appropriate antituberculosis chemotherapy and manage the inflammation in the early stages. Because it is difficult to isolate the organism in a patient with tuberculous meningitis, initial therapy is usually empirical based on the clinical, laboratory, and radiographic data. It is important to start therapy before the diagnosis is proven because any delay may worsen the outcome substantially.

The four drugs used most often to treat drug-susceptible tuberculosis are isoniazid, rifampin, pyrazinamide, and ethambutol. While isoniazid and pyrazinamide penetrate well into the CSF, rifampin and ethambutol do not [39]. The penetration of many anti-tuberculosis drugs is enhanced by meningeal inflammation. Pyrazinamide and isoniazid penetrate into the CSF in the presence and absence of meningeal inflammation, and their use has significantly improved the prognosis of tuberculous meningitis. There is emerging evidence that the traditional rifampin dose of 10–15 mg/kg/day, maximum of 450–600 mg, is inadequate, and many experts now recommend using rifampin doses of at least 20–30 mg/kg/day, maximum of 1200 mg or higher. There is no evidence that the major adverse reactions to rifampin are dose-dependent. The selection of a fourth drug is problematic as no comparative controlled trials have been conducted. A fourth drug likely has little influence on outcomes of drug-susceptible tuberculous meningitis but may be beneficial when the organism is resistant to isoniazid. Ethambutol has poor CSF penetration, and even though its use is recommended in several guidelines, including those of the World Health Organization, consideration should be given to replacing this drug in the initial regimen with either oral ethionamide or a fluoroquinolone or an injectable agent such as amikacin in patients with suspected tuberculous meningitis.

There are few clinical trials of the treatment of tuberculous meningitis because the condition is rare in places where clinical trials can be performed. Early studies showed that treatment with isoniazid and rifampin for 12 months was generally effective in patients with drug-susceptible tuberculous meningitis. Recent studies have shown that when pyrazinamide has been added to the regimen for the first 2 months, a 6–9-month course of therapy with isoniazid and rifampin is curative [40, 41]. Unfortunately, the incidence of drug-resistant tuberculosis is increasing in many areas of the world. In the United States, as many as 10% of *M. tuberculosis* isolates are resistant to at least one antituberculosis drug, and rates of drug resistance may be as high as 30–40% in other areas of the world. Treatment of drug-resistant tuberculous meningitis is challenging and outcomes are far worse even in the most experienced and technically advanced centers [42]. Experts recommend that four antituberculosis drugs be given in the initial regimen for tuberculous meningitis in adults and children; the fourth drug provides additional coverage in the event the patient has an isoniazid-resistant organism. The three drugs that are virtually always used are isoniazid, rifampin, and pyrazinamide. A fourth drug traditionally was chosen from among ethionamide or injectable agents (amikacin, capreomycin, kanamycin, or streptomycin). Recent clinical trials among adults with tuberculous meningitis have demonstrated mixed outcomes when the initial treatment regimen included high-dose rifampin and a fluoroquinolone, either moxifloxacin or levofloxacin, along with isoniazid and pyrazinamide [43–45]. The four-drug regimen may be narrowed after drug susceptibility testing is available if the patient is responding well to therapy. Assuming a drug-susceptible *M. tuberculosis* isolate is found, pyrazinamide may be stopped after 2 months, and the fourth drug (e.g., injectable agent or ethionamide) may be stopped when a pansusceptible isolate is found. Isoniazid and rifampin are continued to complete a 6–9-month course.

The optimal medical treatment of tuberculoma has never been established. Superficial tuberculomas may be treated by surgery or the combination of surgical excision and chemotherapy. However, many tuberculomas have been cured with medical therapy alone. Most experts recommend an initial three- or four-drug regimen with a total length of treatment of 9–12 months.

Tuberculous meningitis may present with signs of increased intracranial pressure due to hydrocephalus. When acute hydrocephalus develops, insertion of a ventriculostomy may be lifesaving [46]. In industrialized countries, hydrocephalus is most often managed by placement of a permanent ventriculoperitoneal shunt (VPS) or a temporary endoscopic third ventriculostomy (ETV) [47]. Studies have implied that the risk of recurrent hydrocephalus is lower with VPS, but the ETV is associated with fewer long-term complications, especially in patients with HIV coinfection [48]. In many high-incidence countries, the hydrocephalus is managed medically using acetazolamide with or without furosemide for 4–6 weeks. There have been no controlled clinical trials comparing outcomes of medical versus surgical management.

While antimicrobial therapy of tuberculous meningitis has received almost all of the previous attention, it is becoming clear that management of the inflammation is also critically important and often inadequate [49]. Corticosteroid therapy has been routinely recommended for patients with tuberculous meningitis, although large controlled studies of the effectiveness of corticosteroid therapy are not available [50–52]. Available evidence examined in a recent Cochran study suggests that corticosteroids reduce cerebral edema and inflammation, reduce mortality, lead to more rapid radiographic resolution, and improve outcomes and mortality in non-HIV-infected persons; unfortunately, there seems to be little benefit for people who also have HIV infection [53]. Most experts have agreed that it is best to use corticosteroids early in treatment, especially if the diagnosis has been reasonably established and the patient's condition is critical [34]. Corticosteroids should never be administered to a patient with suspected tuberculous meningitis without also starting antituberculosis therapy. Corticosteroids are usually given for 3–6 weeks and then tapered over a period of several weeks as the patient improves. All forms of corticosteroids (dexamethasone, prednisone, prednisolone, and hydrocortisone) seem to be effective. Corticosteroids also are used in the management of CNS manifestations of IRIS.

Other anti-inflammatory agents have been studied. Aspirin has antithrombotic and anti-inflammatory properties. While a trial in adults with tuberculous meningitis showed a significant reduction in mortality at 3 months with the use of aspirin [54], a study in children demonstrated no benefit in mortality but did seem to limit development of hemiparesis [55]. Thalidomide has been used in trials involving South African children who had evidence of extreme inflammation, often in response to the large number of organisms found in tuberculous abscesses of the CNS [56, 57]. In these patients, there is a strong CNS cytokine response often including tumor necrosis factor-α [58, 59]. Thalidomide has improved outcomes in children with life-threatening tuberculous mass lesions, including those arising during IRIS, when corticosteroids have been inadequate to control the inflammation; it seems to be particularly helpful when there is visual compromise caused by optochiasmic arachnoiditis [56, 57, 60, 61]. The anti-TNF-α biologic agent infliximab has been used to reduce IRIS in two patients with neurotuberculosis [62].

The current mortality rate of tuberculous meningitis with adequate therapy is 10–20% in developed countries, but it may be as high as 30–40% in developing countries. In general, the prognosis is worse for infants and the very old, immunocompromised patients, malnourished patients, patients with associated disseminated disease, and patients who present with increased intracranial pressure.

The prognosis of meningitis correlates somewhat with the clinical stage of disease when antituberculosis chemotherapy is started [63–65]. The majority of patients diagnosed and treated in stage 1 have a normal outcome. Unfortunately, few patients are diagnosed at this stage. The majority of patients diagnosed in stage 3 will either die or have severe neurological sequelae. Some patients diagnosed in stage 2 have a good outcome, whereas others have persistent neurological deficits, sometimes severe. Some residual physical or cognitive deficit has been reported in 10–50% of young children with tuberculous meningitis. Visual and auditory impairments are the most common sequelae. The frequency of motor deficits after tuberculous meningitis has been reported to be 10–25%. Seizures are common in the early stages of the illness but are less common later, occurring in fewer than 10% of patients. Global developmental delay and impairment of intellect and judgment, dementia, or some degree of behavior or learning disorder are common problems in patients presenting with stage 2 or 3 disease. Endocrinopathies may become evident months or years after tuberculous meningitis. The most common forms cause obesity, hypogonadism, sexual precocity, diabetes insipidus, and growth retardation.

Predicting which patients will have sequelae can be challenging [30]. Young age, advanced state of tuberculous meningitis, presence of infarcts on CT at 1 month, and Glasgow Coma Scale scores may correlate with neurodevelopmental and behavioral outcomes [66]. The plasticity of the pediatric brain leads to many children having better neurodevelopmental outcomes than one would anticipate. However, clinicians should be cautious about estimating future developmental capacity. Often, the true developmental potential of a young child is not evident until they begin school. As with any form of bacterial meningitis, children should receive audiologic screening prior to hospital discharge. In adult patients, the presence of seizures and coma are predictors of mortality. Predictors of neurologic sequelae in this population included cranial nerve palsies and hemiparesis and hemiplegia.

Prevention (Box 6.3)

Box 6.3 Challenges and Research Needs in Prevention
- BCG vaccines can prevent 50–80% of cases of tuberculous meningitis. However, there may be large variation in effectiveness among the various available strains of BCG, but this is largely unstudied. BCG vaccine rates are suboptimal in many high incidence locales. New, more effective tuberculosis vaccines are needed.
- Most children who develop tuberculous meningitis do so rapidly—within weeks to a few months—after acquiring the infection. While treatment of recent tuberculosis infection is extremely effective in preventing tuberculous meningitis, it is not carried out in most high-burden settings. Contact tracing and treatment of children less than 5 years of age who are asymptomatic household contacts is recommended and should be carried out.

CNS tuberculosis will continue to occur as long as untreated tuberculosis infection occurs in adults and children. In the United States, the major methods of preventing tuberculosis infection and disease center on the public health activities of contact tracing with tests of tuberculosis infection. Identifying recently infected persons, particularly infants and toddlers and immunocompromised persons of all ages, and rapidly treating them are the best ways to prevent additional cases of tuberculosis in all its forms.

In many areas of the world, treatment of tuberculosis infection is not available. All countries of the world except the Netherlands and the United States have used BCG vaccines to prevent complications of tuberculosis infection, particularly in children. While universal BCG vaccination is still undertaken in most high-burden countries, the vaccination is more selective for specific high-risk groups in most middle- to low-burden countries. This vaccine is not very effective for preventing tuberculosis infection but is 50–80% effective in preventing serious forms of tuberculosis, such as meningitis, for at least 5 years after vaccination. Although BCG vaccines have had little impact on the control of tuberculosis globally, they have prevented countless cases of tuberculous meningitis, particularly in children, and this vaccination remains a cornerstone of the World Health Organization tuberculosis prevention programs. However, the disease will persist until a more effective vaccine is discovered [67].

References

1. van Well GT, Paes BF, Terwee CB, et al. Twenty years of pediatric tuberculous meningitis: a retrospective cohort study in the western cape of South Africa. Pediatrics. 2009;123:e1–8.
2. van Toorn R, Solomons R. Update on the diagnosis and management of tuberculous meningitis in children. Semin Pediatr Neurol. 2014;21:12–8.
3. World Health Organization. Global tuberculosis report – 2017. Geneva: World Health Organization; 2017.
4. Doerr CA, Starke JR, Ong LT. Clinical and public health aspects of tuberculous meningitis in children. J Pediatr. 1995;127:27–33.
5. Donald PR, Schaaf HS, Schoeman JF. Tuberculous meningitis and miliary tuberculosis: the rich focus revisited. J Infect. 2005;50:193–5.
6. Rich AR, McCordock HA. The pathogenesis of tuberculous meningitis. Bull Johns Hopkins Hosp. 1933;52:5–35.
7. Wolzak NK, Cooke ML, Orth H, et al. The changing profile of pediatric meningitis at a referral centre in Cape Town, South Africa. J Trop Pediatr. 2012;58:491–5.
8. Yaramis A, Gurkan F, Elevli M, et al. Central nervous system tuberculosis in children: a review of 254 cases. Pediatrics. 1998;102:e49.
9. Checkley AM, Njalale Y, Scarborough M, et al. Sensitivity and specificity of an index for the diagnosis of TB meningitis in patients in an urban teaching hospital in Malawi. Trop Med Int Health. 2008;13:1042–6.
10. Lammie GA, Hewlett RH, Schoeman JF, et al. Tuberculous cerebrovascular disease: a review. J Infect. 2009;59:156–66.
11. Wiseman CA, Gie RP, Starke JR, et al. A proposed comprehensive classification of tuberculosis disease severity in children. Pediatr Infect Dis J. 2012;31:347–52.
12. Marais S, Meintjes G, Pepper DJ, et al. Frequency, severity, and prediction of tuberculous meningitis immune reconstitution inflammatory syndrome. Clin Infect Dis. 2013;56:450–60.
13. Meintjes G, Lawn S, Scano F, et al. Tuberculosis-associated immune reconstitution inflammatory syndrome: case definitions for use in resource-limited settings. Lancet Infect Dis. 2008;8:516–23.

14. Meintjes G, Lawn SD, Scano F, et al. International network for the study of HIV-associated IRIS. Tuberculosis-associated immune reconstitution inflammatory syndrome: case definitions for use in resource-limited settings. Lancet Infect Dis. 2008;8:516–23.
15. Post MJ, Thurnher MM, Clifford DB, et al. CNS- immune reconstitution inflammatory syndrome in the setting of HIV infection, Part 2: discussion of neuro-immune reconstitution inflammatory syndrome with and without other pathogens. AJNR Am J Neuroradiol. 2013;34:1308–18.
16. Pepper DJ, Marais S, Maartens G, et al. Neurologic manifestations of paradoxical tuberculosis-associated immune reconstitution inflammatory syndrome: a case series. Clin Infect Dis. 2009;48:e96–107.
17. Marais BJ, Heemskerk AD, Marais SS, et al. Standardized methods for enhance quality and comparability of tuberculous meningitis studies. Clin Infect Dis. 2017;64:501–9.
18. Marais S, Thwaites G, Schoeman J, et al. Tuberculous meningitis: a uniform case definition for use in clinical research. Lancet Infect Dis. 2010;10:803–12.
19. Solomons RS, Visser DH, Marais BJ, Schoeman JF, van Furth AM. Diagnostic accuracy of a uniform research case definition for TBM in children: a prospective study. Int J Tuberc Lung Dis. 2016;20:903–8.
20. Metcalfe JZ, Everett CK, Steingart KR, et al. Interferon-gamma release assays for active pulmonary tuberculosis diagnosis in adults in low- and middle income countries: systematic review and meta-analysis. J Infect Dis. 2011;204:S1120–9.
21. Xu HB, Jiang RH, Li L, Sha W, Xiao HP. Diagnostic value of adenosine deaminase in cerebrospinal fluid for tuberculous meningitis: a meta-analysis. Int J Tuberc Lung Dis. 2010;14:1382–7.
22. Pai M, Flores LL, Pai N, et al. Diagnostic accuracy of nucleic acid amplification tests for tuberculous meningitis: a systematic review and meta-analysis. Lancet Infect Dis. 2003;3:633–43.
23. Tortoli E, Russo C, Piersimoni C, et al. Clinical validation of Xpert MTB/RIF for the diagnosis of extrapulmonary tuberculosis. Eur Respir J. 2012;40:442–7.
24. Patel VB, Theron G, Lenders L, et al. Diagnostic accuracy of quantitative PCR (Xpert MTB/RIF) for tuberculous meningitis in a high burden setting: A prospective study. PLoS Med. 2013;10:e1001536.
25. Rohlwink UK, Mauff K, Wilkinson KA, et al. Biomarkers of cerebral injury and inflammation in pediatric tuberculous meningitis. Clin Infect Dis. 2017;65:1298–307.
26. Tobin DM, Roca FJ, Oh SF, et al. Host genotype-specific therapies can optimize the inflammatory response to mycobacterial infections. Cell. 2012;148:434–46.
27. Andronikou S, Smith B, Hatherhill M, Douis H, Wilmshurst J. Definitive neuroradiological diagnostic features of tuberculous meningitis in children. Pediatr Radiol. 2004;34:876–85.
28. Gupta RK, Kumar S. Central nervous system tuberculosis. Neuroimaging Clin N Am. 2011;21:795–814.
29. Bruwer GE, van der Westhuizen S, Lombard CJ, et al. Can CT predict the level of CSF block in tuberculous hydrocephalus? Childs Nerv Syst. 2004;20:183–7.
30. Schoeman JF, Van Zyl LE, Laubscher JA, et al. Serial CT scanning in childhood tuberculous meningitis: prognostic features in 198 cases. J Child Neurol. 1995;10:320–9.
31. Janse van Rensburg P, Andronikou S, van Toorn R, et al. Magnetic resonance imaging of the central nervous system in children with tuberculous meningitis. Pediatr Radiol. 2008;38:1306–13.
32. Pienaar M, Andronikou S, van Toorn R. MRI to demonstrate features and complications of TBM not seen with CT. Childs Nerv Syst. 2009;25:941–7.
33. van Toorn R, Rabie H, Dramowski A, et al. Neurological manifestations of TB-IRIS: a report of 4 children. Eur J Paediatr Neurol. 2012;16:676–82.
34. Thwaites GE, Mac-Mullin-Price J, Tran TH, et al. Serial MRI to determine the effect of dexamethasone on the cerebral pathology of tuberculous meningitis: an observational study. Lancet Neurol. 2007;6:230–6.
35. Thwaites G, Chau T, Stepniewska K, et al. Diagnosis of adult tuberculous meningitis by use of clinical and laboratory features. Lancet. 2002;360:1287–92.

36. Thwaites GE, Nguyen DB, Nguyen HD, et al. The influence of HIV infection on clinical presentation, response to treatment, and outcome in adults with tuberculous meningitis. J Infect Dis. 2005;192:2134–41.
37. Youssef F, Afifi S, Azab A, et al. Differentiation of tuberculous meningitis from acute bacterial meningitis using simple clinical and laboratory parameters. Diagn Microbiol Infect Dis. 2006;55:275–8.
38. Thwaites GE. Advances in the diagnosis and treatment of tuberculous meningitis. Curr Opin Neurol. 2013;26:295–300.
39. Donald PR. Cerebrospinal fluid concentrations of antituberculous agents in adults and children. Tuberculosis (Edinb). 2010;90:279–92.
40. Donald PR, Schoeman JF, Vanzyl LE, et al. Intensive short-course chemotherapy in the management of tuberculous meningitis. Int J Tuberc Lung Dis. 1998;2:704–11.
41. van Toorn R, Schaaf HS, Laubscher JA, et al. Short intensified treatment in children with drug-susceptible tuberculous meningitis. Pediatr Infect Dis J. 2014;33:248–52.
42. Seddon JA, Visser DH, Bartens M, et al. Impact of drug resistance on clinical outcome in children with tuberculous meningitis. Pediatr Infect Dis J. 2012;31:711–6.
43. Heemskerk AD, Bang ND, Mai NT, et al. Intensified antituberculosis therapy in adults with tuberculous meningitis. N Engl J Med. 2016;374:124–34.
44. Heemskerk AD, Nguyen MTH, Dang HTM, et al. Clinical outcomes of patients with drug-resistant tuberculous meningitis treated with an intensified antituberculosis regimen. Clin Infect Dis. 2017;65:20–8.
45. Ruslami R, Ganiem AR, Dian S, et al. Intensified regimen containing rifampicin and moxifloxacin for tuberculous meningitis: an open-label, randomised controlled phase 2 trial. Lancet Infect Dis. 2013;13:27–35.
46. Rizvi I, Garg RK, Malhotra HS, et al. Ventriculo-peritoneal shunt surgery for tuberculous meningitis: a systematic review. J Neurol Sci. 2017;375:255–63.
47. Yadav YR, Parihar VS, Todorov M, et al. Role of endoscopic third ventriculostomy in tuberculous meningitis with hydrocephalus. Asian J Neurosurg. 2016;11:325–9.
48. Goyal P, Srivastava C, Ojha BK, et al. A randomized study of ventriculoperitoneal shunt versus endoscopic third ventriculostomy for the management of tubercular meningitis with hydrocephalus. Childs Nerv Syst. 2014;30:851–7.
49. Wilkinson RJ, Rohlwink U, Misra UK, et al. Tuberculous meningitis. Nat Rev Neurol. 2017;13:581–98.
50. Dooley DP, Carpenter JL, Rademachen S. Adjunctive corticosteroid therapy for tuberculosis: a critical reappraisal of the literature. Clin Infect Dis. 1997;25:872–87.
51. Schoeman JF, Van Zyl LE, Laubscher JA, Donald PR. Effect of corticosteroids on intracranial pressure, computed tomographic findings, and clinical outcome in young children with tuberculous meningitis. Pediatrics. 1997;99:226–31.
52. Thwaites GE, Nguyen DB, Nguyen HD, et al. Dexamethasone for the treatment of tuberculous meningitis in adolescents and adults. N Engl J Med. 2004;351:1741–51.
53. Prasad K, Singh MB. Corticosteroids for managing tuberculous meningitis. Cochrane Database Syst Rev. 2016;4:CD002244. https://doi.org/10.1002/14651858.CD002244.pub4.
54. Misra UK, Kalita J, Nair PP. Role of aspirin in tuberculous meningitis: a randomized open label placebo controlled trial. J Neurol Sci. 2010;293:12–7.
55. Schoeman JF, Janse van Rensburg A, Laubsher JA, et al. The role of aspirin in childhood tuberculous meningitis. J Child Neurol. 2011;26:956–62.
56. Schoeman JF, Springer P, Ravenscroft A, et al. Adjuvant thalidomide therapy of childhood tuberculous meningitis: possible anti-inflammatory role. J Child Neurol. 2000;15:497–503.
57. van Toorn R, du Plessis A-M, Schaaf HS, Buys H, Hewlett RH, Schoeman JF. Clinicoradiologic response of neurologic tuberculous mass lesions in children treated with thalidomide. Pediatr Infect Dis J. 2015;34:214–8.
58. McHugh SM, Rifkin IR, Deighton J, et al. The immunosuppressive drug thalidomide induces T helper cell type 2 (Th2) and concomitantly inhibits Th1 cytokine production in mitogen- and

antigen-stimulated human peripheral blood mononuclear cell cultures. Clin Exp Immunol. 1995;99:160–7.

59. Paravar T, Lee DJ. Thalidomide: mechanisms of action. Int Rev Immunol. 2008;27:111–35.
60. Schoeman JF, Andronikou S, Stefan DC, et al. Tuberculous meningitis related optic neuritis: recovery of vision with thalidomide in 4 consecutive cases. J Child Neurol. 2010;25:822–8.
61. Schoeman JF, Fieggen G, Seller N, et al. Intractable intracranial tuberculous infection responsive to thalidomide: report of four cases. J Child Neurol. 2006;21:301–8.
62. Molton JS, Huggan PJ, Archuleta S. Infliximab therapy in two cases of severe neurotuberculosis paradoxical reaction. Med J Aust. 2015;202:156–7.
63. Hosoglu S, Gevik MF, Balik I, et al. Predictors of outcome in patients with tuberculous meningitis. Int J Tuberc Lung Dis. 2002;6:64–70.
64. Thwaites GE, Simmons CP, Than Ha Quyen N, et al. Pathophysiology and prognosis in Vietnamese adults with tuberculous meningitis. J Infect Dis. 2003;188:1105–15.
65. van Toorn R, Springer P, Laubscher JA, et al. Value of different staging systems for predicting neurological outcome in childhood tuberculous meningitis. Int J Tuberc Lung Dis. 2012;16:628–32.
66. Wait JW, Schoeman JF. Behavioural profiles after tuberculous meningitis. J Trop Pediatr. 2010;56:166–71.
67. Hokey DA, Ginsberg A. The current state of tuberculosis vaccines. Hum Vaccine Immunother. 2013;9:2142–6.

Neurobrucellosis

7

Mushira Abdulaziz Enani

Introduction

Brucellosis, also known as "undulant fever," "Mediterranean fever," or "Malta fever," is an important human zoonosis and a major public health issue in many parts of the world especially in the Mediterranean countries of Europe, North and East Africa, the Middle East, South and Central Asia, and Central and South America [1].

Among Mediterranean countries, it has been reported that Syria has 16,034 cases followed by Iraq (2784), Turkey (2622), and the Kingdom of Saudi Arabia (KSA) (2144) per million population [2]. *Brucella* are aerobic gram-negative intracellular coccobacilli, four species of which are known to cause disease in humans, namely, *B. melitensis*, *B. suis*, *B. canis*, and *B. abortus*. More recently, marine mammals have been recognized as additional animal reservoirs for *Brucella* species with zoonotic potential. *B. ceti* and *B. pinnipedialis* are the newly proposed species names.

The most severe form is caused by *B. melitensis* that is predominant in KSA and the Middle East. It is transmitted from animals indirectly via consumption of raw milk and milk products, butchering of raw meat or directly by contact with livestock (sheep, goat, camels), milking, and handling parturient of animals such as contact with placenta membrane. In Al Medina region alone, the prevalence of brucellosis was 2.6% and was shown to increase with age in rural communities and low socioeconomic status. The overall prevalence of brucellosis among livestock as assessed by examining blood from a random sample of animals was estimated at 17.4% [3]. A recently published study from KSA reported a significant reduction of incidence rate from 22.9 in 2004 to 12.5 in 2012 per 100,000 persons for the total population [4].

M. A. Enani
Department of Medicine, Section of Infectious Diseases, King Fahad Medical City, Riyadh, Saudi Arabia
e-mail: menani@kfmc.med.sa

© Springer International Publishing AG, part of Springer Nature 2018
R. Hasbun (ed.), *Meningitis and Encephalitis*,
https://doi.org/10.1007/978-3-319-92678-0_7

Clinical Manifestation

Brucellosis can involve any system of the body including the central nervous system.

Most of the studies report that an element of CNS is involved in 4–13% of brucellosis patients [5].

Neurobrucellosis (NB) is defined as isolation of *Brucella* species from CSF of patients with suspected findings for brucellosis, or isolation of *Brucella* species from bone marrow or blood cultures of patients with abnormal CSF findings, with or without standard tube agglutination (STA) positivity of any titer in CSF with abnormal findings [6].

In another series of 128 patients with laboratory-confirmed brucellosis and neurological signs and symptoms, 48 (37.5%) were diagnosed with NB according to any one of the following diagnostic criteria: (1) symptoms and signs suspecting NB; (2) isolation of *Brucella* species from cerebrospinal fluid (CSF) and/or presence of anti-*Brucella* antibodies in CSF; (3) the presence of lymphocytosis, increased protein, and decreased glucose levels in the CSF; or (4) findings in cranial magnetic resonance imaging (MRI) or computed tomography (CT) [7].

Neurobrucellosis is a rare but severe complication occurring in about 5% of systemic brucellosis. It poses a diagnostic challenge, often resembling a variety of other neurologic disorders.

It can manifest in various forms, the most common being meningitis and/or meningoencephalitis-meningomyelitis (acute, subacute, or chronic) and polyradiculoneuropathy with or without cranial nerve involvement (most often the eighth nerve) which is subacute or chronic. Cerebrovascular accidents may present in the following ways: transient ischemic attacks; occlusive episodes; venous thrombosis, either sudden or progressive; thrombophlebitis of the brain and the eye; or subarachnoid and intracerebral hemorrhage due to rupture of mycotic aneurysms.

The clinical picture may be much more subtle and often deceptive, resembling demyelinating, multisystem degenerative, and other localized or diffuse central and/or peripheral nervous system disorders. A patient with recurrent episodes of diplopia and pyramidal symptoms would most likely direct diagnostic probabilities toward multiple sclerosis, which is rampant in Saudi Arabia. Similarly, a young patient with slowly progressive ataxia, polyradiculoneuropathy, and deafness is most likely to suffer from a degenerative, probably inherited disease or may present with Guillain-Barre syndrome. An obese young lady with papilledema and sixth nerve palsy may suffer from benign intracranial hypertension, but CSF shows findings of chronic meningitis, without overt clinical evidence.

In another young patient, with transient and recurrent alternating hemiplegia, NB would be the most implausible choice in the diagnostic list of the experienced neurologist. In addition, a patient with NB may appear with acute confusional episodes or a motor neuron disease-like syndrome or a unilateral brachial neuropathy reminiscent of neuralgic amyotrophy. Other more common presentations may be due to spinal nerve root and/or cord involvement secondary to spinal disc and bone infection (spodylodiscitis) [8].

Studies from Saudi Arabia show that approximately half of clinically diagnosed brucellosis patients have osteoarticular involvement with sacroiliitis, peripheral arthritis, and destructive spondylitis as common presentations [9]. Clinical manifestations and CSF abnormality are similar to tuberculosis, and NB must be kept in mind when approaching patients with acute or chronic lymphocytic meningitis with increased protein and low glucose level in CSF and risk factors of brucellosis [10].

Thwaites and Lancet scoring systems are widely used to aid clinicians practicing in resource-poor countries to predict TB meningitis. Since *Brucella* meningoencephalitis is clinically and biochemically indistinguishable from TB meningitis, the validity of Thwaites and Lancet prediction scoring systems was assessed in a large retrospective Turkish cohort where 294 confirmed *Brucella* meningoencephalitis patients were compared to 190 cases of confirmed TB meningitis selected from Hydarpasa studies database. Interestingly those scoring systems have falsely identified *Brucella* meningoencephalitis patients as TB meningitis; therefore, the authors concluded that *Brucella* meningoencephalitis should be excluded by every diagnostic microbiologic modality when such prediction systems suggest TB meningitis [11].

Further, it is important to think about the diagnosis of NB in patients with subacute-chronic and obscure neurologic involvement, especially living in endemic regions, because NB may potentially cause irreversible neurologic disability.

Diagnosis

The diagnosis of brucellosis is based on serological and microbiological laboratory tests. Full blood count would reveal normal to low leukocyte counts. Minor changes in liver enzymes are noticeable [12]. CSF shows pleocytosis with predominant mononuclear cells. Elevated CSF adenosine deaminase (ADA) is suggestive of *Brucella* meningitis but may also indicate TB meningitis. In a study by Karsen et al., the mean ADA values in CSF of TB meningitis cases were 28.34 compared to 8.71 IU/L in *Brucella* meningoencephalitis. A cutoff value of 12.5 IU/L for the differential diagnosis of TB versus *Brucella* meningoencephalitis has a sensitivity of 92% and a specificity of 88% [13].

In *Brucella* arthritis, leukocytosis with lymphocytic predominance is dominant [12].

Microbial culture is the ideal method in making a diagnosis of brucellosis by culturing the organism from blood, bone marrow, liver biopsy specimen, and/or other body fluids or tissues [14, 15].

Serological tests detect antibodies to the antigens of *Brucella* species in blood. The antigens include smooth lipopolysaccharide (S-LPS) and cytosolic protein. The serological tests such as *serum agglutination testing (SAT)* and enzyme-linked immunosorbent assay (ELISA) detect antibodies against the S-LPS antigen [16].

The Rose Bengal test (RBT) is a rapid, slide-type agglutination assay performed with a stained *Brucella abortus* suspension at a low pH (3.6–3.7) and plain serum. It is a simple and ideal screening test for small laboratories with limited resources that is based on reactivity of antibodies against smooth lipopolysaccharide (LPS)

[17]. *The microagglutination test (MAT)* is a variant of the SAT or ELISA recommended for the serodiagnosis of brucellosis that is rapid and requires less volumes of serum and reagents (antigen and serum) than SAT and can test multiple samples at the same time but has high false-negative rates in complicated and chronic cases.

Coombs test is good for complicated and chronic cases but misses about 7% of cases compared with ELISA [18].

Dipstick assay is a good test to detect IgM antibodies to S-LPS in brucellosis of less than 3 months duration. IgM dipstick assay offers higher sensitivity and easier manipulation than IgM ELISA to detect IgM antibodies to *Brucella* species and improves the interpretation of results, thus establishing cutoff points. It could be used as a rapid and simple alternative to the ELISA IgM for the serodiagnosis of patients with acute brucellosis. The combined results of SAT and IgM dipstick assays can provide an indication of the stage of disease for those patients, in whom the onset of clinical manifestations is unknown [19].

The rapid slide agglutination test (RSAT) could be a suitable screening test for the diagnosis of *B. canis* human brucellosis, and a supplementary technique, such as ELISA, performed on all positive RSAT samples that were negative by *B. abortus* antigen could ensure diagnostic specificity and confirm the diagnosis [20]. Immunochromatographic *Brucella* IgM/IgG lateral flow assay (LFA), a simplified version of ELISA, has a great potential as a rapid point-of-care assay. It has high sensitivity and specificity for *Brucella* IgM and IgG. It is a rapid and simple diagnostic test for confirmation of brucellosis in an endemic area [21].

New Brucella markers can be detected by flow cytometry on CD4+ and CD8+ cells in seronegative patients with brucellosis that can be utilized as a novel diagnostic test for the detection of brucellosis in seronegative individuals [22].

Brucella immunocapture-agglutination test (Brucellacapt), which is based on sandwich ELISA system, is performed with Coombs antiserum and determines the three antibodies that form against *Brucella* (IgM, IgA, IgG). The advantage of this test is that it shows existence of blocking antibodies that is a reason for a false negative test by SAT and RBT. At a cutoff value of 1/160 and 1/320, Brucellacapt sensitivity is 95–100% and has a specificity of 55–59%. It is useful to diagnose disease in patients with long-standing evolution of brucellosis and in the follow-up of treatment; therefore it is considered as a second-level serological test [23].

Molecular Diagnosis of Brucellosis

Standard PCR has excellent sensitivity for the diagnosis of acute and relapsed cases of brucellosis where serology is often negative [19, 24]. It can be applied on blood, serum, or synovial fluid. The standard PCR assays include one pair of primers which is used to amplify the target genomic sequence of *Brucella* spp. Pairs used include the primers for sequences encoding 16S rRNA, outer membrane protein (omp2a, omp2b, and omp31), 31 kDa immunogenic *Brucella abortus* protein (BCSP 31 B4/B5), 16S–23S ribosomal DNA interspace region (ITS66/ITS279), and insertion sequence (IS711).

Real-time PCR seems to be highly reproducible, rapid (final result in 30 min), sensitive, and specific. Additionally, the risk of infection in laboratory workers is minimal. Samples that have been tested by real-time PCR include cultured *Brucella* cells, serum, blood, and paraffin-embedded tissues. The IS711-based assay was the most sensitive, specific, efficient, and reproducible method to detect *Brucella* spp.

Several multiplex PCRs have been reported which identify the genus *Brucella* at the species and partly at the biovar level using different primer combinations [21, 24, 25].

It has a great utility in chronic and atypical cases. The most interesting use of multiplex PCR is that it simultaneously detects *Brucella* spp. and *Mycobacterium tuberculosis* complex in countries where both diseases are endemic. The procedure targeted the IS711, bcsp31, and omp2a genes for *Brucella* spp. and the IS6110, senX3-regX3, and cfp31 genes for *M. tuberculosis* complex.

Angiography is used for detection of vascular changes. *Neurophysiologic elec-tromyographic* and *nerve conduction* studies are reserved for cases with peripheral and cranial nerve involvement [26].

Neuroimaging

A recent multicenter study has evaluated 263 adults with NB and reviewed their CT and MRI images. They categorized the finding into five groups. Group 1 had normal CT and MRI (143 patients, 54.3%), and group 2 had inflammatory changes (72 patients, 27.4%), diffuse inflammation (59 patients) including leptomeningeal involvement (44 patients), basal meningeal enhancement (30 patients), and local-ized inflammation (24 patients), in the form of cranial nerve involvement (14 patients), spinal nerve root enhancement (8 patients), brain abscess (7 patients), granuloma (6 patients), and arachnoiditis (4 patients); 11 patients had co-existent diffuse inflammation. Group 3 had white matter abnormalities (32 patients, 12.2%) and demyelinating lesions (7patients), while group 4 had vascular insults (42 patients, 16%), of which 37 patients had chronic cerebral ischemic changes, two patients had acute cerebral ischemia, two had subdural hematomas, and one patient had a subarachnoid hemorrhage. Group 5 had cerebral edema/hydrocephalus (48 patients, 18.2%), and 20 patients (7.6%) had hydrocephalus; cerebral edema was seen in 40 out of 263 patients (15%), while coexistent cerebral edema and hydro-cephalus were seen in 12 patients. The authors concluded that diffuse inflammation is the primary neuroimaging abnormality which is most commonly seen with longer duration of symptoms, higher CSF protein, lower CSF/serum glucose ratio, and with the presence of polyneuropathy or radiculopathy on clinical examination [27].

Focal cord expansion and poorly delineated increased signal in spinal cord on T2 W images may be seen in case of myelopathy due to involvement of spinal cord. In *Brucella* spondylitis, the lumbar spine is the most commonly involved site, par-ticularly the L4–L5 and L5–S1 junctions. In the majority of patients (98%), a soli-tary lesion was identified. However, the incidence of multiple site involvement has been reported as high as 9–30% in some studies. Abscess formation has become a common finding (21–42%) following the development of highly sensitive diagnostic techniques such as CT and MRI [26].

Among 20 patients with spondylodiscitis, it was complicated with paravertebral or epidural abscess in seven, radiculitis in six, and psoas abscess in five of cases [28, 29]. The demonstration of IgG/oligoclonal bands in CSF and serum is a rapid test which can be used as an important index in the diagnosis of NB at the time of presentation, as it may be confused with CNS infections with mycobacteria, treponema, or fungi [30].

Treatment and Prevention Challenges

The optimal drug treatment and duration are both controversial. The treatment of central nervous system complications of brucellosis poses a special problem because of the need to achieve high concentrations of drugs in the CSF. Although doxycycline is the best among tetracyclines in penetrating the blood-brain barrier, it is recommended to add other drugs which achieve this, such as rifampicin or co-trimoxazole in the treatment regimen of patients with NB [1].

Some studies showed the benefit of adding third-generation cephalosporin such as ceftriaxone in NB as it achieves concentrations in CSF higher than the MIC against *Brucella* species. In the Istanbul study, adult patients treated for NB were retrospectively reviewed in 28 healthcare institutions from four different countries. It was found that ceftriaxone-based regimens are more successful in terms of less clinical failure and relapse, and they require shorter therapy than the oral treatment protocol alone [31].

The usual span of treatment is as short as 6–8 weeks up to 18 months if patients have residual disease [32].

Although adding steroids in NB has not been proved to be consistently beneficial, adjunctive corticosteroid therapy has been used for concurrent vasculitis or demyelinating disease [33].

In a series of patients with spondylitis, antibiotic regimens included two or three antibiotics with combination of doxycycline, rifampin, and streptomycin. The mean duration of antimicrobial therapy was 18 weeks (range 12–56 weeks). Prolonged duration of treatment is important especially in complicated cases in order to avoid possible sequelae [28, 30].

Doxycycline, 100 mg twice daily, for at least 12 weeks combined with streptomycin, 1 g daily, for the first 2 or 3 weeks remains the first choice of antibiotic therapy in *Brucella* spondylitis [29, 30]. The use of streptomycin in CNS brucellosis is discouraged owing to its questionable ability to penetrate into the cerebrospinal fluid and its potential neurotoxicity that may perplex the clinical presentation [32, 33].

The Saudi Pediatric Infectious Diseases Society recommends treating NB in children above 8 years with doxycycline and trimethoprim-sulfamethoxazole (TMP-SMX), while for those younger than 8 years, rifampicin, TMP-SMX, and ciprofloxacin for 3–6 months up to 1 year in complicated cases. Gentamicin is added in the initial 14 days with the option of adding ceftriaxone in the initial 2–4 weeks [34].

There are no randomized trials for brucellosis in pregnancy. The most extended series support the use of TMP-SMX alone or in combination with rifampicin [35].

Surgical intervention should be carried out in NB if indicated as in other CNS infections. The challenge lies in establishing guidelines for diagnosis and treatment as each case is unique and the clinical manifestations vary from individual to individual. Not all forms of NB are the same nor they carry a similar prognosis. Relapses are also not unusual. Further adverse effects due to drug therapy or due to the complications of the disease itself needs careful monitoring over a period of time. Early clinical and laboratory diagnosis followed by ideal and prompt treatment for adequate period of time is indispensable to prevent lifelong residual deficits.

Establishment of National Brucellosis control program is recommended not only for KSA but also for all endemic regions. Animal husbandry should be properly practiced.

Detailed information on frequency and distribution of infection is required to estimate cost effective options for control.

Consumption of raw milk should be avoided in all age groups until regular screening services can be provided.

Strategic vaccination of ruminants combined with public health education programs may help in controlling the disease.

Through national and international collaboration well-designed epidemiological studies should be conducted to bridge the gap in the management of brucellosis [36].

Importation of *Brucella* spp. especially into non-endemic areas, or areas which have achieved recent control of both animal and human brucellosis, may have public health repercussions, and timely recognition is essential [37]. In pediatric brucellosis cases, family history has been reported in 33% of cases in Turkey. So screening of family members when a patient with brucellosis is diagnosed is very important [38]. Effective vaccines are currently available and it is important to find means and resources for their effective use in resource-poor countries in conjunction with sustained control efforts that incorporate local farming practices, dietary habits, and traditional beliefs [39].

Mixing different herds of animals together should be avoided as this practice facilitates the transmission of disease among animals. The government should stress the screening of animals, the vaccination of seronegative animals, and slaughtering diseased ones. A collaborative team to implement a brucellosis control program should be arranged and maintained among the concerned government sectors including the Ministry of Health, the Ministry of Agriculture, the Custom Department, and the Municipal Department [34].

Indeed, with such extraordinary advancement in healthcare system and general awareness, brucellosis should be eradicated from this region.

Conclusion

Zoonotic brucellosis remains widespread and neglected in many areas despite notable advances in science, technology, and management in the nineteenth and twentieth centuries [40].

Neurobrucellosis is not readily identified because of its variable picture and must be prioritized in the list of differential diagnosis of any neurological disorder in patients living in or returning from endemic area.

Diagnosis depends on keen awareness of possible infection and a thorough occupational and travel history. A definitive diagnosis requires isolation of the organism by culture of blood, CSF, bone marrow, or other clinical samples. However, a diagnosis of brucellosis is often made serologically, most frequently by standard tube agglutination measuring antibody to *B. abortus* antigen or ELISA, which is more sensitive and specific. The mortality rate of brucellosis is very low (0.1%) and is associated with late diagnosis and late therapy, especially when *Brucella* affects the central nervous system, resulting in meningitis or cerebral abscess. Therapeutic intensity is obviously higher in focal disease, some cases requiring surgery and/or a longer duration of antibiotic therapy. Combination antimicrobial therapy with more than two agents for a prolonged duration that may extend to 6–9 months is necessary to control NB and prevent relapse.

Patients with persistent symptoms following extended antibiotic therapy, for whom focal disease or relapse have been ruled out pose a difficult clinical management problem. This disabling syndrome, sometimes called chronic brucellosis, is similar to chronic fatigue syndrome and must be treated symptomatically [41].Since there is no human vaccine and no significant human-to-human transmission, control of animal brucellosis, milk pasteurization, and other food hygiene measures are the only options to reduce its occurrence in humans. The challenges and opportunities for brucellosis management must be recognized as fundamentally multivariate, multifaceted, and integrative; it is crucial for veterinary, public health, and wildlife/conservation professions to collaboratively develop, adopt and declare brucellosis one health paradigm [40].

References

1. Corbel MJ, et al. Brucellosis in humans and animals. WHO/CDS/EPR/2006.7.
2. Pappas G, Papadimitriou P, Akritidis N, Christou L, Tsianos EV. The new global map of human brucellosis. Lancet Infect Dis. 2006;6(2):91–9.
3. Al-Sekait MA. Epidemiology of brucellosis in Al Medina region, Saudi Arabia. J Fam Community Med. 2000;7(1):47–53.
4. Aloufi A, Memish Z, Assiri M, McNabb S. Trends of reported human cases of brucellosis, Kingdom of Saudi Arabia, 2004–2012. J Epidemiol Glob Health. 2016;6:11–8.
5. Alhedaithy A, Aldubayan N, Alqurashi D, Aldubayan S. Clinical-features, serological patterns and long-term complications of 22 patients with neurobrucellosis. Int J Adv Res. 2016;4(10):1682–9.
6. Buzgan T, Karahocagil MK, Irmak H, Baran AI, Evirgen O, Akdeniz H. Clinical manifestations and complications in 1028 cases of brucellosis: a retrospective evaluation and review of the literature. Int J Infect Dis. 2010;14:e469–78.
7. Guven T, Ugurlu K, Ergonul O, Celikbas AK, Gok SE, Comoglu S, et al. Neurobrucellosis: clinical and diagnostic features. Clin Infect Dis. 2013;56(10):1407–12.
8. Panayiotopoulos CP. Neurobrucellosis: a cause for concern and action. Ann Saudi Med. 1988;8(30):167–8.

9. Paul E, Abdelkareem M, Malik S. Overview of human brucellosis in Aseer region, Saudi Arabia. AMJ. 2017;10(3):202–10.
10. Pourhassan A. Clinical and laboratory findings in neurobrucellosis: a study of 43 cases. Iran J Clin Infect Dis. 2007;2(2):71–6.
11. Erdem H, Senbayrak S, Gencer S, Hasbun R, Karahocagil M, Sengoz G. Tuberculous and brucellosis meningitis differential diagnosis. Travel Med Infect Dis. 2015;13(2):185–91.
12. Pappas G, Akritidis N, Bosilkovski M, Tsianos E. Brucellosis. N Engl J Med. 2005;352:2325.
13. Karsen H, Koruk S, Karahocagil M, Calisir C, Baran F. Comparative analysis of cerebrospinal fluid adenosine deaminase activity in meningitis. Swiss Med Wkly. 2011;141:w13214.
14. Young EJ. Brucellosis: current epidemiology, diagnosis, and management. Curr Clin Top Infect Dis. 1995;15:115.
15. Aliskan H. The value of culture and serological methods in the diagnosis of human brucellosis. Mikrobiyol Bul. 2008;42:185–95.
16. Shenoy B, Jaiswal A, Vinod A. Lab diagnosis of brucellosis. Pediatr Infect Dis. 2016;8:40–4.
17. Serra J, Viñas M. Laboratory diagnosis of brucellosis in a rural endemic area in northeastern Spain. Int Microbiol. 2004;7:53.
18. Araj GF. Update on laboratory diagnosis of human brucellosis. Int J Antimicrob Agents. 2010;36:12–7.
19. Geresu MA, Kassa GM. A review on diagnostic methods of brucellosis. J Vet Sci Technol. 2016;7:323.
20. Lucero NE, Escobar GI, Ayala SM, Jacob N. Diagnosis of human brucellosis caused by Brucella canis. J Med Microbiol. 2005;54:457–61.
21. Christopher S, Umapathy BL, Ravikumar KL. Brucellosis: review on the recent trends in pathogenicity and laboratory diagnosis. J Lab Physicians. 2010;2:55–60.
22. Sun Y-H, Rolan HG, den Hartigh AB, Sondervan D, Tsolis RM. Brucella abortus VirB12 is expressed during infection but is not an essential component of the type IV secretion system. Infect Immun. 2005;73:6048–54.
23. Özdemir M, Feyzioglu B, Kurtoglu MG, et al. A comparison of immunocapture agglutination and ELISA methods in serological diagnosis of brucellosis. Int J Med Sci. 2011;8(5):428–32.
24. Andriopoulos P, Tsironi M. Molecular diagnosis of brucellosis: a brief report. Adv Mol Diag. 2016;1:108.
25. Sanjuuan-Jimenez R, Colmenero J, Bermudez P, Alonso A, Morata P. Amplicon DNA melting analysis for the simultaneous detection of Brucella spp and Mycobacterium tuberculosis complex. Potential use in rapid differential diagnosis between extrapulmonary tuberculosis and focal complication of brucellosis. PLoS One. 2013;8(3):e58353.
26. Kizilkilic O. Neurobrucellosis. Neuroimaging Clin N Am. 2011;21:927–37.
27. Erdem H, Senbayrak S, Meriç K, Batirel A, Karahocagil MK, Hasbun R, et al. Cranial imaging findings in neurobrucellosis: results of Istanbul-3 study. Infection. 2016;44(5):623–3127.
28. Ulu-Kilic A, Sayar MS, Tutuncu E, Sezen F, Sencan I. Complicated brucellar spondylodiscitis: experience from an endemic area. Rheumatol Int. 2013;33(11):2909–12.
29. Alp E, Doganay M. Current therapeutic strategy in spinal brucellosis. Int J Infect Dis. 2008;12:573–7.
30. Daif AK. The value of oligoclonal bands in neurobrucellosis. Ann Saudi Med. 1991;11(4):411–3.
31. Erdem H, Ulu-Kilic A, Kilic S, et al. Efficacy and tolerability of antibiotic combinations in neurobrucellosis: results of the Istanbul study. Antimicrob Agents Chemother. 2012;56(3):1523–8.
32. Pappas G, Akritidis N, Christou L. Treatment of neurobrucellosis: what is known and what remains to be answered. Expert Rev Anti Infect Ther. 2007;5(6):983–90.
33. Madjdinasab N, Naieni AR. Neurobrucellosis and steroid therapy. Iran J Clin Infect Dis. 2006;1(2):103–7.
34. Alshaalan MA, Alalola SA, Almuneef M, Albanyan EA, Balkhy HH, AlShahrani DA, AlJohani S. Brucellosis in children: prevention, diagnosis and management guidelines for general pediatricians endorsed by the Saudi Pediatric Infectious Diseases Society (SPIDS). Int J Pediatr Adolesc Med. 2014;1:40e46.

35. Ariza J, Bosilkovski M, Cascio A, et al. Perspectives for the treatment of brucellosis in the 21st century: the Ioannina recommendations. PLoS Med. 2007;4(12):e317.
36. Musallam I, Abo-Shehada M, Hegazy Y, Holt H, Guitian F. Systematic review of brucellosis in the Middle East: disease frequency in ruminants and humans and risk factors for human infection. Epidemiol Infect. 2016;144(4):671–85.
37. Norman FF, Monge-Maillo B, Chamorro-Tojeiro S, Pérez-Molina JA, Lopez-Velez R. Imported brucellosis: a case series and literature review. Travel Med Infect Dis. 2016;14(3):182–99.
38. Yoldas T, Tezer H, Ozkaya-Parlakay A, Sayli TR. Clinical and laboratory findings of 97 pediatric brucellosis patients in Central Turkey. J Microbiol Immunol Infect. 2015;48:446–9.
39. Franco MP, Mulder M, Gilman RH, Smits HL. Human brucellosis. Lancet Infect Dis. 2007;7:775–6.
40. Plumb GE, Olsen SC, Buttke D. Brucellosis: 'one health' challenges and opportunities. Rev Sci Tech. 2013;32(1):271–8.
41. Solera J. Update on brucellosis: therapeutic challenges. Int J Antimicrob Agents. 2010;36(Suppl 1):S18–20.

West Nile Encephalitis

Megan McKenna, Shannon E. Ronca, Melissa S. Nolan, and Kristy O. Murray

Introduction

West Nile virus (WNV) is a mosquito-borne illness found worldwide, with manifestations ranging from asymptomatic infection to neuroinvasive disease (WNND), characterized by encephalitis, meningitis, and acute flaccid paralysis. First isolated in Uganda, the virus has spread globally, and transmission has now been documented on all six inhabited continents. The public health impact of WNV is considerable, with greater than six million people estimated to have been infected in the United States alone. This vector-borne disease is propagated in nature between the mosquito vector and birds, while horses and humans act as incidental, dead-end hosts. Diagnostic tests are widely available, but detection of antibodies, antibody cross-reactivity with other flaviviruses, and virus isolation in biological samples continue to pose challenges to clinical diagnosis. With limited treatment options and no FDA-approved vaccines, decreasing one's personal vector exposure is the most effective way to prevent disease. This widespread disease continues to be an annual public health threat, resulting in high morbidity, prolonged sequelae, and excessive mortality, thus warranting further study to improve diagnostics, treatments, and prevention to increase patient quality of life.

M. McKenna
Department of Infectious Diseases, Baylor College of Medicine, Harris County Hospital District, Houston, TX, USA

S. E. Ronca · M. S. Nolan · K. O. Murray (✉)
Department of Pediatrics, Baylor College of Medicine, Texas Children's Hospital, Houston, TX, USA
e-mail: kmurray@bcm.edu

© Springer International Publishing AG, part of Springer Nature 2018
R. Hasbun (ed.), *Meningitis and Encephalitis*,
https://doi.org/10.1007/978-3-319-92678-0_8

Epidemiology

First isolated in 1937 in the West Nile district of Uganda, WNV was one of the first arthropod-borne viruses (arboviruses) to be identified [1]. Since the mid-1990s, there has been an increase in human and equine outbreaks coinciding to large culling of avian populations [2]. WNV was first detected in North America in 1999, during an epidemic of meningoencephalitis in New York City [3]. Following its introduction into North America, a rapid geographic spread occurred between 2000 and 2004 followed by annual outbreaks in endemic areas [4, 5]. To date, millions are estimated to have been infected with WNV in the United States [6]. Similar rapid geographic expansions have been documented in other naïve populations globally. Diagnosis of human WNV cases is complicated by the potential for cross-reactivity in regions where other flavivirus infections are endemic: dengue virus in South America, Kunjin virus in Australia, Japanese encephalitis in Asia, and St. Louis encephalitis in North America. Cost estimates indicate that up to $400,000 are spent caring for each individual suffering from WNV sequelae [7]. With a robust vector range and sustained annual transmission internationally, this infection continues to present a significant health concern.

Transmission

Culex sp. mosquitoes are the principal vectors of WNV, with *Culex pipiens* (northern United States), *C. quinquefasciatus* (southern United States), and *C. tarsalis* (western United States) the most common in the United States [8–10]. However, these are not the only vectors, as the virus has been identified in at least 65 different mosquito species [9–11].

Birds are the natural reservoir and amplifying host, with WNV identified in over 300 different species. WNV is maintained through a bird-mosquito-bird transmission cycle. Dead-end hosts, such as horses and humans, can be infected through the bite of an infected mosquito but do not reach levels of viremia necessary for transmission back to the mosquito population. However, WNV can be transmitted from human-to-human through blood transfusions, organ transplant, intrauterine infection, and breastfeeding [12–16].

Transmission via organ transplantation was first reported in 2002 [17]. The same year in Toronto, community-acquired cases revealed an increased rate of WNND among transplant recipients (200/100,000 people) compared to the general population (5/100,000 people) [18]. In addition, chronically immune-suppressed solid organ transplant recipients have an increased risk for severe meningoencephalitis compared to the general population [19, 20].

The first intrauterine infection of WNV was documented when an infected mother gave birth to an infant with chorioretinitis and cerebral tissue damage [14]. Although the exact mechanisms involved in intrauterine infections remain unclear, mouse models indicate that infection of placental trophoblast cells can progress to infection of the embryo and that the timing of pregnancy plays a role [18]. Other infected mothers have given birth to children without defects, although there is one report of premature birth [19, 21]. There is a clear risk of transmission between mother and child, but the extent of the risk and associated outcomes require further study. Multiple body fluids are potentially infectious during peak viremia, as documented by case reports of transmission from mothers to their infants via infectious breast milk [22].

Viral Characteristics and Pathogenesis

WNV is a member of the family *Flaviviridae*, genus *Flavivirus* (Fig. 8.1). Flaviviruses are positive-sense RNA viruses divided by their antigenic cross-reactivity into different serocomplexes. WNV is a member of the Japanese encephalitis serocomplex, which also includes St. Louis encephalitis virus, Japanese encephalitis virus, and Murray Valley encephalitis virus. The diversity of WNV strains has been studied in great detail, with four lineages being described [23–25], although lineage II strains are often attributed to severe neuroinvasive disease. The RNA genome is made up of structural genes C, prM, E, and nonstructural genes (NS1, NS2A, NS2B, NS3, NS4A, NS4B, and NS5). These genes play different roles in the virus life cycle, virulence, and pathogenicity of infection.

Methods of immune evasion increase the pathogenicity of WNV. WNV enhances viral replication once in the host by blocking type-I interferons and evading the antiviral activity of IFN-stimulated genes (ISGs) [26, 27]. NS1, NS2A, NS4B, and NS5 may contribute to controlling this signaling cascade [28–30]. Interestingly, the IFN-inducible gene 20,50-oligoadenylate synthetase (OAS) has been shown to protect against flavivirus infection [31–33]. OAS is involved in the RNA decay pathway, known as the OAS/RNase L pathway, indicating it may promote antiviral activity of the immune system. Polymorphisms of OAS1 have indicated an increased

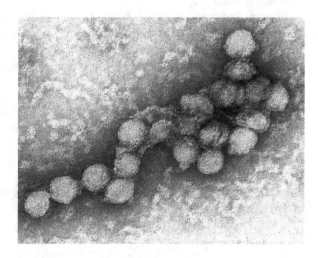

Fig. 8.1 West Nile virions. Digitally colored transmission electron microscope (TEM) image of West Nile virions. Photo credit: Cynthia Goldsmith. Provided by CDC/P.E. Rollin

susceptibility to WNV infection in horses and humans [34, 35]. Identification of other viral and host factors that affect WNV infection is critical to understanding, preventing, and treating future infections.

Pathology of Infection

After a blood meal, the mosquito vectors initiate host responses that drive the spread of infection. The mosquito injects saliva-containing virus within the dermis of the host, where the saliva acts as a potent enhancer of the host immune response, causing inflammation and edema. This drives the recruitment of leukocytes that become infected and allow for viral replication in additional target cells. Ultimately, virus migrates to the lymph nodes [36, 37]. Once in the lymph tissue, additional viral replication leads to viremia and infection of other organ systems (Fig. 8.2). Viremia peaks 2–4 days after infection and declines by the time of symptom onset [38], complicating the detection of viral particles for isolation and diagnosis. Viral persistence has been described in the kidneys and CNS [39–45]; however, the exact immune modulation is unknown.

Once in the brain, the virus directly infects neurons in nearly all regions but most commonly in the basal ganglia, thalamus, and brain stem (predominantly the medulla and pons) [46–48]. In cases of encephalitis and meningoencephalitis, the gross appearance of the brain is normal. Neuronal death, necrosis, mononuclear inflammation, and microglial nodules composed of lymphocytes and histiocytes are observed microscopically [47, 49]. Leptomeningeal mononuclear inflammatory infiltrates are present in cases of meningitis, with CD8 T lymphocytes the predominant inflammatory cell type in the nodules and infiltrates [48, 49]. Spinal cord infection primarily involves the ventral and dorsal gray and white matter, as well as the nerve roots, most commonly affecting the spinal cord anterior horn cells [47, 49–51]. Radiculitis caused by involvement of spinal and cranial nerve roots has also been documented [52].

Exact pathogenesis of CNS invasion in humans is unknown. Originally, neurovirulence was thought to depend on initial viral spread prior to the establishment of an immune response. Other theories include endocytosis into the CNS across vascular endothelium, as was previously demonstrated [53, 54], and CNS entry by infection of olfactory neurons, which are unprotected by the blood-brain barrier (BBB) [55–57]. Other hypothesized entry routes include WNV-infected leukocyte migration through tight junctions; direct viral shedding through the choroid plexus, across the cerebral endothelial cell to the brain parenchyma [58]; and transportation through peripheral nerve axons in a retrograde fashion [55, 59]. Animal models suggest viral entry into the CNS is facilitated by peripheral production of tumor necrosis factor alpha, leading to increased permeability of the BBB [60]. Highly neurovirulent flaviviruses have been shown to exhibit an upregulation of genes involved in IFN signaling, T-cell recruitment, MHC class I and II antigen presentation, and apoptosis [61, 62].

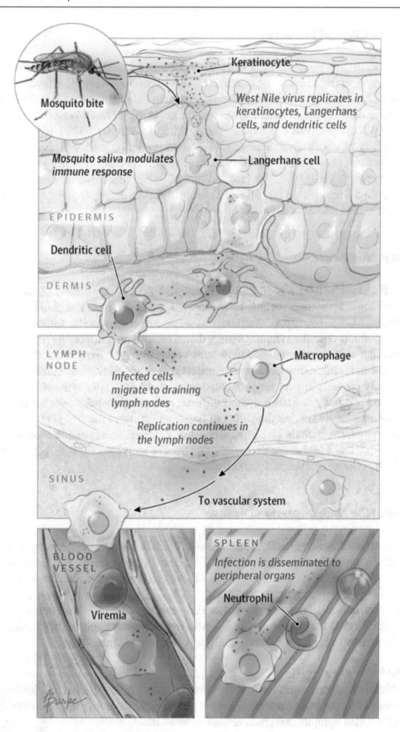

Fig. 8.2 Pathogenesis of WNV infection. From West Nile Virus: Review of the Literature. Petersen LR, Brault AC, and Nasci RS. JAMA 2013;310(3):308–315. doi: https://doi.org/10.1001/jama.2013.8042

Acute Clinical Features

Incubation time ranges from 2 to 14 days, with an estimated 80% of human cases remaining asymptomatic. Approximately 20% develop West Nile fever (WNF), generally a mild febrile illness [63, 64]. Less than 1% of patients progress to neuro-invasive disease, which includes West Nile meningitis (WNM), West Nile encepha-litis (WNE), and WNV-associated acute flaccid paralysis (AFP) [64, 65]. The frequency of neuroinvasive cases varies based on region [66], with North Dakota having the highest percentage of neuroinvasive clinical cases compared to febrile or asymptomatic cases [67]. The inherent bias of syndromic surveillance reporting in the United States makes it challenging to elucidate the exact percentage of neuroin-vasive versus febrile or asymptomatic cases.

West Nile Fever

WNF can range from a mild flu-like illness to a severe, debilitating illness lasting for months. Symptoms include headache, fatigue, fever, myalgia, chills, rash, and emesis [64, 68, 69]. Most symptoms of acute infection resolve within days, but some patients describe symptoms more than 6 months after infection [70]. It is theo-rized that febrile patients with long-term sequelae may have presented with sub-clinical neurologic disease that was misclassified upon initial examination. Rash typically presents in younger patients, persists 5–14 days after symptom onset [71, 72], and is usually nonpruritic, morbilliform, and maculopapular over the torso and extremities while sparing the palms of hands and soles of the feet [71]. Less com-mon symptoms include eye pain, arthralgia, diarrhea, and lymphadenopathy [68, 69]. WNF has a higher incidence among younger individuals [68, 69] and females [69] than the other clinical forms of disease.

West Nile Neuroinvasive Disease

Progressing from a general, febrile illness, WNND leads to severe symptoms and death in approximately 10% of WNND cases. Previous serosurveillance studies have found age to be the most important host risk factor for the development of WNND [73, 74]. Advanced age greatly increases the risk of WNND, especially encephalitis, with a risk of 1:50 in those 65 years or older [67]. Additional risk fac-tors for WNND are found in Table 8.1, with hypertension, immune suppression, and male gender being the most commonly reported after advanced age.

West Nile Meningitis
WNM clinically manifests with abrupt onset of fever, headache, nuchal rigidity, and photophobia, but these symptoms are not distinguishable from other causes of men-ingitis. Other symptoms include nausea, emesis, myalgia, muscle jerking, and trem-ors [43, 44]. For patients with severe meningeal symptoms, some patients may need hospitalization for pain control due to severe headaches or antiemetics and

Table 8.1 Risk factors for WNND and mortality

Risk factors	References
Neuroinvasive disease risk factors	
Increased age	[73–84]
Male sex	[67, 73, 81, 82, 84]
Diabetes	[77–79, 84]
Hypertension	[77, 78, 81, 84, 85]
Cardiovascular disease	[77, 78, 81]
Alcohol abuse	[77–79]
Chronic renal disease	[77, 78, 81, 83]
Chronic obstructive pulmonary disease	[77, 78]
Solid organ transplant	[17, 86]
Cancer	[77, 78, 83]
Immunosuppression	[79, 81, 83]
Chemokine CCR5 receptor deficiency	[87]
SNP in the *OAS1* gene	[88]
Mortality risk factors	[73–84]
Increased age	[67, 73, 81, 82, 84]
Neuroinvasive disease	[77–79, 84]
Male sex	[77, 78, 81, 84, 85]
Hypertension	[77, 78, 81]
Diabetes	[77–79]
Cardiovascular disease	[77, 78, 81, 83]
Chronic renal disease	[77, 78]
Previous stroke	[17, 82]
Chronic obstructive pulmonary disease	[77, 78, 83]
Hepatitis C	[79, 81, 83]
Alcohol abuse	[87]
Immunosuppression	[88]
Cancer	[73–84]
Anemia on admission	[67, 73, 81, 82, 84]
Change in level of consciousness	[77–79, 84]
Chemokine CCR5 receptor deficiency	[77, 78, 81, 84, 85]

rehydration for nausea and vomiting [89]. WNM makes up the largest percentage of WNND cases in younger age groups (age <65 years) [43, 44, 66].

West Nile Encephalitis

WNE can present with a wide range of symptoms, including those described in WNF, and with altered mental status (i.e., confusion, disorientation, and/or coma) lasting more than 24 h, which is the primary clinical indicator for encephalitis. The most common symptoms include fever (84–95%), altered mentation or somnolence (59–100%), fatigue (27%), myalgia (27%), headache (41–83%), stiff neck (19–49%), rash

(19–39%), vomiting (23–47%), diarrhea (19%), abdominal pain (17%), dizziness (12%), blurred vision (12%), slurred speech (17%), and weakness (22–55%) [66, 85, 90]. An abnormal neurological exam is found in almost all patients [85]. Seizures (10%), hypo- or hyperreflexia [44, 72, 75], neuromuscular weakness (59%), AFP (13%), loss of consciousness (20%), and somnolence (23%) can occur, sometimes requiring intubation and ventilator support for patient survival [85, 90]. Patients diagnosed with WNE have a mortality rate of approximately 15–18.6% [67, 68].

Acute Flaccid Paralysis

AFP occurs in 5–15% of patients with WNND, presenting as a poliomyelitis-like (anterior myelitis) or a Guillain-Barre-like syndrome (GBS) [44, 91, 92]. Paralysis can present more symmetrically, sometimes resulting in quadriplegia if there is extensive spinal cord involvement, and can be associated with areflexia or hyporeflexia without sensory deficits [44, 93, 94]. The poliomyelitis-like presentation is the most common form of WNV AFP (84%) and is caused by viral injury to lower motor neurons, leading to an asymmetrical paralysis and possibly permanent weakness or paralysis [93]. Nerve conduction studies revealed axonopathy with no significant demyelination [44, 95] or pronounced anterior horn cell or motor axonal injury [90, 96]. Spinal MRI may reveal anterior horn damage or ventral root enhancement [90, 93, 95]. Symptoms of AFP usually develop abruptly, with pain presenting in affected limb prior to symptom onset [44, 93, 97]. Approximately 80% of cases with AFP also present with encephalitis or meningitis [93]. Parkinsonian-like symptoms and bowel/bladder dysfunction have also been described [44, 96, 98]. When innervations to the respiratory muscles are involved, including the diaphragm and intercostal muscle, paralysis can result in respiratory failure. Consequential endotracheal intubation may last for months [90, 93, 96]. MRI findings reveal enhancement of the cauda equina and lumbosacral nerve roots and increased intensity of the spinal cord [44, 46, 97, 99, 100].

The Guillain-Barre-like presentation occurs less commonly (13%) [93] and radiculopathy-associated WNV infection very rarely. Weakness associated with the Guillain-Barre-like presentation is characterized by ascending and more symmetric weakness, pain in affected limb prior to weakness onset, and sensory and autonomic dysfunction [93, 98]. Weakness onset and nadir appear to occur later in the disease process compared to the poliomyelitis-like presentation [93], and nerve conduction studies reveal a predominantly demyelinating sensorimotor neuropathy [93].

Outcomes and Sequelae

Hospital stays are variable for those with WNV infection, but for WNND, this can last from days to months, depending on the degree of impairment, and some patients require discharge to long-term care or rehabilitation facilities [101, 102]. Among those with WNND, only 25–68% patients are discharged home [79]. Case fatality ranges from 4.3 to 47.6% [44, 46, 66, 72, 74–77, 79, 80, 85, 90, 93, 97, 102–108] and appears to be more common in the elderly [104] and among those with WNND, especially WNE [106]. The most common sequelae are found in Table 8.2. Overall, survival analysis indicates that recovery plateaus after the second year, with WNE patients having the worst outcome [106].

Recovery of neurological deficits is variable among affected individuals, but persistent weakness and functional disability are common, which usually requires physical rehabilitation. Limb strength appears to improve within the first 6–8 months [111, 118], and generally, those presenting with less weakness during clinical presentation have a more rapid and complete recovery of muscle strength [93]. Patients presenting with WNE and over the age of 50 usually have a prolonged or poor recovery time [106]. In the 1999 New York outbreak, only 37% achieved full recovery at 1 year [110]. Some also report a possible occurrence of relapse or delayed-onset of AFP symptoms from WNV infection [119]. Neuromuscular, depression, and cognitive long-term outcomes have been noted several years postinfection, particularly among those with neuroinvasive disease [45, 100, 120]. Excessive mortality has also been documented among those in a Colorado cohort, in which those diagnosed with WNV patients had 2.0 standard mortality ratios at 4 years postinfection, indicating two times greater prevalence of death than the average population [78]. Individual prognosis for improvement is difficult to predict, but new evidence for patient outcomes for WNND continues to emerge.

Ocular manifestations have also been identified in WNV infection, but ocular involvement usually has a self-limited course. Bilateral multifocal chorioretinitis is the most common ocular manifestation, occurring in nearly 80% of patients with severe systemic disease, but other ocular findings include anterior uveitis, retinal vasculitis, optic neuritis, and retinal scarring [116]. Retinopathy is seen more in the elderly and those with encephalitis, and it is associated with a great likelihood of

Table 8.2 Common sequelae of WNV infection

Condition	References
Abnormal reflexes	[45, 109]
Altered mental status	[44, 104, 106, 110–112]
Ataxia	[93, 106, 111, 113]
Balance disturbance	[43, 112]
Debilitating fatigue	[43, 44, 106, 110–112]
Depression	[43, 106, 110–112]
Dizziness	[106, 110, 112]
Headache	[43, 44, 93, 106, 110–112]
Insomnia	[43, 110, 112]
Language disorder	[112, 114, 115]
Myalgias and/or arthralgias	[43, 44, 106, 110–112]
Ocular manifestations	[43, 109, 116]
Renal insufficiency	[40, 85, 117]
Tremors	[43–45, 93, 111–113]

abnormal reflexes, poorer learning, greater dependence for activities of daily living, and a lower quality of life [109].

Hepatitis [121], pancreatitis [122], myocarditis [123], autonomic dysfunction [98], neuropsychiatric symptoms (depression, anxiety, and apathy) [106, 124], and rhabdomyolysis [97] have also been attributed to WNV infection. Renal insufficiency has been noted in 12% of acutely infected WNE patients [125], and one study observed that 40% of patients went on to develop chronic kidney disease years postinfection, with neuroinvasive WNV being significantly associated with any stage of chronic kidney disease based on multivariate analysis [40]. Studies detecting viral RNA in human urine after infection have yielded contradictory results [39, 126–130], but this may be due to the low levels of virus excretion, the time points of urine collection, and the need for more sensitive diagnostic methods.

Diagnosis

Diagnosis of WNV infection can be a challenging process, as the clinical symptoms are generally nonspecific; however, seasonality can be an indicator based on peak transmission, but incidence has been documented year-round in the United States [131]. In 2003, clinical criteria for assessing patients with suspected WNND were released [44]. For WNM, criteria include signs of meningeal inflammation, evidence of acute infection characterized by fever or hypothermia, and/or CSF pleocytosis. For WNE, criteria include encephalopathy defined by depressed or altered consciousness, lethargy, and/or personality changes lasting at least 24 h and at least two symptoms evident of CNS inflammation including fever or hypothermia, increased peripheral leukocyte counts, CSF pleocytosis, acute demyelination, focal neurological deficits, and seizures. AFP criteria include acute onset of limb weakness with clear progression over 48 h, asymmetry of weakness, absence of pain, numbness in affected limbs, CSF pleocytosis and raised protein levels, and/or spinal cord MRI with increased signal in the anterior gray matter. Even with this information on WNND criteria, many cases go unidentified.

Diagnosis requires recognition of a combination of clinical features and positive laboratory tests. If WNV is suspected, patient serum and/or cerebrospinal fluid should be tested for IgM and IgG antibodies to WNV using an FDA-approved enzyme-linked immunosorbent assay (ELISA). Generally, a patient being IgM+ and IgG− can be an indicator of acute infection versus past infection; yet, extended IgM antibody titers have been well documented within the first year postinfection [132–135] and possibly up to 8 years postinfection [136]. Diagnostics are commercially available in the United States, and some health departments offer reference testing for clinicians. Processing these samples can take up to 7 days if using a referral laboratory, delaying a timely diagnosis while continuing unnecessary empirical antibiotic and acyclovir treatment. In addition, antibodies may not be present at the time of symptom onset for WNF cases. In fact, one study identified that only 58% of WNF cases had detectable IgM levels when they presented to the clinic at the onset of symptoms [137]. Additional studies have identified that 90% of WNND cases have detectable IgM antibodies in the CSF within 8 days of symptom onset; however, there are rare accounts of patients that never develop IgM antibodies [136]. The laboratory test most commonly used to detect WNV antibodies is the IgM-capture enzyme-linked immunosorbent assay (MAC-ELISA) [138], but other FDA-approved methods, like the lateral-flow IgM strip assay, can provide rapid, simpler means of diagnosis with less training and instrumentation [139].

It is important to note that although detection of antibodies provides evidence of WNV infection, it can also be an indication of a cross-reaction with another endemic flaviviruses, such as St. Louis encephalitis virus, dengue virus, Kunjin virus, and/or Japanese encephalitis virus. Travel history should be considered to determine potential cross-reactive flavivirus species. To determine the specific flavivirus causing infection, plaque reduction neutralization assays (PRNTs) can be done in reference laboratories. In some cases, PRNTs can be used to diagnose an acute infection if a fourfold or greater change is detected from acute and convalescent samples. However, using PRNTs for acute infection can delay diagnosis as it can take at least 5 days to perform depending on the capacities of the laboratory. Other diagnostics include viral cultures and PCR to detect virus in whole blood, serum, or CSF, but it is unlikely that a patient would present with clinical disease when these samples would still have detectable virus levels. Physicians should be aware that blood banks in the United States test for viremia via polymerase chain reaction (PCR) in asymptomatic blood donors, and patients might receive their blood bank results prior to symptom onset. Detailed information regarding testing through reference laboratories can be found on the CDC's website.

Treatment and Prevention

Currently, there are no FDA-approved treatments or vaccines for WNV infections in humans, although an equine vaccine is available. Current management focuses on supportive care. Anecdotal reports of effective alternative agents have been reported, including antiviral agents, immunomodulating agents, angiotensin-receptor blockers, and nucleic acid analogues. Given the lack of random controlled trials and varied outcomes in case reports and animal models, there are no official recommendations to use such agents in clinical practice [58, 140]. Ribavirin was used during an outbreak of WNV in Israel but was associated with a higher risk of death; however, this experimental intervention was only used in severe cases [76]. The use of intravenous immunoglobulin (IVIG) containing high anti-WNV antibody in patients with WNND led to improvement, even in cases where IVIG was administered several days after onset of symptoms [141], but randomized, placebo-controlled trials are lacking. The use of corticosteroids for WNND remains controversial, but previous studies have shown intravenous steroids administered during acute infection may have led to a shorter clinical syndrome with decreased recovery time [142] or a decrease in mortality [79].

Preclinical vaccines tested in animal models have explored the success of DNA-vectored vaccines, live chimeric/recombinant vaccines, live-attenuated vaccines, inactivated whole virus vaccines, and recombinant subunit vaccines [143]. DNA, live chimeric, and recombinant subunit vaccines have made it to phase I and phase II clinical trials, but when and if these will be licensed and available to the general public remains to be seen. Tracking of the status of these vaccines can be done at https://clinicaltrials.gov/.

Conclusions

Without a preventative vaccine or therapeutic options available, WNV will continue to be a significant threat to public health. WNV has resulted in more than 41,000 reported clinical cases of disease and more than 1900 deaths since its introduction into the United States in 1999 [144]. It is estimated that greater than three million people in the United States have been infected [6]. Although many advancements have been made, many gaps in the understanding of the pathology, diagnostics, management, and prevention of the WNV disease process still exist. With continued study and research into these challenges, we can continue to work toward the goal of controlling future epidemics and improving morbidity and mortality associated with WNV infections worldwide.

References

1. Smithburn KC, Hughes TP, Burke AW, Paul JH. A neurotropic virus isolated from the blood of a native of Uganda1. Am J Trop Med Hyg. 1940;1(4):471–92.
2. Petersen LR, Roehrig JT. West Nile virus: a reemerging global pathogen. Emerg Infect Dis. 2001;7(4):611–4.
3. Centers for Disease Control and Prevention (CDC). Outbreak of West Nile-like viral encephalitis—New York, 1999. MMWR Morb Mortal Wkly Rep. 1999;48(38):845–9.
4. Centers for Disease Control and Prevention (CDC). West Nile virus activity—United States, 2001. MMWR Morb Mortal Wkly Rep. 2002;51(23):497–501.
5. Marfin AA, Petersen LR, Eidson M, Miller J, Hadler J, Farello C, et al. Widespread West Nile virus activity, eastern United States, 2000. Emerg Infect Dis. 2001;7(4):730–5.
6. Petersen LR, Carson PJ, Biggerstaff BJ, Custer B, Borchardt SM, Busch MP. Estimated cumulative incidence of West Nile virus infection in US adults, 1999–2010. Epidemiol Infect. 2013;141(3):591–5.
7. Staples JE, Shankar MB, Sejvar JJ, Meltzer MI, Fischer M. Initial and long-term costs of patients hospitalized with West Nile virus disease. Am J Trop Med Hyg. 2014;90(3):402–9.
8. Crockett RK, Burkhalter K, Mead D, Kelly R, Brown J, Varnado W, et al. Culex flavivirus and West Nile virus in Culex quinquefasciatus populations in the southeastern United States. J Med Entomol. 2012;49(1):165–74.
9. Turell MJ, Dohm DJ, Sardelis MR, Oguinn ML, Andreadis TG, Blow JA. An update on the potential of North American mosquitoes (Diptera: Culicidae) to transmit West Nile virus. J Med Entomol. 2005;42(1):57–62.
10. Komar N. West Nile virus: epidemiology and ecology in North America. Adv Virus Res. 2003;61:185–234.
11. Komar N, Panella NA, Burns JE, Dusza SW, Mascarenhas TM, Talbot TO. Serologic evidence for West Nile virus infection in birds in the New York City vicinity during an outbreak in 1999. Emerg Infect Dis. 2001;7(4):621–5.

12. Biggerstaff BJ, Petersen LR. Estimated risk of West Nile virus transmission through blood transfusion during an epidemic in queens, New York City. Transfusion. 2002;42(8):1019–26.
13. Centers for Disease Control and Prevention (CDC). Investigations of West Nile virus infections in recipients of organ transplantation and blood transfusion—Michigan, 2002. MMWR Morb Mortal Wkly Rep. 2002;51(39):879.
14. Centers for Disease Control and Prevention (CDC). Intrauterine West Nile virus infection—New York, 2002. MMWR Morb Mortal Wkly Rep. 2002;51(50):1135–6.
15. Centers for Disease Control and Prevention (CDC). Investigations of West Nile virus infections in recipients of blood transfusions. MMWR Morb Mortal Wkly Rep. 2002;51(43):973–4.
16. Hinckley AF, O'Leary DR, Hayes EB. Transmission of West Nile virus through human breast milk seems to be rare. Pediatrics. 2007;119(3):e666–71.
17. Kumar D, Drebot MA, Wong SJ, Lim G, Artsob H, Buck P, et al. A seroprevalence study of West Nile virus infection in solid organ transplant recipients. Am J Transplant. 2004;4(11):1883–8.
18. Julander JG, Winger QA, Rickords LF, Shi PY, Tilgner M, Binduga-Gajewska I, et al. West Nile virus infection of the placenta. Virology. 2006;347(1):175–82.
19. Chapa JB, Ahn JT, DiGiovanni LM, Ismail MA. West Nile virus encephalitis during pregnancy. Obstet Gynecol. 2003;102(2):229–31.
20. Iwamoto M, Jernigan DB, Guasch A, Trepka MJ, Blackmore CG, Hellinger WC, et al. Transmission of West Nile virus from an organ donor to four transplant recipients. N Engl J Med. 2003;348(22):2196–203.
21. Hayes EB, O'Leary DR. West Nile virus infection: a pediatric perspective. Pediatrics. 2004;113(5):1375–81.
22. Hinckley AF, O'Leary DR, Hayes EB. Transmission of West Nile virus through breast milk seems to be rare. Pediatrics. 2007;119(3):e666–e71.
23. Jia XY, Briese T, Jordan I, Rambaut A, Chi HC, Mackenzie JS, et al. Genetic analysis of West Nile New York 1999 encephalitis virus. Lancet. 1999;354(9194):1971–2.
24. Lanciotti RS, Roehrig JT, Deubel V, Smith J, Parker M, Steele K, et al. Origin of the West Nile virus responsible for an outbreak of encephalitis in the northeastern United States. Science. 1999;286(5448):2333–7.
25. Lvov DK, Butenko AM, Gromashevsky VL, Larichev VP, Gaidamovich SY, Vyshemirsky OI, et al. Isolation of two strains of West Nile virus during an outbreak in southern Russia, 1999. Emerg Infect Dis. 2000;6(4):373–6.
26. Guo JT, Hayashi J, Seeger C. West Nile virus inhibits the signal transduction pathway of alpha interferon. J Virol. 2005;79(3):1343–50.
27. Jones M, Davidson A, Hibbert L, Gruenwald P, Schlaak J, Ball S, et al. Dengue virus inhibits alpha interferon signaling by reducing STAT2 expression. J Virol. 2005;79(9):5414–20.
28. Liu WJ, Wang XJ, Mokhonov VV, Shi PY, Randall R, Khromykh AA. Inhibition of interferon signaling by the New York 99 strain and Kunjin subtype of West Nile virus involves blockage of STAT1 and STAT2 activation by nonstructural proteins. J Virol. 2005;79(3):1934–42.
29. Munoz-Jordan JL, Laurent-Rolle M, Ashour J, Martinez-Sobrido L, Ashok M, Lipkin WI, et al. Inhibition of alpha/beta interferon signaling by the NS4B protein of flaviviruses. J Virol. 2005;79(13):8004–13.
30. Munoz-Jordan JL, Sanchez-Burgos GG, Laurent-Rolle M, Garcia-Sastre A. Inhibition of interferon signaling by dengue virus. Proc Natl Acad Sci U S A. 2003;100(24):14333–8.
31. Kajaste-Rudnitski A, Mashimo T, Frenkiel MP, Guenet JL, Lucas M, Despres P. The 2′,5′-oligoadenylate synthetase 1b is a potent inhibitor of West Nile virus replication inside infected cells. J Biol Chem. 2006;281(8):4624–37.
32. Mashimo T, Lucas M, Simon-Chazottes D, Frenkiel MP, Montagutelli X, Ceccaldi PE, et al. A nonsense mutation in the gene encoding 2′-5′-oligoadenylate synthetase/L1 isoform is associated with West Nile virus susceptibility in laboratory mice. Proc Natl Acad Sci U S A. 2002;99(17):11311–6.
33. Perelygin AA, Scherbik SV, Zhulin IB, Stockman BM, Li Y, Brinton MA. Positional cloning of the murine flavivirus resistance gene. Proc Natl Acad Sci U S A. 2002;99(14):9322–7.

34. Rios JJ, Fleming JG, Bryant UK, Carter CN, Huber JC, Long MT, et al. OAS1 polymorphisms are associated with susceptibility to West Nile encephalitis in horses. PLoS One. 2010;5(5):e10537.

35. Lim JK, Lisco A, McDermott DH, Huynh L, Ward JM, Johnson B, et al. Genetic variation in OAS1 is a risk factor for initial infection with West Nile virus in man. PLoS Pathog. 2009;5(2):e1000321.

36. Pingen M, Schmid MA, Harris E, McKimmie CS. Mosquito biting modulates skin response to virus infection. Trends Parasitol. 2017;33(8):645–57.

37. Lim PY, Behr MJ, Chadwick CM, Shi PY, Bernard KA. Keratinocytes are cell targets of West Nile virus in vivo. J Virol. 2011;85(10):5197–201.

38. Goldblum N, Sterk VV, Jasinskaklingberg W. The natural history of West Nile fever. II. Virological findings and the development of homologous and heterologous antibodies in West Nile infection in man. Am J Hyg. 1957;66(3):363–80.

39. Murray K, Walker C, Herrington E, Lewis JA, McCormick J, Beasley DW, et al. Persistent infection with West Nile virus years after initial infection. J Infect Dis. 2010;201(1):2–4.

40. Nolan MS, Podoll AS, Hause AM, Akers KM, Finkel KW, Murray KO. Prevalence of chronic kidney disease and progression of disease over time among patients enrolled in the Houston West Nile virus cohort. PLoS One. 2012;7(7):e40374.

41. Sejvar JJ. The long-term outcomes of human West Nile virus infection. Clin Infect Dis. 2007;44(12):1617–24.

42. Sejvar JJ. Clinical manifestations and outcomes of West Nile virus infection. Viruses. 2014;6(2):606–23.

43. Sejvar JJ, Curns AT, Welburg L, Jones JF, Lundgren LM, Capuron L, et al. Neurocognitive and functional outcomes in persons recovering from West Nile virus illness. J Neuropsychol. 2008;2(Pt 2):477–99.

44. Sejvar JJ, Haddad MB, Tierney BC, Campbell GL, Marfin AA, Van Gerpen JA, et al. Neurologic manifestations and outcome of West Nile virus infection. JAMA. 2003;290(4):511–5.

45. Weatherhead JE, Miller VE, Garcia MN, Hasbun R, Salazar L, Dimachkie MM, et al. Long-term neurological outcomes in West Nile virus-infected patients: an observational study. Am J Trop Med Hyg. 2015;92(5):1006–12.

46. Ali M, Safriel Y, Sohi J, Llave A, Weathers S. West Nile virus infection: MR imaging findings in the nervous system. AJNR Am J Neuroradiol. 2005;26(2):289–97.

47. Guarner J, Shieh WJ, Hunter S, Paddock CD, Morken T, Campbell GL, et al. Clinicopathologic study and laboratory diagnosis of 23 cases with West Nile virus encephalomyelitis. Hum Pathol. 2004;35(8):983–90.

48. Kelley TW, Prayson RA, Ruiz AI, Isada CM, Gordon SM. The neuropathology of West Nile virus meningoencephalitis. A report of two cases and review of the literature. Am J Clin Pathol. 2003;119(5):749–53.

49. Sampson BA, Ambrosi C, Charlot A, Reiber K, Veress JF, Armbrustmacher V. The pathology of human West Nile virus infection. Hum Pathol. 2000;31(5):527–31.

50. Kleinschmidt-DeMasters BK, Marder BA, Levi ME, Laird SP, McNutt JT, Escott EJ, et al. Naturally acquired West Nile virus encephalomyelitis in transplant recipients: clinical, laboratory, diagnostic, and neuropathological features. Arch Neurol. 2004;61(8):1210–20.

51. Agamanolis DP, Leslie MJ, Caveny EA, Guarner J, Shieh WJ, Zaki SR. Neuropathological findings in West Nile virus encephalitis: a case report. Ann Neurol. 2003;54(4):547–51.

52. Park M, Hui JS, Bartt RE. Acute anterior radiculitis associated with West Nile virus infection. J Neurol Neurosurg Psychiatry. 2003;74(6):823–5.

53. Liou ML, Hsu CY. Japanese encephalitis virus is transported across the cerebral blood vessels by endocytosis in mouse brain. Cell Tissue Res. 1998;293(3):389–94.

54. German AC, Myint KS, Mai NT, Pomeroy I, Phu NH, Tzartos J, et al. A preliminary neuropathological study of Japanese encephalitis in humans and a mouse model. Trans R Soc Trop Med Hyg. 2006;100(12):1135–45.

55. Hunsperger EA, Roehrig JT. Temporal analyses of the neuropathogenesis of a West Nile virus infection in mice. J Neurovirol. 2006;12(2):129–39.

56. Matthews V, Robertson T, Kendrick T, Abdo M, Papadimitriou J, McMinn P. Morphological features of Murray Valley encephalitis virus infection in the central nervous system of Swiss mice. Int J Exp Pathol. 2000;81(1):31–40.
57. Monath TP, Cropp CB, Harrison AK. Mode of entry of a neurotropic arbovirus into the central nervous system. Reinvestigation of an old controversy. Lab Investig. 1983;48(4):399–410.
58. Sejvar JJ. West Nile virus infection. Microbiol Spectr. 2016;4(3) https://doi.org/10.1128/microbiolspec.EI10-0021-2016.
59. Samuel MA, Wang H, Siddharthan V, Morrey JD, Diamond MS. Axonal transport mediates West Nile virus entry into the central nervous system and induces acute flaccid paralysis. Proc Natl Acad Sci U S A. 2007;104(43):17140–5.
60. Diamond MS, Klein RS. West Nile virus: crossing the blood-brain barrier. Nat Med. 2004;10(12):1294–5.
61. Venter M, Myers TG, Wilson MA, Kindt TJ, Paweska JT, Burt FJ, et al. Gene expression in mice infected with West Nile virus strains of different neurovirulence. Virology. 2005;342(1):119–40.
62. Wacher C, Muller M, Hofer MJ, Getts DR, Zabaras R, Ousman SS, et al. Coordinated regulation and widespread cellular expression of interferon-stimulated genes (ISG) ISG-49, ISG-54, and ISG-56 in the central nervous system after infection with distinct viruses. J Virol. 2007;81(2):860–71.
63. Goldblum N, Sterk VV, Paderski B. West Nile fever, the clinical features of the disease and the isolation of West Nile virus from the blood of nine human cases. Am J Hyg. 1954;59(1):89–103.
64. Mostashari F, Bunning ML, Kitsutani PT, Singer DA, Nash D, Cooper MJ, et al. Epidemic West Nile encephalitis, New York, 1999: results of a household-based seroepidemiological survey. Lancet. 2001;358(9278):261–4.
65. Craven RB, Roehrig JT. West Nile virus. JAMA. 2001;286(6):651–3.
66. Huhn GD, Austin C, Langkop C, Kelly K, Lucht R, Lampman R, et al. The emergence of West Nile virus during a large outbreak in Illinois in 2002. Am J Trop Med Hyg. 2005;72(6):768–76.
67. Carson PJ, Borchardt SM, Custer B, Prince HE, Dunn-Williams J, Winkelman V, et al. Neuroinvasive disease and West Nile virus infection, North Dakota, USA, 1999–2008. Emerg Infect Dis. 2012;18(4):684–6.
68. Brown JA, Factor DL, Tkachenko N, Templeton SM, Crall ND, Pape WJ, et al. West Nile viremic blood donors and risk factors for subsequent West Nile fever. Vector Borne Zoonotic Dis. 2007;7(4):479–88.
69. Zou S, Foster GA, Dodd RY, Petersen LR, Stramer SL. West Nile fever characteristics among viremic persons identified through blood donor screening. J Infect Dis. 2010;202(9):1354–61.
70. Cook RL, Xu X, Yablonsky EJ, Sakata N, Tripp JH, Hess R, et al. Demographic and clinical factors associated with persistent symptoms after West Nile virus infection. Am J Trop Med Hyg. 2010;83(5):1133–6.
71. Ferguson DD, Gershman K, LeBailly A, Petersen LR. Characteristics of the rash associated with West Nile virus fever. Clin Infect Dis. 2005;41(8):1204–7.
72. Brilla R, Block M, Geremia G, Wichter M. Clinical and neuroradiologic features of 39 consecutive cases of West Nile virus meningoencephalitis. J Neurol Sci. 2004;220(1–2):37–40.
73. O'Leary DR, Marfin AA, Montgomery SP, Kipp AM, Lehman JA, Biggerstaff BJ, et al. The epidemic of West Nile virus in the United States, 2002. Vector Borne Zoonotic Dis. 2004;4(1):61–70.
74. Nash D, Mostashari F, Fine A, Miller J, O'Leary D, Murray K, et al. The outbreak of West Nile virus infection in the New York City area in 1999. N Engl J Med. 2001;344(24):1807–14.
75. Tsai TF, Popovici F, Cernescu C, Campbell GL, Nedelcu NI. West Nile encephalitis epidemic in southeastern Romania. Lancet. 1998;352(9130):767–71.
76. Chowers MY, Lang R, Nassar F, Ben-David D, Giladi M, Rubinshtein E, et al. Clinical characteristics of the West Nile fever outbreak, Israel, 2000. Emerg Infect Dis. 2001;7(4):675–8.
77. Lindsey NP, Staples JE, Lehman JA, Fischer M. Medical risk factors for severe West Nile virus disease, United States, 2008–2010. Am J Trop Med Hyg. 2012;87(1):179–84.

78. Lindsey NP, Sejvar JJ, Bode AV, Pape WJ, Campbell GL. Delayed mortality in a cohort of persons hospitalized with West Nile virus disease in Colorado in 2003. Vector Borne Zoonotic Dis. 2012;12(3):230–5.
79. Bode AV, Sejvar JJ, Pape WJ, Campbell GL, Marfin AA. West Nile virus disease: a descriptive study of 228 patients hospitalized in a 4-county region of Colorado in 2003. Clin Infect Dis. 2006;42(9):1234–40.
80. Riabi S, Gaaloul I, Mastouri M, Hassine M, Aouni M. An outbreak of West Nile virus infection in the region of Monastir, Tunisia, 2003. Pathog Glob Health. 2014;108(3):148–57.
81. Murray K, Baraniuk S, Resnick M, Arafat R, Kilborn C, Cain K, et al. Risk factors for encephalitis and death from West Nile virusinfection. Epidemiol Infect. 2006;134(6):1325–32.
82. Lindsey NP, Staples JE, Lehman JA, Fischer M, Centers for Disease Control and Prevention (CDC). Surveillance for human West Nile virus disease—United States, 1999–2008. MMWR Surveill Summ. 2010;59(2):1–17.
83. Patnaik JL, Harmon H, Vogt RL. Follow-up of 2003 human West Nile virus infections, Denver, Colorado. Emerg Infect Dis. 2006;12(7):1129–31.
84. Jean CM, Honarmand S, Louie JK, Glaser CA. Risk factors for West Nile virus neuroinvasive disease, California, 2005. Emerg Infect Dis. 2007;13(12):1918–20. https://doi.org/10.3201/eid1312.061265.
85. Murray KO, Baraniuk S, Resnick M, Arafat R, Kilborn C, Shallenberger R, et al. Clinical investigation of hospitalized human cases of West Nile virus infection in Houston, Texas, 2002–2004. Vector Borne Zoonotic Dis. 2008;8(2):167–74.
86. Kumar D, Prasad GV, Zaltzman J, Levy GA, Humar A. Community-acquired West Nile virus infection in solid-organ transplant recipients. Transplantation. 2004;77(3):399–402.
87. Glass WG, Lim JK, Cholera R, Pletnev AG, Gao JL, Murphy PM. Chemokine receptor CCR5 promotes leukocyte trafficking to the brain and survival in West Nile virus infection. J Exp Med. 2005;202(8):1087–98.
88. Bigham AW, Buckingham KJ, Husain S, Emond MJ, Bofferding KM, Gildersleeve H, et al. Host genetic risk factors for West Nile virus infection and disease progression. PLoS One. 2011;6(9):e24745. https://doi.org/10.1371/journal.pone.0024745.
89. Centers for Disease Control and Prevention (CDC) West Nile virus for healthcare providers treatment and prevention 2015. Available from: https://www.cdc.gov/westnile/healthcareproviders/healthCareProviders-TreatmentPrevention.html.
90. Pepperell C, Rau N, Krajden S, Kern R, Humar A, Mederski B, et al. West Nile virus infection in 2002: morbidity and mortality among patients admitted to hospital in southcentral Ontario. CMAJ. 2003;168(11):1399–405.
91. Ahmed S, Libman R, Wesson K, Ahmed F, Einberg K. Guillain-Barre syndrome: an unusual presentation of West Nile virus infection. Neurology. 2000;55(1):144–6.
92. Centers for Disease Control and Prevention (CDC). Acute flaccid paralysis syndrome associated with West Nile virus infection—Mississippi and Louisiana, July–August 2002. MMWR Morb Mortal Wkly Rep. 2002;51(37):825–8.
93. Sejvar JJ, Bode AV, Marfin AA, Campbell GL, Ewing D, Mazowiecki M, et al. West Nile virus-associated flaccid paralysis. Emerg Infect Dis. 2005;11(7):1021–7.
94. Glass JD, Samuels O, Rich MM. Poliomyelitis due to West Nile virus. N Engl J Med. 2002;347(16):1280–1.
95. Al-Shekhlee A, Katirji B. Electrodiagnostic features of acute paralytic poliomyelitis associated with West Nile virus infection. Muscle Nerve. 2004;29(3):376–80.
96. Leis AA, Stokic DS, Polk JL, Dostrow V, Winkelmann M. A poliomyelitis-like syndrome from West Nile virus infection. N Engl J Med. 2002;347(16):1279–80.
97. Jeha LE, Sila CA, Lederman RJ, Prayson RA, Isada CM, Gordon SM. West Nile virus infection: a new acute paralytic illness. Neurology. 2003;61(1):55–9.
98. Fratkin JD, Leis AA, Stokic DS, Slavinski SA, Geiss RW. Spinal cord neuropathology in human West Nile virus infection. Arch Pathol Lab Med. 2004;128(5):533–7.
99. Petropoulou KA, Gordon SM, Prayson RA, Ruggierri PM. West Nile virus meningoencephalitis: MR imaging findings. AJNR Am J Neuroradiol. 2005;26(8):1986–95.

100. Athar P, Hasbun R, Garcia MN, Salazar L, Woods S, Sheikh K, et al. Long-term neuromuscular outcomes of West Nile virus infection: a clinical and Electromyograph evaluation of patients with a history of infection. Muscle Nerve. 2017;57(1):77–82.
101. Crichlow R, Bailey J, Gardner C. Cerebrospinal fluid neutrophilic pleocytosis in hospitalized West Nile virus patients. J Am Board Fam Pract. 2004;17(6):470–2.
102. Weiss D, Carr D, Kellachan J, Tan C, Phillips M, Bresnitz E, et al. Clinical findings of West Nile virus infection in hospitalized patients, New York and New Jersey, 2000. Emerg Infect Dis. 2001;7(4):654–8.
103. Platonov AE, Shipulin GA, Shipulina OY, Tyutyunnik EN, Frolochkina TI, Lanciotti RS, et al. Outbreak of West Nile virus infection, Volgograd region, Russia, 1999. Emerg Infect Dis. 2001;7(1):128–32.
104. Berner YN, Lang R, Chowers MY. Outcome of West Nile fever in older adults. J Am Geriatr Soc. 2003;50(11):1844–6.
105. Gottfried K, Quinn R, Jones T. Clinical description and follow-up investigation of human West Nile virus cases. South Med J. 2005;98(6):603–6.
106. Murray KO, Garcia MN, Rahbar MH, Martinez D, Khuwaja SA, Arafat RR, et al. Survival analysis, long-term outcomes, and percentage of recovery up to 8 years post-infection among the Houston West Nile virus cohort. PLoS One. 2014;9(7):e102953.
107. Platonov AE. West Nile encephalitis in Russia 1999–2001: were we ready? Are we ready? Ann N Y Acad Sci. 2001;951:102–16.
108. Weinberger M, Pitlik SD, Gandacu D, Lang R, Nassar F, Ben David D, et al. West Nile fever outbreak, Israel, 2000: epidemiologic aspects. Emerg Infect Dis. 2001;7(4):686–91.
109. Hasbun R, Garcia MN, Kellaway J, Baker L, Salazar L, Woods SP, et al. West Nile virus retinopathy and associations with long term neurological and neurocognitive Sequelae. PLoS One. 2016;11(3):e0148898.
110. Klee AL, Maidin B, Edwin B, Poshni I, Mostashari F, Fine A, et al. Long-term prognosis for clinical West Nile virus infection. Emerg Infect Dis. 2004;10(8):1405–11.
111. Sejvar JJ, Bode AV, Marfin AA, Campbell GL, Pape J, Biggerstaff BJ, et al. West Nile virus-associated flaccid paralysis outcome. Emerg Infect Dis. 2006;12(3):514–6.
112. Carson PJ, Konewko P, Wold KS, Mariani P, Goli S, Bergloff P, et al. Long-term clinical and neuropsychological outcomes of West Nile virus infection. Clin Infect Dis. 2006;43(6):723–30.
113. Bosanko CM, Gilroy J, Wang AM, Sanders W, Dulai M, Wilson J, et al. West nile virus encephalitis involving the substantia nigra: neuroimaging and pathologic findings with literature review. Arch Neurol. 2003;60(10):1448–52.
114. Mickail N, Klein NC, Cunha BA. West Nile virus aseptic meningitis and stuttering in woman. Emerg Infect Dis. 2011;17(8):1567–8. https://doi.org/10.3201/eid1708.101691.
115. Fromm NM, Salisbury DB, Driver SJ, Dahdah MN, Monden KR. Functional recovery from neuroinvasive West Nile virus: A tale of two courses. Rehabil Psychol. 2015;60(4):383–90. https://doi.org/10.1037/rep0000058.
116. Khairallah M, Ben Yahia S, Kahloun R. West Nile virus. In: Zierhut M, Pavesio C, Ohno S, Orefice F, Rao NA, editors. Intraocular inflammation. Heidelberg: Springer; 2016. p. 1239–46.
117. Saxena V, Xie G, Li B, Farris T, Welte T, Gong B, et al. A hamster-derived West Nile virus isolate induces persistent renal infection in mice. PLoS Negl Trop Dis. 2013;7(6):e2275. https://doi.org/10.1371/journal.pntd.0002275.
118. Cao NJ, Ranganathan C, Kupsky WJ, Li J. Recovery and prognosticators of paralysis in West Nile virus infection. J Neurol Sci. 2005;236(1–2):73–80.
119. Sejvar JJ, Davis LE, Szabados E, Jackson AC. Delayed-onset and recurrent limb weakness associated with West Nile virus infection. J Neurovirol. 2010;16(1):93–100.
120. Nolan MS, Hause AM, Murray KO. Findings of long-term depression up to 8 years post infection from West Nile virus. J Clin Psychol. 2012;68(7):801–8.
121. Georges AJ, Lesbordes JL, Georges-Courbot MC, Meunier DMY, Gonzalez JP. Fatal hepatitis from West Nile virus. Ann l'Institut Pasteur/Virol. 1987;138(2):237–44.
122. Perelman A, Stern J. Acute pancreatitis in West Nile fever. Am J Trop Med Hyg. 1974;23(6):1150–2.

123. Kushawaha A, Jadonath S, Mobarakai N. West Nile virus myocarditis causing a fatal arrhythmia: a case report. Cases J. 2009;2:7147.
124. Berg PJ, Smallfield S, Svien L. An investigation of depression and fatigue post West Nile virus infection. S D Med. 2010;63(4):127–9. 31–3.
125. Murray KO, Koers E, Baraniuk S, Herrington E, Carter H, Sierra M, et al. Risk factors for encephalitis from West Nile virus: a matched case-control study using hospitalized controls. Zoonoses Public Health. 2009;56(6–7):370–5.
126. Gibney KB, Lanciotti RS, Sejvar JJ, Nugent CT, Linnen JM, Delorey MJ, et al. West Nile virus RNA not detected in urine of 40 people tested 6 years after acute West Nile virus disease. J Infect Dis. 2011;203(3):344–7.
127. Baty SA, Gibney KB, Staples JE, Patterson AB, Levy C, Lehman J, et al. Evaluation for West Nile virus (WNV) RNA in urine of patients within 5 months of WNV infection. J Infect Dis. 2012;205(9):1476–7.
128. Barzon L, Pacenti M, Franchin E, Pagni S, Martello T, Cattai M, et al. Excretion of West Nile virus in urine during acute infection. J Infect Dis. 2013;208(7):1086–92.
129. Papa A, Testa T, Papadopoulou E. Detection of West Nile virus lineage 2 in the urine of acute human infections. J Med Virol. 2014;86(12):2142–5.
130. Nagy A, Ban E, Nagy O, Ferenczi E, Farkas A, Banyai K, et al. Detection and sequencing of West Nile virus RNA from human urine and serum samples during the 2014 seasonal period. Arch Virol. 2016;161(7):1797–806.
131. Nolan MS, Schuermann J, Murray KO. West Nile virus infection among humans, Texas, USA, 2002–2011. Emerg Infect Dis. 2013;19(1):137–9.
132. Roehrig JT, Nash D, Maldin B, Labowitz A, Martin DA, Lanciotti RS, et al. Persistence of virus-reactive serum immunoglobulin m antibody in confirmed West Nile virus encephalitis cases. Emerg Infect Dis. 2003;9(3):376–9.
133. Kapoor H, Signs K, Somsel P, Downes FP, Clark PA, Massey JP. Persistence of West Nile virus (WNV) IgM antibodies in cerebrospinal fluid from patients with CNS disease. J Clin Virol. 2004;31(4):289–91.
134. Papa A, Danis K, Athanasiadou A, Delianidou M, Panagiotopoulos T. Persistence of West Nile virus immunoglobulin M antibodies, Greece. J Med Virol. 2011;83(10):1857–60.
135. Prince HE, Tobler LH, Yeh C, Gefter N, Custer B, Busch MP. Persistence of West Nile virus-specific antibodies in viremic blood donors. Clin Vaccine Immunol. 2007;14(9):1228–30.
136. Murray KO, Garcia MN, Yan C, Gorchakov R. Persistence of detectable immunoglobulin M antibodies up to 8 years after infection with West Nile virus. Am J Trop Med Hyg. 2013;89(5):996–1000.
137. Tilley PA, Walle R, Chow A, Jayaraman GC, Fonseca K, Drebot MA, et al. Clinical utility of commercial enzyme immunoassays during the inaugural season of West Nile virus activity, Alberta, Canada. J Clin Microbiol. 2005;43(9):4691–5.
138. Malan AK, Martins TB, Hill HR, Litwin CM. Evaluations of commercial West Nile virus immunoglobulin G (IgG) and IgM enzyme immunoassays show the value of continuous validation. J Clin Microbiol. 2004;42(2):727–33.
139. Sambol AR, Hinrichs SH. Evaluation of a new West Nile virus lateral-flow rapid IgM assay. J Virol Methods. 2009;157(2):223–6.
140. Penn RG, Guarner J, Sejvar JJ, Hartman H, McComb RD, Nevins DL, et al. Persistent neuroinvasive West Nile virus infection in an immunocompromised patient. Clin Infect Dis. 2006;42(5):680–3.
141. Walid MS, Mahmoud FA. Successful treatment with intravenous immunoglobulin of acute flaccid paralysis caused by West Nile virus. Perm J. 2009;13(3):43–6.
142. Narayanaswami P, Edwards L, Hyde C, Page C, Hastings NE. West Nile meningitis/encephalitis: experience with corticosteroid therapy. Neurology. 2004;62:A404.
143. Pletnev AG, Claire MS, Elkins R, Speicher J, Murphy BR, Chanock RM. Molecularly engineered live-attenuated chimeric West Nile/dengue virus vaccines protect rhesus monkeys from West Nile virus. Virology. 2003;314(1):190–5.
144. CDC. Preliminary maps & data for 2016–2017. Available from: https://www.cdc.gov/westnile/statsmaps/preliminarymapsdata/index.html.

Herpes Simplex and Varicella Zoster Virus

9

Karen C. Bloch

Herpes simplex virus (HSV) and *varicella zoster* virus (VZV) are DNA viruses in the family *Herpesviridae*, subfamily *Alphaherpesvirinae*. These viruses are common causes of human mucocutaneous infections and, although central nervous system (CNS) infection occurs in only a minority of cases, are among the most common causes of meningoencephalitis in the United States [1]. The spectrum of CNS disease for both HSV and VZV ranges from a mild, self-limited meningitis to fulminant and sometimes fatal encephalitis. While these viruses share many commonalities, the epidemiology, clinical presentation, and, to some extent, treatment are distinct; therefore HSV and VZV CNS infections will be discussed separately in this chapter.

Herpes Simplex Virus Causing CNS Infection

Epidemiology

Herpes simplex virus (HSV) mucosal infection is common among adults in the United States. Large cross-sectional studies among American teenagers and adults have identified a seroprevalence of 54–68% for HSV-1 and 16–24% for HSV-2 [2, 3]. HSV-1 infection is frequently asymptomatic but may cause self-limited oro-labial lesions ("fever blisters" or "cold sores"). HSV-2, typically spread through sexual transmission, is associated with genital ulcers. Recently, however, this strict viral tropism for specific mucocutaneous sites has been called into question. HSV-1 is increasingly recognized as a cause of genital ulcers in younger patients, with transmission in this population believed due to changing sexual practices and increased

K. C. Bloch, MD, MPH
Vanderbilt University Medical Center, Department of Infectious Diseases,
Nashville, TN, USA
e-mail: karen.bloch@Vanderbilt.Edu

© Springer International Publishing AG, part of Springer Nature 2018
R. Hasbun (ed.), *Meningitis and Encephalitis*,
https://doi.org/10.1007/978-3-319-92678-0_9

frequency of oral-genital intercourse [4]. Following acute infection, both HSV 1 and 2 survive latently in nerve tissue, allowing the potential for viral reactivation manifested as asymptomatic shedding of virus or recurrent symptomatic infection.

While CNS involvement is an infrequent complication of HSV infection, HSV, and in particular HSV-1, is a leading cause of meningoencephalitis. The incidence of HSV encephalitis (HSE) is 1–1.2 cases/100,000 population [5], making this the single most common cause of endemic encephalitis in the United States. HSV encephalitis accounts for approximately 15% of all encephalitis cases, 74% of all diagnosed viral causes of encephalitis, and 21.8% of all encephalitis deaths [5, 6]. In contrast, most cases of HSV meningitis are caused by HSV-2, accounting for 17–23% of cases of aseptic meningitis in adults [7, 8].

Pathophysiology

Neurologic infection with HSV can occur at the time of initial infection or with reactivation of latent virus. Serologic studies indicate that HSE is associated with acute HSV-1 infection in a third of cases and with reactivation in the remainder [9]. Following infection, the virus survives in a latent state in the trigeminal ganglion. Travel of the virus retrograde via the trigeminal or olfactory nerves results in focal infection of the adjacent temporal lobe [10].

In contrast, most cases of HSV-2 meningitis occur at the time of primary infection. Meningitis symptoms are present in 36% of women and 13% of men during the initial HSV-2 genital infection [11]. Following primary infection, HSV-2 persists latently in sacral ganglion and can cause aseptic meningitis either in association with recurrent genital outbreaks or in the absence of visible genital lesions.

Risk Factors

An important, but unanswered question is why CNS involvement is relatively rare given the ubiquity of HSV infection among adults. HSE has been anecdotally reported in patients with HIV [12, 13] and those receiving anti-TNF alpha inhibitors [14, 15], but the majority of patients with HSE are immunocompetent. There is an increasing body of literature suggesting CNS malignancy, intracranial radiation, and recent neurosurgical intervention may be risk factors for HSE [16–20]; whether this is due to immunosuppression from concurrent chemotherapy or high-dose corticosteroid treatment is uncertain.

Reports of multiple family members with HSE or individuals with recurrent episodes of HSE support the possibility of a genetic predisposition for this disease. Genetic mutations that effect the production or activity of interferon, particularly defects in *TLR*3 function, have been identified as risk factors for HSE in childhood [21, 22]. Studies in adults with HSE have also identified genetic mutations that impair the innate immune response and likely contribute to an increased risk for HSE [23, 24].

Clinical Presentation of CNS Infections

Encephalitis

Herpes simplex viruses can cause a multitude of CNS syndromes, including encephalitis, meningitis, myelitis, radiculopathy, cranial neuropathy, and acute retinal necrosis. Outside of the neonatal period, >90% of HSE cases are caused by HSV-1 [25]. HSV-2 encephalitis typically presents with milder neurologic impairment and does not display focal temporal lobe tropism [26].

The clinical presentation of HSE is generally subacute and nonspecific (Table 9.1), precluding differentiation from other causes of meningoencephalitis at presentation. Similarly, routine laboratory testing does not differentiate HSE from other causes of encephalitis. The cerebrospinal fluid typically shows a lymphocytic pleocytosis. CSF red blood cells may be elevated when there is significant parenchymal necrosis [27].

Neuroimaging studies showing unilateral or bilateral temporal lobe inflammation are suggestive of HSE (Fig. 9.1); however, this finding is by no means pathognomonic. In a large prospective study of 251 cases of temporal lobe encephalitis, a quarter of cases were caused by HSV-1, 19% by other infectious etiologies, and 16% by noninfectious causes; in the remainder (41%), no etiology was identified [28]. MRI with diffusion-weighted images (DWI) is the most sensitive study for detecting temporal lobe changes due to HSV infection, particularly early in the disease course [29]. Immunocompromised patients may lack the classic temporal

Table 9.1 Clinical manifestations of herpes simplex and varicella zoster virus encephalitis

Variable	HSV (% or value, range)	VZV (% or value, range)
Signs/symptoms		
Fever	80% (70–97)	45–90%
Altered mentation	72% (54–81)	70–82%
Headache	58% (42–70)	83%
Seizures	54% (35–65)	11–20%
Focal neurologic deficits	41% (26–79)	12–55%
Nausea and/or vomiting	40% (19–46)	31%
Aphasia or dysphasia	40% (12–65)	30%
Coma	33% (4–48)	n/a
Meningismus	28% (13–38)	31–60%
Rash	0%	64–85%
Laboratory findings		
CSF WBC/mm^3	70 (5–500)	150 (0–1240)
CSF lymphocytes	80% (60–98)	82–86%
CSF protein mg/dl	80 (50–200)	99 (22–500)
Neurodiagnostics		
Abnormal CT scan	50% (25–80)	75%
Abnormal MRI	95%	65%
Abnormal EEG	45%	92%

Adapted from Refs. [10, 27, 32, 62, 66]

Fig. 9.1 MRI of patient with
HSE showing temporal lobe
enhancement on T2 FLAIR
imaging (Image courtesy of
Karen C Bloch, MD, MPH)

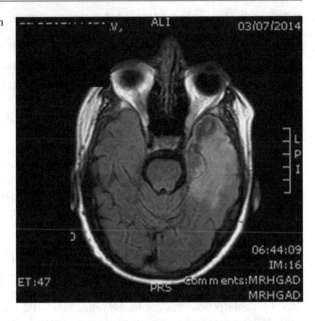

lobe radiographic findings [30], and a high level of suspicion should be maintained
in this population.

Meningitis

In contrast to HSE, herpes meningitis is almost universally caused by HSV-2. The
presence of genital ulcers is often suggestive of this diagnosis, but these are present
in a minority of patients at the time of CNS involvement [31]. Patients with HSV
meningitis are significantly younger and significantly less likely to have medical
comorbidities than those with HSE; however, CSF findings between these two
groups are indistinguishable [32].

HSV-2 is a well-recognized cause of recurrent meningitis, sometimes termed
"Mollaret's meningitis" after the pathologist who first described this condition. The
frequency of recurrence following an initial episode of HSV-2 meningitis ranges from
10% to 20% [31, 33] and may occur years after the initial episode of meningitis.

Diagnosis of HSV Meningoencephalitis

Laboratory confirmation of HSV meningoencephalitis is by direct detection of the
virus in the CNS. Historically this was performed by culture or staining of brain
tissue. Brain biopsy has been replaced by HSV PCR of CSF, which allows rapid
diagnosis through a minimally invasive procedure. In a seminal study comparing
HSV CSF PCR to brain biopsy, the sensitivity of the latter was found to be 98%,
with a specificity of 94% [34]. These performance characteristics hold true even
after 7 days of acyclovir therapy. False negatives may occur early in the course of
disease [35, 36]; therefore, when there is a high suspicion for HSE, continuation of
empiric therapy pending a repeat test on a CSF sample obtained 3–7 days later is

indicated [37, 38]. CSF viral culture and intrathecal HSV serologic testing are quite insensitive, and these studies are not recommended for diagnostic purposes [39].

Treatment

HSV is one of the few treatable viral causes of encephalitis, and the initiation of empiric therapy with acyclovir is uniformly recommended for all patients with encephalitis at the time of presentation [37, 38, 40–42]. Dosing of acyclovir for adults with preserved renal function is 10 mg/kg intravenously every 8 h for 14–21 days [37, 40]. Higher doses (e.g., 20 mg/kg intravenously every 8 h) are associated with improved outcomes in neonatal HSE, but have not shown a survival benefit outside of this age group [27, 43]. Acyclovir resistance, while rare, has been identified in both immunocompromised and immunocompetent patients with HSE, and should be considered in patients who do not show clinical improvement on therapy [44–46]. A recently published multicenter randomized controlled trial found no clinical benefit among patients who received terminal therapy with a 3-month course of oral valacyclovir following completion of parenteral acyclovir [47].

The use of adjunctive corticosteroids for HSE is an area of ongoing research. Case reports have suggested improved outcomes when initiated in conjunction with antiviral therapy [48]. A clinical trial designed to investigate the efficacy of acyclovir plus adjuvant therapy with 4-day course of dexamethasone versus placebo suffered from inadequate enrollment and was not completed [49, 50]. Currently, a randomized controlled clinical trial, the DEX-ENCEPH study, is enrolling patients in Europe in an attempt to answer this question. Pending publication of these results, most authorities restrict the use of adjuvant corticosteroids to patients with a clear indication such as evidence of increased intracranial pressure or cerebral edema [10, 27].

Acyclovir therapy may decrease symptoms and hasten recovery in patients with severe HSV-2 meningitis. However, unlike with HSE, there is no consensus on the route or duration of antiviral treatment for this syndrome. A retrospective study of 60 patients hospitalized with HSV meningitis found no difference in the frequency of adverse clinical outcomes among patients who received no antiviral therapy, those who received solely oral treatment, and those who were treated with parenteral acyclovir [32]. In this study, the median duration of either oral or intravenous antiviral therapy was 4 days. HSV-2 meningitis has been associated with sustained neurologic impairment in immunocompromised individuals, and antiviral treatment is recommended in this population [51].

Complications

Refractory or relapsing symptoms of encephalitis among patients with HSE has long been thought to be due to recrudescent virus. However, more recently antibodies against a neuronal protein, the anti-*N*-Methyl-D-aspartate receptor (NMDAR), have been identified in patients with worsening symptoms despite appropriate antiviral therapy. It is hypothesized that HSV infection may serve as an antigenic stimulus for secondary development of these antibodies, causing a post-infectious autoimmune encephalitis [52, 53].

These patients typically present with a bimodal illness, characterized by the development of new or recurrent neurological symptoms 1–2 months following the diagnosis of HSE and an initial clinical response to acyclovir therapy. There is significant clinical overlap between these syndromes, although movement disorders are more common with anti-NMDAR encephalitis and seizures with HSE [54]. Diagnosis of anti-NMDAR encephalitis is through detection of serum or CSF antibodies in patients with a compatible clinical presentation. Development of anti-neuronal antibodies has been documented in up to 25% of patients following HSE in the absence of symptoms, and the significance is uncertain in this population [55]. Identification of post-HSE anti-NMDAR encephalitis is critical, as these patients typically respond to treatment with immunotherapy rather than prolongation of acyclovir.

Outcomes

Untreated, the mortality of HSE approaches 70%, with the majority of survivors experiencing severe neurologic sequelae [56]. Acyclovir therapy combined with supportive neurocritical care has led to a decrease in the case fatality rate to 10–19% [6, 47]. Delay in initiation of acyclovir, age >30 years, and Glasgow Coma Score <10 at presentation have been identified as independent predictors of an adverse outcome [57, 58]. Immunocompromise also appears to be a predictor of a poor prognosis [30]. In contrast, HSV-2 meningitis is almost universally associated with complete recovery, even in the absence of treatment [32].

Prevention

There is no commercially available vaccine to prevent herpes simplex virus, and given the rarity of CNS involvement, prophylaxis is not indicated following mucocutaneous infection. A randomized controlled clinical trial evaluating secondary prophylaxis with oral valacyclovir following HSV-2 meningitis found no difference in the frequency of recurrence during treatment but identified a statistically significant rebound effect after discontinuation of antiviral therapy [59]. Based on these data, secondary prophylaxis following HSV meningitis is not recommended.

Varicella Zoster Virus Neurologic Infections

Epidemiology

Primary varicella infection causes chicken pox, which was a nearly universal infection of childhood prior to the availability of the live attenuated varicella vaccine in 1995. With the decline in the incidence of primary varicella infections, there has

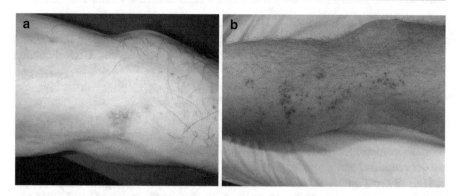

Fig. 9.2 Zoster cutaneous lesions (Photos courtesy of Patty Wright, MD). (**a**) Early lesions presenting as clustered vesicles on an erythematous base. (**b**) Progression of infection with shallow ulcerations in a dermatomal distribution

been a proportional reduction in the frequency of pediatric CNS disease due to VZV. A cohort study from a large tertiary care pediatric hospital reported a decrease in VZV-associated CNS admissions from 55 to 20 per 100,000 after the widespread implementation of vaccination, with the majority of cases occurring in non-immunized children [60].

Reactivation of latent VZV is associated with a vesicular skin eruption termed herpes zoster or shingles (Fig. 9.2: PW). Immunization of adults ≥60 years of age with the zoster vaccine is recommended by the US Advisory Committee on Immunization Practices to decrease the risk of herpes zoster. Until recently, the most widely available formulation of the herpes zoster vaccine was also a live attenuated virus; however, CNS infections have not been documented with zoster vaccine-associated strains of VZV, likely due to pre-existing host immunity limiting neuronal spread [61]. A recent population-based study of patients hospitalized for encephalitis in the United States found VZV accounted for <1% of encephalitis cases hospitalized between 2000 and 2010 [6].

Pathophysiology

Following natural infection, the varicella virus persists latently in dorsal root and cranial nerve ganglia. Reactivation of virus presents as herpes zoster, with eruptions occuring in a unilateral dermatomal eruption, although dissemination may occur in immunocompromised patients.

The exact mechanism of CNS infection with either primary VZV infection or reactivation has not been elucidated. Virus is detectable in the CSF of most patients with VZV meningitis and encephalitis, and these syndromes are therefore presumed to involve direct infection of the meninges and brain parenchyma [62]. Conversely, with VZV vasculopathy, infection of intracranial arteries with associated inflammatory cells and intimal thickening has been demonstrated, and direct detection of virus in the CSF is uncommon [61]. Molecular typing has demonstrated intraparenchymal infection can occur with varicella vaccine-associated strains; therefore, a history of varicella vaccination doesn't preclude subsequent CNS infection [62–64].

Risk Factors

Immunocompromise and advanced age are both independent risk factors for herpes zoster eruptions and may also increase the risk of CNS infection [65]. In one case series, 82% patients with VZV encephalitis were ≥60 years of age or immunocompromised, compared to 31% with VZV meningitis [62]. Genotyping of VZV isolates from patients with meningoencephalitis has identified heterogeneous strains causing CNS infection, arguing against a particularly neurotropic variant [62].

Clinical Manifestations

A diffuse or dermatomal vesicular rash in the presence of neurological symptoms is suggestive of VZV CNS infection. However, caution should be used in attributing causality, as zoster skin eruptions may be precipitated by other infections or illnesses [37]. Similarly, the absence of cutaneous findings does not exclude this diagnosis, as skin findings may lag behind, or even be absent in up to 45% of VZV encephalitis cases, a syndrome termed *zoster sine herpete* [62, 66]. In addition to meningitis and encephalitis, VZV can cause a broad array of CNS manifestations, including cerebellitis, myelitis, optic neuritis, acute disseminated encephalomyelitis (ADEM), stroke, and vasculopathy [60, 62, 66, 67].

Encephalitis

Encephalitis may occur with either primary VZV infection or with reactivation of latent virus. Often these can be differentiated based on the history and dermatologic exam. A diffuse vesicular eruption is more consistent with primary varicella infection, although may also be seen with disseminated zoster, particularly in an immunocompromised host.

Clinically, patients with VZV encephalitis resemble those with HSE (Table 9.1), although skin lesions and elevated CSF RBC count are significantly more common in the former group [32, 68]. In one case series, 40% of patients with VZV encephalitis exhibited cranial neuropathy [66], most commonly facial nerve palsy. Patients with VZV encephalitis are often critically ill, with up to a third requiring intensive care admission [66].

Neuroimaging with VZV encephalitis is frequently normal, and when abnormalities are detected, these are often nonspecific [60, 62]. VZV encephalitis may be associated with vascular lesions on imaging, including vessel stenosis and intraparenchymal or intraventricular bleeding [66]. Occasionally VZV causes localized temporal lobe abnormalities on neuroimaging or EEG, mimicking HSE [62, 66].

Acute Cerebellar Ataxia

A syndrome termed acute cerebellar ataxia, associated with ataxia and nystagmus, occurs exclusively with primary VZV infection [69]. In one large pediatric case series, acute cerebellar ataxia was the most common VZV-associated CNS complication, accounting for 31% of VZV-associated CNS hospitalizations [60]. These patients have normal sensorium and therefore do not fit the case criteria for encephalitis [38], although they have focal abnormalities on MRI including enhancement of the posterior occipital and cerebellar regions.

Meningitis

VZV meningitis does not differ substantially from other forms of aseptic meningitis. A history of cutaneous vesicular lesions in the preceding month is suggestive of this diagnosis, with one study finding that patients with involvement of facial or cervical dermatomes had a >5-fold increased risk for subsequent VZV meningitis [70]. However, cutaneous lesions are absent in >50% of cases at the time of presentation [62, 71], necessitating a high level of suspicion even in the absence of a compatible rash. CSF profiles are similar in patients with VZV meningitis, HSV meningitis, and VZV encephalitis and are not useful in differentiating these syndromes [32, 62, 72].

Vasculopathy

VZV has been associated with infection of the cerebral arteries, causing a variety of vascular syndromes including vasculitis, vascular stenosis, aneurysm, and strokes, collectively termed VZV vasculopathy. The clinical presentation of VZV vasculopathy is often characterized by symptoms related to vascular ischemia or hemorrhage. Differentiation from VZV encephalitis may be challenging as altered mentation or focal neurologic deficits can be present in both syndromes [65], and VZV parenchymal and vascular involvement may coexist, causing an overlap syndrome [66]. VZV vasculopathy tends to have a subacute onset, and neurological symptoms may persist for many years prior to diagnosis [73, 74]. Fever is uncommon and skin lesions and pleocytosis are absent in >1/3 of patients, further obscuring the diagnosis [65, 75]. Abnormalities on neuroimaging are almost universal with this syndrome, most commonly involving lesions at the gray-white matter junction [61]. MRA or angiography is positive in up to 70% of patients, with involvement of both large and small cerebral arteries reported [76].

Diagnosis

VZV infection is suggested by the presence of a characteristic skin eruption. Scraping of cutaneous vesicles allows confirmation of VZV infection through Tzanck stain, direct fluorescent antibody testing, or VZV PCR. However, zoster may occur in the setting of other illnesses, and therefore testing of CSF is necessary to confirm the diagnosis. Similarly, VZV CNS infection may occur in the absence of cutaneous lesions [62, 66, 71]. For this reason, encephalitis guidelines published by the Infectious Diseases Society of America [37] and multiple international groups [38, 40–42] recommend VZV PCR on CSF as part of the standard workup for all patients with encephalitis.

Detection of VZV in the CSF by PCR is highly specific for CNS infection, but the sensitivity of this test varies by syndrome. In a series of pediatric patients with CNS complications of acute VZV infection, CSF PCR was positive in 83% of meningitis cases, 25% of encephalitis cases, and 11% of acute cerebellar ataxia cases [60]. Similarly, only 30% of patients with VZV vasculopathy have detectable VZV DNA in the CSF and when present, virus is often detectable for only a short duration early in the course of infection [75]. Studies have found an inconsistent association between CSF VZV viral load, severity of infection, and outcome [71, 77].

Given the limitations of PCR, ancillary testing for VZV antibodies in the CSF is recommended by many authorities [38]. Intrathecal production of VZV IgG antibody is confirmed by an elevated VZV index, namely, when the serum-to-CSF ratio of anti-VZV IgG antibody is reduced compared to that of serum-to-CSF ratio of albumin and total IgG [78]. Detectable anti-VZV IgG antibody is present in >90% of patients with VZV vasculopathy [61, 65] and is the most sensitive test in this population. The presence of anti-VZV IgM antibody in CSF is also diagnostic of CNS infection, as this large molecule does not passively diffuse into the CSF. The sensitivity of intrathecal antibody testing for other forms of CNS VZV infection is uncertain.

Treatment

In the absence of evidence-based studies evaluating treatment of VZV CNS infection, recommendations for treatment are based on anecdotal reports of clinical response to therapy [79]. There is consensus for treating VZV encephalitis with intravenous acyclovir, although some authorities recommend use of a higher dose (15 mg/kg three times per day) compared to therapy for HSE for this infection [40, 42]. Immunocompromised patients or those with recurrent infections may require prolonged or repeated courses of acyclovir therapy, followed by oral therapy [76]. Anecdotal reports suggest improvement in symptomatology with intravenous acyclovir may occur even when initiated more than 6 years after onset of symptoms [73, 74].

The role of corticosteroids for VZV CNS infection is less clear, especially as iatrogenic immunosuppression is a well-recognized risk factor for zoster and subsequent dissemination. VZV vasculopathy is associated with arterial inflammation, and many authorities recommend a short course (e.g., 5 days) of prednisone 1 mg/kg daily be given concurrently with parenteral acyclovir [65]. British and Australian consensus guidelines on encephalitis suggest consideration of adjunct steroids in patients with VZV encephalitis due to the inflammatory nature of these infections [41, 42].

Complications

VZV encephalitis has been associated with subsequent development of anti-NMDAR encephalitis, although this appears to less common than with HSE [80, 81]. VZV vasculopathy may lead to the development of cerebral aneurysms, with the potential for rupture with catastrophic consequences [61, 82].

Outcomes

Outcomes following VZV CNS infection vary based on the specific syndrome. In patients with acute cerebellar ataxia, complete recovery is the rule [60], even in the absence of antiviral therapy. VZV meningitis is typically a self-limited illness, although has been associated with residual facial palsy in up to 25% of cases [72]. In contrast, encephalitis is a much more morbid disease, with 60% of patients having an adverse clinical outcome in one series [32]. VZV encephalitis is associated with prolonged hospitalization (median duration of 14–23 days) and residual neurologic deficits in many patients that persist at 3-year follow-up [32, 66]. In one series, patients with CNS symptoms in the absence of skin lesions had significant delays in initiation of acyclovir therapy (6 days versus 2.5 days), but this was not clearly associated with adverse outcome [71].

Prevention

Since licensure of the varicella vaccine, VZV CNS infections in pediatric patients have declined precipitously [60]. In the United States, varicella vaccine is recommended for all children at age 12–15 months of age, with a repeat dose at age 4–6 years. Herpes zoster vaccine has been shown to decrease the risk of cutaneous outbreaks in adults ≥60 years of age, but data on the impact of vaccination on VZV CNS infection is lacking.

References

1. Hasbun R, Rosenthal N, Balada-Llasat JM, Chung J, Duff S, Bozzette S, et al. Epidemiology of meningitis and encephalitis in the United States from 2011–2014. Clin Infect Dis. 2017;65(3):359–63. https://doi.org/10.1093/cid/cix319.
2. Delaney S, Gardella C, Saracino M, Magaret A, Wald A. Seroprevalence of herpes simplex virus type 1 and 2 among pregnant women, 1989–2010. JAMA. 2014;312:746–8. https://doi.org/10.1001/jama.2014.4359.
3. Bradley H, Markowitz LE, Gibson T, McQuillan GM. Seroprevalence of herpes simplex virus types 1 and 2—United States, 1999–2010. J Infect Dis. 2014;209(3):325–33. https://doi.org/10.1093/infdis/jit458.
4. Looker KJ, Magaret AS, May MT, Turner KM, Vickerman P, Gottlieb SL, et al. Global and regional estimates of prevalent and incident herpes simplex virus type 1 infections in 2012. PLoS One. 2015;10:e0140765. https://doi.org/10.1371/journal.pone.0140765.

5. Vora NM, Holman RC, Mehal JM, Steiner CA, Blanton J, Sejvar J. Burden of encephalitis-associated hospitalizations in the United States, 1998–2010. Neurology. 2014;82:443–51. https://doi.org/10.1212/WNL.0000000000000086.
6. George BP, Schneider EB, Venkatesan A. Encephalitis hospitalization rates and inpatient mortality in the United States, 2000–2010. PLoS One. 2014;9:e104169. https://doi.org/10.1371/journal.pone.0104169.
7. Jarrin I, Sellier P, Lopes A, Morgand M, Makovec T, Delcey V, et al. Etiologies and management of aseptic meningitis in patients admitted to an internal medicine department. Medicine (Baltimore). 2016;95:e2372. https://doi.org/10.1097/MD.0000000000002372.
8. Shukla B, Aguilera EA, Salazar L, Wootton SH, Kaewpoowat Q, Hasbun R. Aseptic meningitis in adults and children: diagnostic and management challenges. J Clin Virol. 2017;94:110–4. https://doi.org/10.1016/j.jcv.2017.07.016.
9. Nahmias AJ, Whitley RJ, Visintine AN, Takei Y, Alford CA Jr. Herpes simplex virus encephalitis: laboratory evaluations and their diagnostic significance. J Infect Dis. 1982;145(6):829–36.
10. Bradshaw MJ, Venkatesan A. Herpes simplex virus-1 encephalitis in adults: pathophysiology, diagnosis, and management. Neurotherapeutics. 2016;13:493–508. https://doi.org/10.1007/s13311-016-0433-7.
11. Corey L, Adams HG, Brown ZA, Holmes KK. Genital herpes simplex virus infections: clinical manifestations, course, and complications. Ann Intern Med. 1983;98:958–72.
12. Li JZ, Sax PE. HSV-1 encephalitis complicated by cerebral hemorrhage in an HIV-positive person. AIDS Read. 2009;19:153–5.
13. Grover D, Newsholme W, Brink N, Manji H, Miller R. Herpes simplex virus infection of the central nervous system in human immunodeficiency virus-type 1-infected patients. Int J STD AIDS. 2004;15:597–600.
14. Crusio RH, Singson SV, Haroun F, Mehta HH, Parenti DM. Herpes simplex virus encephalitis during treatment with etanercept. Scand J Infect Dis. 2014;46:152–4. https://doi.org/10.3109/00365548.2013.849816.
15. Bradford RD, Pettit AC, Wright PW, Mulligan MJ, Moreland LW, McLain DA, et al. Herpes simplex encephalitis during treatment with tumor necrosis factor-alpha inhibitors. Clin Infect Dis. 2009;49:924–7. https://doi.org/10.1086/605498.
16. Sermer DJ, Woodley JL, Thomas CA, Hedlund JA. Herpes simplex encephalitis as a complication of whole-brain radiotherapy: a case report and review of the literature. Case Rep Oncol. 2014;7:774–9. https://doi.org/10.1159/000369527.
17. Berzero G, Di Stefano AL, Dehais C, Sanson M, Gaviani P, Silvani A, et al. Herpes simplex encephalitis in glioma patients: a challenging diagnosis. J Neurol Neurosurg Psychiatry. 2015;86:374–7. https://doi.org/10.1136/jnnp-2013-307198.
18. Graber JJ, Rosenblum MK, DeAngelis LM. Herpes simplex encephalitis in patients with cancer. J Neurooncol. 2011;105:415–21. https://doi.org/10.1007/s11060-011-0609-2.
19. Koudriavtseva T, Onesti E, Tonachella R, Pelagalli L, Vidiri A, Jandolo B. Fatal herpetic encephalitis during brain radiotherapy in a cerebral metastasized breast cancer patient. J Neurooncol. 2010;100:137–40. https://doi.org/10.1007/s11060-010-0134-8.
20. Jaques DA, Bagetakou S, L'Huillier AG, Bartoli A, Vargas MI, Fluss J, et al. Herpes simplex encephalitis as a complication of neurosurgical procedures: report of 3 cases and review of the literature. Virol J. 2016;13:83. https://doi.org/10.1186/s12985-016-0540-4.
21. Zhang SY, Abel L, Casanova JL. Mendelian predisposition to herpes simplex encephalitis. Handb Clin Neurol. 2013;112:1091–7. https://doi.org/10.1016/B978-0-444-52910-7.00027-1.
22. Lim HK, Seppänen M, Hautala T, Ciancanelli MJ, Itan Y, Lafaille FG, et al. TLR3 deficiency in herpes simplex encephalitis: high allelic heterogeneity and recurrence risk. Neurology. 2014;83:1888–97. https://doi.org/10.1212/WNL.0000000000000999.
23. Sironi M, Peri AM, Cagliani R, Forni D, Riva S, Biasin M, et al. TLR3 mutations in adult patients with herpes simplex virus and varicella-zostervirus encephalitis. J Infect Dis. 2017;215:1430–4. https://doi.org/10.1093/infdis/jix166.

24. Mørk N, Kofod-Olsen E, Sørensen KB, Bach E, Ørntoft TF, Østergaard L, et al. Mutations in the TLR3 signaling pathway and beyond in adult patients with herpes simplex encephalitis. Genes Immun. 2015;16:552–66. https://doi.org/10.1038/gene.2015.46.
25. Aurelius E, Johansson B, Sköldenberg B, Forsgren M. Encephalitis in immunocompetent patients due to herpes simplex virus type 1 or 2 as determined by type-specific polymerase chain reaction and antibody assays of cerebrospinal fluid. J Med Virol. 1993;39:179–86.
26. Moon SM, Kim T, Lee EM, Kang JK, Lee SA, Choi SH. Comparison of clinical manifestations, outcomes and cerebrospinal fluid findings between herpes simplex type 1 and type 2 central nervous system infections in adults. J Med Virol. 2014;86:1766–71. https://doi.org/10.1002/jmv.23999.
27. Gnann JW Jr, Whitley RJ. Herpes simplex encephalitis: an update. Curr Infect Dis Rep. 2017;19:13. https://doi.org/10.1007/s11908-017-0568-7.
28. Chow FC, Glaser CA, Sheriff H, Xia D, Messenger S, Whitley R, et al. Use of clinical and neuroimaging characteristics to distinguish temporal lobe herpes simplex encephalitis from its mimics. Clin Infect Dis. 2015;60:1377–83. https://doi.org/10.1093/cid/civ051.
29. Renard D, Nerrant E, Lechiche C. DWI and FLAIR imaging in herpes simplex encephalitis: a comparative and topographical analysis. J Neurol. 2015;262:2101–5. https://doi.org/10.1007/s00415-015-7818-0.
30. Tan IL, McArthur JC, Venkatesan A, Nath A. Atypical manifestations and poor outcome of herpes simplex encephalitis in the immunocompromised. Neurology. 2012;79:2125–32. https://doi.org/10.1212/WNL.0b013e3182752ceb.
31. Miller S, Mateen FJ, Aksamit AJ Jr. Herpes simplex virus 2 meningitis: a retrospective cohort study. J Neurovirol. 2013;19:166–71. https://doi.org/10.1007/s13365-013-0158-x.
32. Kaewpoowat Q, Salazar L, Aguilera E, Wootton SH, Hasbun R. Herpes simplex and varicella zoster CNS infections: clinical presentations, treatments and outcomes. Infection. 2016;44:337–45. https://doi.org/10.1007/s15010-015-0867-6.
33. Aurelius E, Forsgren M, Gille E, Sköldenberg B. Neurologic morbidity after herpes simplex virus type 2 meningitis: a retrospective study of 40 patients. Scand J Infect Dis. 2002;34:278–83.
34. Lakeman FD, Whitley RJ. Diagnosis of herpes simplex encephalitis: application of polymerase chain reaction to cerebrospinal fluid from brain-biopsied patients and correlation with disease. National Institute of Allergy and Infectious Diseases Collaborative Antiviral Study Group. J Infect Dis. 1995;171:857–63.
35. Weil AA, Glaser CA, Amad Z, Forghani B. Patients with suspected herpes simplex encephalitis: rethinking an initial negative polymerase chain reaction result. Clin Infect Dis. 2002;34:1154–7.
36. Buerger KJ, Zerr K, Salazar R. An unusual presentation of herpes simplex encephalitis with negative PCR. BMJ Case Rep. 2015;2015. https://doi.org/10.1136/bcr-2015-210522.
37. Tunkel AR, Glaser CA, Bloch KC, Sejvar JJ, Marra CM, Roos KL, Infectious Diseases Society of America, et al. The management of encephalitis: clinical practice guidelines by the Infectious Diseases Society of America. Clin Infect Dis. 2008;47:303–27. https://doi.org/10.1086/589747.
38. Venkatesan A, Tunkel AR, Bloch KC, Lauring AS, Sejvar J, Bitnun A, International Encephalitis Consortium, et al. Case definitions, diagnostic algorithms, and priorities in encephalitis: consensus statement of the international encephalitis consortium. Clin Infect Dis. 2013;57(8):1114–28. https://doi.org/10.1093/cid/cit458.
39. Sauerbrei A, Wutzler P. Laboratory diagnosis of central nervous system infections caused by herpesviruses. J Clin Virol. 2002;25:S45–51.
40. Stahl JP, Azouvi P, Bruneel F, De Broucker T, Duval X, Fantin B, et al. Guidelines on the management of infectious encephalitis in adults. Med Mal Infect. 2017;47:179–94. https://doi.org/10.1016/j.medmal.2017.01.005.
41. Britton PN, Eastwood K, Paterson B, Durrheim DN, Dale RC, Cheng AC, Australasian Society of Infectious Diseases (ASID); Australasian College of Emergency Medicine (ACEM); Australian and New Zealand Association of Neurologists (ANZAN); Public Health Association of Australia (PHAA), et al. Consensus guidelines for the investigation and management of

encephalitis in adults and children in Australia and New Zealand. Intern Med J. 2015;45:563–76. https://doi.org/10.1111/imj.12749.

42. Solomon T, Michael BD, Smith PE, Sanderson F, Davies NW, Hart IJ, National Encephalitis Guidelines Development and Stakeholder Groups, et al. Management of suspected viral encephalitis in adults—Association of British Neurologists and British Infection Association National Guidelines. J Infect. 2012;64:347–73. https://doi.org/10.1016/j.jinf.2011.11.014.

43. Stahl JP, Mailles A, De Broucker T, Steering Committee and Investigators Group. Herpes simplex encephalitis and management of acyclovir in encephalitis patients in France. Epidemiol Infect. 2012;140:372–81. https://doi.org/10.1017/S0950268811000483.

44. Gateley A, Gander RM, Johnson PC, Kit S, Otsuka H, Kohl S. Herpes simplex virus type 2 meningoencephalitis resistant to acyclovir in a patient with AIDS. J Infect Dis. 1990;161:711–5.

45. Schepers K, Hernandez A, Andrei G, Gillemot S, Fiten P, Opdenakker G, et al. Acyclovir-resistant herpes simplex encephalitis in a patient treated with anti-tumor necrosis factor-α monoclonal antibodies. J Clin Virol. 2014;59:67–70. https://doi.org/10.1016/j.jcv.2013.10.025.

46. Schulte EC, Sauerbrei A, Hoffmann D, Zimmer C, Hemmer B, Mühlau M. Acyclovir resistance in herpes simplex encephalitis. Ann Neurol. 2010;67:830–3. https://doi.org/10.1002/ana.21979.

47. Gnann JW Jr, Sköldenberg B, Hart J, Aurelius E, Schliamser S, Studahl M, National Institute of Allergy and Infectious Diseases Collaborative Antiviral Study Group, et al. Herpes simplex encephalitis: lack of clinical benefit of long-term valacyclovir therapy. Clin Infect Dis. 2015;61:683–91. https://doi.org/10.1093/cid/civ369.

48. Kamei S, Sekizawa T, Shiota H, Mizutani T, Itoyama Y, Takasu T, et al. Evaluation of combination therapy using acyclovir and corticosteroid in adult patients with herpes simplex virus encephalitis. J Neurol Neurosurg Psychiatry. 2005;76:1544–9.

49. Martinez-Torres F, Menon S, Pritsch M, Victor N, Jenetzky E, Jensen K, GACHE Investigators, et al. Protocol for German trial of acyclovir and corticosteroids in herpes-simplex-virus-encephalitis (GACHE): a multicenter, multinational, randomized, double-blind, placebo-controlled German, Austrian and Dutch trial [ISRCTN45122933]. BMC Neurol. 2008;8:40. https://doi.org/10.1186/1471-2377-8-40.

50. Tyler KL. Editorial commentary: failure of adjunctive Valacyclovir to improve outcomes in herpes simplex encephalitis. Clin Infect Dis. 2015;61:692–4. https://doi.org/10.1093/cid/civ373.

51. Noska A, Kyrillos R, Hansen G, Hirigoyen D, Williams DN. The role of antiviral therapy in immunocompromised patients with herpes simplex virus meningitis. Clin Infect Dis. 2015;60:237–42. https://doi.org/10.1093/cid/ciu772.

52. Prüss H, Finke C, Höltje M, Hofmann J, Klingbeil C, Probst C, et al. N-methyl-D-aspartate receptor antibodies in herpes simplex encephalitis. Ann Neurol. 2012;72:902–11. https://doi.org/10.1002/ana.23689.

53. Armangue T, Moris G, Cantarín-Extremera V, Conde CE, Rostasy K, Erro ME, et al. Spanish prospective multicentric study of autoimmunity in herpes simplex encephalitis. Autoimmune post-herpes simplex encephalitis of adults and teenagers. Neurology. 2015;85:1736–43. https://doi.org/10.1212/WNL.0000000000002125.

54. Nosadini M, Mohammad SS, Corazza F, Ruga EM, Kothur K, Perilongo G, et al. Herpes simplex virus-induced anti-N-methyl-D-aspartate receptor encephalitis: a systematic literature review with analysis of 43 cases. Dev Med Child Neurol. 2017;59:796–805. https://doi.org/10.1111/dmcn.13448.

55. Westman G, Studahl M, Ahlm C, Eriksson BM, Persson B, Rönnelid J, et al. N-methyl-D-aspartate receptor autoimmunity affects cognitive performance in herpes simplex encephalitis. Clin Microbiol Infect. 2016;22:934–40. https://doi.org/10.1016/j.cmi.2016.07.028.

56. Whitley RJ, Soong SJ, Dolin R, Galasso GJ, Ch'ien LT, Alford CA. Adenine arabinoside therapy of biopsy-proved herpes simplex encephalitis. National Institute of Allergy and Infectious Diseases collaborative antiviral study. N Engl J Med. 1977;297:289–94.

57. Whitley RJ, Alford CA, Hirsch MS, Schooley RT, Luby JP, Aoki FY, et al. Vidarabine versus acyclovir therapy in herpes simplex encephalitis. N Engl J Med. 1986;314:144–9.

58. Erdem H, Cag Y, Ozturk-Engin D, Defres S, Kaya S, Larsen L, et al. Results of a multinational study suggest the need for rapid diagnosis and early antiviral treatment at the onset of herpetic meningoencephalitis. Antimicrob Agents Chemother. 2015;59:3084–9. https://doi.org/10.1128/AAC.05016-14.

59. Aurelius E, Franzen-Röhl E, Glimåker M, Akre O, Grillner L, Jorup-Rönström C, HSV-2 Meningitis Study Group, et al. Long-term valacyclovir suppressive treatment after herpes simplex virus type 2 meningitis: a double-blind, randomized controlled trial. Clin Infect Dis. 2012;54:1304–13. https://doi.org/10.1093/cid/cis031.

60. Science M, MacGregor D, Richardson SE, Mahant S, Tran D, Bitnun A. Central nervous system complications of varicella-zoster virus. J Pediatr. 2014;165:779–85. https://doi.org/10.1016/j.jpeds.2014.06.014.

61. Nagel MA, Gilden D. Developments in varicella zoster virus vasculopathy. Curr Neurol Neurosci Rep. 2016;16:12. https://doi.org/10.1007/s11910-015-0614-5.

62. Pahud BA, Glaser CA, Dekker CL, Arvin AM, Schmid DS. Varicella zoster disease of the central nervous system: epidemiological, clinical, and laboratory features 10 years after the introduction of the varicella vaccine. J Infect Dis. 2011;203:316–23. https://doi.org/10.1093/infdis/jiq066.

63. Levin MJ, DeBiasi RL, Bostik V, Schmid DS. Herpes zoster with skin lesions and meningitis caused by 2 different genotypes of the Oka varicella-zoster virus vaccine. J Infect Dis. 2008;198:1444–7. https://doi.org/10.1086/592452.

64. Goulleret N, Mauvisseau E, Essevaz-Roulet M, Quinlivan M, Breuer J. Safety profile of live varicella virus vaccine (Oka/Merck): five-year results of the European Varicella Zoster Virus Identification Program (EU VZVIP). Vaccine. 2010;28:5878–82. https://doi.org/10.1016/j.vaccine.2010.06.056.

65. Nagel MA, Gilden D. Neurological complications of varicella zoster virus reactivation. Curr Opin Neurol. 2014;27:356–60. https://doi.org/10.1097/WCO.0000000000000092.

66. De Broucker T, Mailles A, Chabrier S, Morand P, Stahl JP. Steering committee and investigators group. Acute varicella zoster encephalitis without evidence of primary vasculopathy in a case-series of 20 patients. Clin Microbiol Infect. 2012;18:808–19. https://doi.org/10.1111/j.1469-0691.2011.03705.x.

67. Gilden D, Nagel MA, Cohrs RJ, Mahalingam R. The variegate neurological manifestations of varicella zoster virus infection. Curr Neurol Neurosci Rep. 2013;13:374. https://doi.org/10.1007/s11910-013-0374-z.

68. Pollak L, Dovrat S, Book M, Mendelson E, Weinberger M. Varicella zoster vs. herpes simplex meningoencephalitis in the PCR era. A single center study. J Neurol Sci. 2012;314:29–36. https://doi.org/10.1016/j.jns.2011.11.004.

69. van der Maas NA, Bondt PE, de Melker H, Kemmeren JM. Acute cerebellar ataxia in the Netherlands: a study on the association with vaccinations and varicella zoster infection. Vaccine. 2009;27:1970–3. https://doi.org/10.1016/j.vaccine.2009.01.019.

70. Kim SH, Choi SM, Kim BC, Choi KH, Nam TS, Kim JT, et al. Risk factors for aseptic meningitis in herpes zoster patients. Ann Dermatol. 2017;29:283–7. https://doi.org/10.5021/ad.2017.29.3.283.

71. Persson A, Bergström T, Lindh M, Namvar L, Studahl M. Varicella-zoster virus CNS disease--viral load, clinical manifestations and sequels. J Clin Virol. 2009;46:249–53. https://doi.org/10.1016/j.jcv.2009.07.014.

72. Choi R, Kim GM, Jo IJ, Sim MS, Song KJ, Kim BJ, et al. Incidence and clinical features of herpes simplex viruses (1 and 2) and varicella-zoster virus infections in an adult Korean population with aseptic meningitis or encephalitis. J Med Virol. 2014;86:957–62. https://doi.org/10.1002/jmv.23920.

73. Gilden D, Grose C, White T, Nagae L, Hendricks RL, Cohrs RJ, et al. Successful antiviral treatment after 6 years of chronic progressive neurological disease attributed to VZV brain infection. J Neurol Sci. 2016;368:240–2. https://doi.org/10.1016/j.jns.2016.07.035.

74. Silver B, Nagel MA, Mahalingam R, Cohrs R, Schmid DS, Gilden D. Varicella zoster virus vasculopathy: a treatable form of rapidly progressive multi-infarct dementia after 2 years' duration. J Neurol Sci. 2012;323:245–7. https://doi.org/10.1016/j.jns.2012.07.059.

75. Nagel MA, Cohrs RJ, Mahalingam R, Wellish MC, Forghani B, Schiller A, et al. The vari-cella zoster virus vasculopathies: clinical, CSF, imaging, and virologic features. Neurology. 2008;70:853–60. https://doi.org/10.1212/01.wnl.0000304747.38502.e8.
76. Nagel MA, Jones D, Wyborny A. Varicella zoster virus vasculopathy: the expanding clini-cal spectrum and pathogenesis. J Neuroimmunol. 2017;308:112–7. https://doi.org/10.1016/j.jneuroim.2017.03.014.
77. Aberle SW, Aberle JH, Steininger C, Puchhammer-Stöckl E. Quantitative real time PCR detec-tion of varicella-zoster virus DNA in cerebrospinal fluid in patients with neurological disease. Med Microbiol Immunol. 2005;194:7–12.
78. Nagel MA, Forghani B, Mahalingam R, Wellish MC, Cohrs RJ, Russman AN, et al. The value of detecting anti-VZV IgG antibody in CSF to diagnose VZV vasculopathy. Neurology. 2007;68:1069–73.
79. Kennedy PG. Issues in the treatment of neurological conditions caused by reactivation of varicella zoster virus (VZV). Neurotherapeutics. 2016;13:509–13. https://doi.org/10.1007/s13311-016-0430-x.
80. Schäbitz WR, Rogalewski A, Hagemeister C, Bien CG. VZV brainstem encephalitis triggers NMDA receptor immunoreaction. Neurology. 2014;83:2309–11. https://doi.org/10.1212/WNL.0000000000001072.
81. Solís N, Salazar L, Hasbun R. Anti-NMDA receptor antibody encephalitis with concomi-tant detection of varicella zoster virus. J Clin Virol. 2016;83:26–8. https://doi.org/10.1016/j.jcv.2016.08.292.
82. Pollak L, Dovrat S, Book M, Mendelson E, Weinberger M. Varicella zoster vs.herpes simplex meningoencephalitis in the PCR era. A single center study. J Neurol Sci. 2012;314(1–2):29–36. https://doi.org/10.1016/j.jns.2011.11.004.

Human Immunodeficiency Virus (HIV)-Associated CD8 Encephalitis

10

Steven Paul Woods and Rodrigo Hasbun

Overview

It is estimated that over 35 million people worldwide are infected by the human immunodeficiency virus (HIV), with nearly two million new infections each year [1]. Despite a modest 10% decrease in the incidence of new HIV infections in the United States (USA) in recent years, the prevalence of HIV continues to rise in conjunction with better survival rates. An estimated 1.1 million people in the USA are currently living with HIV disease [2]. HIV is primarily transmitted by way of unprotected sexual contact with men, as well as by injection drug use: In the USA, HIV transmission rates are highest among men who have sex with men, particularly for young racial and ethnic minorities [3]. The life expectancy for HIV-infected persons in the USA has almost normalized due to the widespread use of effective combination antiretroviral therapy (cART), beginning in the mid-1990s [4]. Nevertheless, HIV persists as a serious public health problem, as there are significant gaps in its detection and treatment across the continuum of care in the USA and worldwide [5]. At the population level, HIV suppression rates remain well below clinical targets, and the disease is associated with elevated rates of mortality and morbidity, including central nervous system (CNS) complications.

This chapter specifically reviews the available research on one such CNS complication of HIV disease: CD8 encephalitis. This chapter begins by providing a historical context for HIV-associated CD8 encephalitis (HIV-CD8E), which is one of the many CNS complications of HIV disease that have evolved in step with the development and widespread availability of effective cART. Next, this chapter briefly

S. P. Woods (✉)
University of Houston, Department of Psychology, Cognitive Neuropsychology of Daily Life (CNDL) Laboratory, Houston, TX, USA
e-mail: spwoods@uh.edu

R. Hasbun
UT Health-McGovern Medical School, Houston, TX, USA

© Springer International Publishing AG, part of Springer Nature 2018
R. Hasbun (ed.), *Meningitis and Encephalitis*,
https://doi.org/10.1007/978-3-319-92678-0_10

outlines the current epidemiology, pathogenesis, and clinical presentation of HIV-associated CNS complications in the era of cART, including immune reconstitution inflammatory syndrome (IRIS). This chapter then provides an in-depth review of the available scientific evidence for HIV-CD8E, which derives from an emerging literature that is almost exclusively based on case studies and series. As such, this chapter attempts to meaningfully stitch together the available threads of evidence regarding the clinical presentation, diagnosis, management, course, and pathophysiology of HIV-CD8E. This chapter concludes by highlighting gaps in the current science and clinical management of HIV-CD8E, which may guide future research efforts.

Historical Context of HIV-Associated CNS Complications

In 1981, a case series from the Centers for Disease Control [6] reported an unusual incidence of cancer (i.e., Kaposi's sarcoma) and opportunistic infections (i.e., Pneumocystis pneumonia) in New York and California among men who had sex with men (MSM). The causal agent for this emergent acquired immunodeficiency syndrome (AIDS) was identified in 1983 as a T-lymphotropic retrovirus [7], which is believed to have evolved from a simian immunodeficiency virus (SIV) that adapted to human hosts in sub-Saharan Africa during the early part of the twentieth century [8]. Clinical reports of CNS symptoms accompanying HIV infection emerged early in the course of the AIDS epidemic in the USA: that is, a subset of affected patients was showing "organic" mental and neurological symptoms [9]. In 1983, Snyder et al. [9] reported the first systematic case series of AIDS-related CNS complications, including frank dementia, which was sometimes the initial manifestation of illness and was often a harbinger of imminent mortality. Whether these striking neurobehavioral syndromes stemmed from the direct CNS effects of HIV infection itself and/or secondary to CNS opportunistic infections was controversial. Indeed, CNS tumors (e.g., lymphoma) and opportunistic infections were quite common in the pre-cART era [10] and included fungal (e.g., cryptococcal meningitis), viral (e.g., encephalitis due to *progressive multifocal leukoencephalopathy* or cytomegalovirus), and parasitic (e.g., toxoplasmic encephalitis) agents. Nevertheless, HIV itself was also associated with a specific neuropathological finding, namely, fused microglia and perivascular macrophages that formed the multinucleated giant cells (aka syncytia) that are now characteristic of HIV encephalitis. Further support for HIV's direct contribution to CNS symptoms arose from studies showing that milder forms of neurobehavioral disturbance (e.g., apathy, neurocognitive impairment) were evident in the absence of CNS opportunistic infections and in otherwise asymptomatic HIV-infected patients [11].

HIV-Associated CNS Complications in the Era of cART

The widespread use of effective cART in the modern era has drastically altered the neurological landscape of HIV disease in developed countries. The incidence and prevalence of frank HIV-associated dementia is currently well below 5% [12], and CNS opportunistic infections are the exception rather than the norm. Nevertheless, the prevalence of CNS complications, including HIV-associated neurocognitive disorders (HAND) remains high and can often represent a serious challenge to clinicians and researchers. In practical terms, a diagnosis of HAND means that an individual shows evidence of impairment (i.e., a significant decline from estimated premorbid levels) in two or more cognitive domains (e.g., attention, executive functions, memory, processing speed, and motor skills) that is at least partly explained by HIV disease [13]. In the modern era, it is estimated that 30–50% of HIV-infected persons meet criteria for HAND. Incidence rates vary between 5% and 20% [14], and the course of HAND is highly variable; that is, unlike many neurodegenerative conditions, HAND is not associated with inevitable progression to dementia and death. In 30–60% of cases, the impairment associated with HAND is mild to moderate and at least partly interferes with daily activities, leading to a diagnosis of HIV-associated minor neurocognitive disorder (MND). In 30–60% of cases, the impairment is mild to moderate and does not interfere with daily activities, which is termed HIV-associated asymptomatic neurocognitive impairment (ANI). In less than 5% of cases, the impairment is severe and markedly interferes with daily activities, thus warranting a diagnosis of HIV-associated dementia (HAD). Of course, these epidemiological estimates vary depending on the criteria [15] and specific diagnostic methods [16].

The neuropathophysiology of HAND remains poorly understood in the cART era, and there are no well-validated diagnostic biomarkers or effective treatments. That said, current models propose that HIV is indeed neurovirulent and crosses the blood-brain barrier early in the course of infection, imbedded in activated monocytes and other white blood cells that traffic into brain parenchyma [17]. HIV does not widely *infect* neurons, but it does carry direct and indirect adverse CNS effects on brain structure and function. In terms of its direct effects, HIV is detectable in brain parenchyma and can replicate in perivascular macrophages, astrocytes, and microglia, which may express neurotoxic viral proteins like gp120 and Tat [18]. HIV's indirect effects on the brain are primarily from neuroinflammatory processes, such as upregulation of cytokines and chemokines that can alter neuronal functioning [19]. Well over half of HIV-infected persons will evidence some form of neuropathology upon autopsy [20]. Unlike the pre-cART era in which HIV-E and CNS opportunistic infections were most prevalent, HIV-associated pathologies in the cART era are quite heterogeneous and include neural apoptosis, synaptodendritic injury, encephalitis, gliosis, and vasculopathy [18]. Such pathological diversity has made the quest for discovering a biomarker of HAND quite challenging. A host of different plasma and CSF biomarkers reflecting these neuropathogenic processes have been examined in the context of HAND, including markers of chemokines (e.g., MCP-1), astrocytosis (e.g., S-100β), neuroinflammation (e.g., tumor necrosis factor-alpha), and neuronal damage (e.g., neurofilament light) [19], with varying levels of success. Similarly, although the prevalence and severity of HAND can increase with the clinical severity of immunovirological disease, this relationship is generally quite weak and nonlinear in the cART era [12]. Nadir (i.e., lowest) CD4$^+$ cell count shows modest correspondence to the level of neurocognitive impairment in the cART era (e.g., [21]), but the value of that historical immune marker may dwindle under evolving cART guidelines in which patients are treated despite high CD4 counts.

Although the effects of HIV can be observed throughout the brain, HIV-associated neural abnormalities are most commonly present in the white and gray matter structures of fronto-striato-thalamo-cortical circuits [22]. Accordingly, the neurobehavioral profile of HAND parallels that which is observed in other primarily frontal systems conditions, such as Parkinson's disease; specifically, HAND is often marked by mild-to-moderate deficits in executive functions, working memory, psychomotor speed/coordination, and the strategic aspects of learning and memory, with relative sparing of memory consolidation (i.e., amnesia is uncommon), visuospatial abilities, and praxis. In recent years, investigators have begun to raise the possibility that as the HIV population ages, HAND is evolving into a more posterior cortical disease, akin to Alzheimer's disease; however, neurobehavioral evidence for such claim is presently scant (e.g., [23]). Effective disease modifying therapies for HAND do not yet exist. The initiation of cART is not strongly neuroprotective or restorative [24], even with regimens that penetrate the CNS [25]. Studies evaluating various nonantiretroviral agents (e.g., selegiline; [26]) and rehabilitation approaches (e.g., [27]) have generally not demonstrated widespread effectiveness in improving or restoring neurocognitive functions in HIV, although a few investigations demonstrate promising early findings [28, 29] that await confirmation in randomized controlled trials.

CNS Immune Reconstitution Inflammatory Syndrome (IRIS)

The incidence and prevalence of CNS opportunistic infections has declined considerably in the cART era [30]. At present, CNS opportunistic infections are estimated to occur in only about 1% of the HIV+ population, particularly in the setting of immune compromise [31]. The most commonly encountered CNS opportunistic infections in the modern era include progressive multifocal leukoencephalopathy (PML) due primarily to John Cunningham (JC) virus, cerebral toxoplasmosis, and cryptococcal meningitis, as well as tuberculosis and cytomegalovirus. Opportunistic infections such as PML and cryptococcal meningitis play a key role in the immune reconstitution inflammatory syndrome (IRIS), which is a pathological inflammatory response that can occur in a variety of organ systems, including the CNS. IRIS is a clinical syndrome in which an unexpected, excessive pro-inflammatory response to a pathogen (usually an opportunistic infection) occurs within weeks or months of ART. The inflammatory response is characterized by a wide range of focal and systemic symptoms that if untreated can lead to death [32]. IRIS is commonly classified as either (1) "paradoxical," meaning that the CNS opportunistic infection is known and treated with some success prior to initiation of ART, after which clinical deterioration occurs secondary to the pathological inflammatory response, or (2) "unmasked," meaning that the diagnosis of the CNS opportunistic infection comes after the initiation of ART, which sparked the clinical deterioration [32]. The general incidence of IRIS is approximately 10% in the USA [32], with risk factors including treatment naïve, immunosuppression, and viremia, as well as some characteristics of the opportunistic infection itself. IRIS is less common in the CNS than it is in other bodily systems and is estimated to occur in only 0.05–2% of HIV⁺ patients. Of course, the incidence of IRIS is much higher among those persons with CNS opportunistic infections; for example, estimates of IRIS incidence are 15–20% among those cryptococcal meningitis and PML who initiate cART [33] for whom the mortality rates are estimated between 5% and 15%. Treatment typically involves corticosteroids, but there are no published guidelines, and interventions are variable depending on the specific diagnosis and clinical context. The CNS pathology of IRIS involves high numbers of CD8⁺ cells in perivascular regions, but with lower than expected rates of CD4⁺ cells, despite the latter increasing in the periphery.

HIV-Associated CD8E

HIV-associated CD8E is an emergent, relatively rare syndrome in which otherwise well-controlled HIV⁺ patients experience an IRIS-like pathological inflammatory response. Unlike classic CNS IRIS cases in which an opportunistic infection and rapid immunovirological recovery are typically key features of the encephalitis, CD8E cases do not have an immediately identifiable pathogen. In 2013, Lescure et al. [34] provided a detailed case series of 14 HIV⁺ patients observed near Paris, France, between 1999 and 2008 (see also Gray et al. [35] for the neuropathological findings from 10 of these patients). The majority of Lescure's [34] patients were under good immunovirological control but nevertheless experienced severe encephalitis for which comprehensive work-ups did not yield any significant precipitant. Indeed, brain biopsies revealed only inconsistent/weak expression of HIV RNA but rather large numbers of CD8⁺ cells in perivascular regions accompanied by activation of astrocytes and microglia. Mortality rates were high in this series, and only 30% of these patients had a positive outcome. Since then, four additional single case reports of CD8E have been published [36–39], along with one case of apparent CD8E transverse myelitis [40]. Subsequent authors (e.g., the accompanying commentary by Langford and Letendre [41]) have noted the clinical and pathological similarities between Lescure's [34] CD8E syndrome and prior case studies of CNS IRIS that were published around the same time as Lescure's patients were being followed in clinic [42–44]. As such, it appears that CD8E, while rare, is not an isolated neurological complication of HIV infection whose incidence has remained steadily low during the cART era.

So, if CD8E occurs in the absence of the typical signs of CNS IRIS and other types of HIV-associated neurological complications (e.g., leukoencephalopathy), what then are its precipitants and underlying mechanisms? Lescure et al. [34] proposed that the driving neurobiological force of CD8E is a "transient disequilibrium between HIV and brain immunity." Specifically, it is posited that peripheral T cells are re/activated and then migrate across the blood-brain barrier. Although the precise source of the re/activation is unknown (and may be multifaceted), possible triggers include HIV DNA reservoirs in the brain or other latent infections. In the published case studies to date, CD8E triggers have included minor infections, virological escape (e.g., high CSF HIV RNA levels without viremia in plasma), CNS IRIS, and cART interruption. Low levels of HIV replication and/or HIV DNA reservoirs may play a role in the re/activation of T cells; in fact, the CD8+ response to covert HIV infection in the brain has even been proposed as a primary mechanism for persistence of HAND in the cART era [41]. The CD8+ cells eventually "overshoot" the original target that triggered their re/activation, now outnumbering CD4+ cells in the brain [34]. CD8+ cells are rare in healthy brains but can be present in gray and white matter in the setting of infection and/or encephalitis and produce direct or indirect injury to neurons, particularly when they outnumber CD4+ cells [45]. In the case of CD8E, pathology shows marked-to-severe CD8 cells and microglial activation, along with marked astrocytosis and white matter changes indicative of edema and myelin loss [35]. There is a weak presence of HIV P24 and CD4+ cells and no evidence of the hallmark multinucleated giant cells.

Clinical Presentation and Diagnosis

Neurological Symptoms

The presenting neurological symptoms of CD8E appear to be fairly diverse, although there are some patterns emerging. One or more of the following four neurological symptoms were evident in approximately 30–45% of CD8E cases reported to date: cognitive impairment, headache, seizures, and/or confusion. Across this small literature, it appears that men may be more likely than women to present with cognitive impairment (56% vs 13%), which includes dementia and memory difficulties. By way of contrast, women may be more likely than men to report headache (75% vs 22%). Less frequent presenting symptoms of CD8E (<15%) have included dizziness, gait abnormalities, imbalance, tremor, facial palsy, coma, or dysarthria.

Laboratory Findings

Flow cytometry reveals a high number of CD8+ cells in the CSF. Protein levels are typically elevated. HIV RNA has been detectable in the CSF of 11 out 12 cases reported thus far, most often in the setting of undetectable (or sometimes much lower) HIV RNA in plasma, suggesting viral escape.

Neuroimaging

FLAIR MRI of CD8E patients tends to show bilateral, diffuse signal intensities that are nonspecific and suggestive of leukoencephalopathy [34, 35] (see Fig. 10.1). However, Lescure et al. [34] observed that postgadolinium contrast (spin-echo T1 with magnetization transfer) revealed a highly sensitive and specific pattern of "multiple punctate or linear gadolinium-enhanced lesions" in the perivascular region. In four patients, these image lesions were confirmed with high-intensity signal on diffusion-weighted scans (see also [39]). The MRI findings in CD8E are usually diffuse but can be focal in their presentation in some instances (see [36]). Interestingly, the case described by Morioka was negative on T1 postgadolinium contrast but nevertheless had positive findings for CD8E on brain biopsy.

Fig. 10.1 MRI of the brain of a patient with biopsy-proven CD8 encephalitis showing bilateral white matter abnormalities

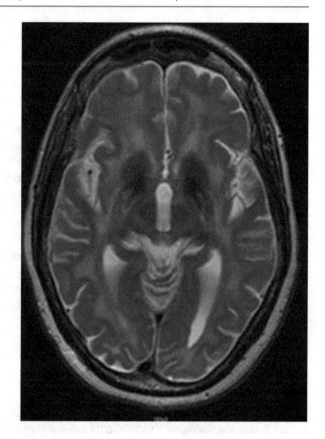

Management

Overall, the prognosis for CD8E patients is poor, but early diagnosis and prompt management are key to increase the likelihood of a positive outcome. Lescure et al. [34] suggest that the clinical features, CSF studies, and MRI (with gadolinium contrast) are sufficient to make a reliable diagnosis of CD8E without a brain biopsy. However, it should be noted that flow cytometry and gadolinium contrast scans are not always available [41]. Timely administration of combination of ART and corticosteroids shows some evidence of effectiveness across the published case studies. In the Lescure cases [34], the authors followed the recommended glucocorticosteroid treatment protocol recommended for patients with acute disseminating encephalomyelitis (ADEM). In those cases, treatment involved intravenous methylprednisolone (1 g/day for 5 days, then tapered for a median of 6 months). Salam et al. [38] detail an instance in which initial treatment with corticosteroids was effective but met with a relapse, which ultimately responded to mycophenolate mofetil. Also of note, the patient described in the Morioka et al. [37] study had a positive response to a switch in cART (i.e., without corticosteroids), which was initiated following the detection of a drug-resistant mutation (M184V).

Future Directions

As is true of many rare conditions, there is much left to learn about the epidemiology, mechanisms, clinical course, and management of CD8E. The case studies reviewed above provide important initial insights and allow for hypothesis generation, but well-designed studies with larger sample sizes and proper comparison groups are needed. For example, what are the predictors of incident CD8E (e.g., why do some minor infections trigger CD8E while others do not and what explains individual patient differences in that regard?)? What are the host and viral genetics of CD8E (e.g., why is such a large proportion of the cases in the literature thus far observed in persons of African descent?). Can CD8E be reliably distinguished from other HIV-associated neurological complications, such as CNS IRIS? What are the most robust clinicopathological correlates in CD8E (e.g., do gadolinium MRI abnormalities reliably map onto CD8+ cells in the CSF and in brain biopsies?)? What is the profile and neurocognitive trajectory of CD8E? Nearly 50% of patients present with neurocognitive impairment (e.g., memory problems) and approximately 50% of those who recovered from CD8E had residual neurocognitive complications. Further downstream, among those who survive and recover, what is the impact of CD8E on daily activities and quality of life?

References

1. United Nations. Global AIDS update. Author. 2016.
2. Johnson SA, Son R, Hall HI. Estimated HIV incidence, prevalence, and undiagnosed infections in US states and Washington, DC, 2010–2014. J Acquir Immune Defic Syndr. 2017;76(2):116–22. https://doi.org/10.1097/QAI.0000000000001495.
3. Centers for Disease Control and Surveillance HIV Surveillance Report. Diagnoses of HIV infection in the United States and dependent areas, vol. 28; 2016.
4. Harrison KM, Song R, Zhang X. Life expectancy after HIV diagnosis based on national HIV surveillance data from 25 states, United States. J Acquir Immune Defic Syndr. 2010;53(1):124–30. https://doi.org/10.1097/QAI.0b013e3181b563e7.
5. Gardner EM, Young B. The HIV care cascade through time. Lancet Infect Dis. 2014;14(1):5–6. https://doi.org/10.1016/S1473-3099(13)70272-X.
6. Centers for Disease Control and Surveillance. Pneumocystis pneumonia—Los Angeles. MMWR Morb Mortal Wkly Rep. 1981;30:250–2.
7. Gallo RC, Montagnier L. The discovery of HIV as the cause of AIDS. N Engl J Med. 2003;349:2283–5. https://doi.org/10.1056/NEJMp038194.
8. Hirsch VM, Olmsted RA, Murphey-Corb M, Purcell RH, Johnson PR. An African primate lentivirus (SIVsm) closely related to HIV-2. Nature. 1989;339(6223):389–92.
9. Snider WD, Simpson DM, Aronyk KE, Nielsen SL. Primary lymphoma of the nervous system associated with acquired immune-deficiency syndrome. N Engl J Med. 1983;308(1):45.
10. Anders HJ, Goebel FD. Neurological manifestations of cytomegalovirus infection in the acquired immunodeficiency syndrome. Int J STD AIDS. 1999;10(3):151–9.
11. Grant I, Atkinson JH, Hesselink JR, Kennedy CJ, Richman DD, Spector SA, McCutchan JA. Evidence for early central nervous system involvement in the acquired immunodeficiency syndrome (AIDS) and other human immunodeficiency virus (HIV) infections. Studies with neuropsychologic testing and magnetic resonance imaging. Ann Intern Med. 1987;107(6):828–36.

12. Heaton RK, Clifford DB, Franklin DR Jr, Woods SP, Ake C, Vaida F, Ellis RJ, Letendre SL, Marcotte TD, Atkinson JH, Rivera-Mindt M, Vigil OR, Taylor MJ, Collier AC, Marra CM, Gelman BB, McArthur JC, Morgello S, Simpson DM, McCutchan JA, Abramson I, Gamst A, Fennema-Notestine C, Jernigan TL, Wong J, Grant I, CHARTER Group. HIV-associated neurocognitive disorders persist in the era of potent antiretroviral therapy: CHARTER study. Neurology. 2010;75(23):2087–96. https://doi.org/10.1212/WNL.0b013e318200d727.
13. Antinori A, Arendt G, Becker JT, Brew BJ, Byrd DA, Cherner M, Clifford DB, Cinque P, Epstein LG, Goodkin K, Gisslen M, Grant I, Heaton RK, Joseph J, Marder K, Marra CM, McArthur JC, Nunn M, Price RW, Pulliam L, Robertson KR, Sacktor N, Valcour V, Wojna VE. Updated research nosology for HIV-associated neurocognitive disorders. Neurology. 2007;69(18):1789–99.
14. Sheppard DP, Woods SP, Bondi MW, Gilbert PE, Massman PJ, Doyle KL, HNRP Group. Does older age confer an increased risk of incident neurocognitive disorders among persons living with HIV disease? Clin Neuropsychol. 2015;29(5):656–77. https://doi.org/10.1080/13854046.2015.1077995.
15. Tierney SM, Sheppard DP, Kordovski VM, Faytell MP, Avci G, Woods SP. A comparison of the sensitivity, stability, and reliability of three diagnostic schemes for HIV-associated neurocognitive disorders. J Neurovirol. 2017;23(3):404–21. https://doi.org/10.1007/s13365-016-0510-z.
16. Blackstone K, Moore DJ, Heaton RK, Franklin DR Jr, Woods SP, Clifford DB, Collier AC, Marra CM, Gelman BB, McArthur JC, Morgello S, Simpson DM, Rivera-Mindt M, Deutsch R, Ellis RJ, Hampton Atkinson J, Grant I, CHARTER Group. Diagnosing symptomatic HIV-associated neurocognitive disorders: self-report versus performance-based assessment of everyday functioning. J Int Neuropsychol Soc. 2012;18(1):79–88. https://doi.org/10.1017/S135561771100141X.
17. Hult B, Chana G, Masliah E, Everall I. Neurobiology of HIV. Int Rev Psychiatry. 2008;20(1):3–13. https://doi.org/10.1080/09540260701862086.
18. Ellis R, Langford D, Masliah E. HIV and antiretroviral therapy in the brain: neuronal injury and repair. Nat Rev Neurosci. 2007;8(1):33–44.
19. González-Scarano F, Martín-García J. The neuropathogenesis of AIDS. Nat Rev Immunol. 2005;5(1):69–81.
20. Everall IP, Hansen LA, Masliah E. The shifting patterns of HIV encephalitis neuropathology. Neurotox Res. 2005;8(1–2):51–61.
21. Ellis RJ, Badiee J, Vaida F, Letendre S, Heaton RK, Clifford D, Collier AC, Gelman B, McArthur J, Morgello S, McCutchan JA, Grant I, CHARTER Group. CD4 nadir is a predictor of HIV neurocognitive impairment in the era of combination antiretroviral therapy. AIDS. 2011;25(14):1747–51. https://doi.org/10.1097/QAD.0b013e32834a40cd.
22. Aylward EH, Henderer JD, McArthur JC, Brettschneider PD, Harris GJ, Barta PE, Pearlson GD. Reduced basal ganglia volume in HIV-1-associated dementia: results from quantitative neuroimaging. Neurology. 1993;43(10):2099–104.
23. Iudicello JE, Woods SP, Deutsch R, Grant I, HIV Neurobehavioral Research Program HNRP Group. Combined effects of aging and HIV infection on semantic verbal fluency: a view of the cortical hypothesis through the lens of clustering and switching. J Clin Exp Neuropsychol. 2012;34(5):476–88. https://doi.org/10.1080/13803395.2011.651103.
24. Al-Khindi T, Zakzanis KK, van Gorp WG. Does antiretroviral therapy improve HIV-associated cognitive impairment? A quantitative review of the literature. J Int Neuropsychol Soc. 2011;17(6):956–69. https://doi.org/10.1017/S1355617711000968.
25. Ellis RJ, Letendre S, Vaida F, Haubrich R, Heaton RK, Sacktor N, Clifford DB, Best BM, May S, Umlauf A, Cherner M, Sanders C, Ballard C, Simpson DM, Jay C, McCutchan JA. Randomized trial of central nervous system-targeted antiretrovirals for HIV-associated neurocognitive disorder. Clin Infect Dis. 2014;58(7):1015–22.
26. Schifitto G, Zhang J, Evans SR, Sacktor N, Simpson D, Millar LL, Hung VL, Miller EN, Smith E, Ellis RJ, Valcour V, Singer E, Marra CM, Kolson D, Weihe J, Remmel R, Katzenstein D, Clifford DB, ACTG A5090 Team. A multicenter trial of selegiline transdermal system for HIV-associated cognitive impairment. Neurology. 2007;69(13):1314–21.

27. Kaur J, Dodson JE, Steadman L, Vance DE. Predictors of improvement following speed of processing training in middle-aged and older adults with HIV: a pilot study. J Neurosci Nurs. 2014;46(1):23–33.
28. Letendre SL, Woods SP, Ellis RJ, Atkinson JH, Masliah E, van den Brande G, Durelle J, Grant I, Everall I, HNRC Group. Lithium improves HIV-associated neurocognitive impairment. AIDS. 2006;20(14):1885–8.
29. Avci G, Woods SP, Verduzco M, Sheppard DP, Sumowski JF, Chiaravalloti ND, DeLuca J, HNRP Group. Effect of retrieval practice on short-term and long-term retention in HIV⁺ individuals. J Int Neuropsychol Soc. 2017;23(3):214–22. https://doi.org/10.1017/S1355617716001089.
30. Garvey L, Winston A, Walsh J, Post F, Porter K, Gazzard B, Fisher M, Leen C, Pillay D, Hill T, Johnson M, Gilson R, Anderson J, Easterbrook P, Bansi L, Orkin C, Ainsworth J, Phillips AN, Sabin CA. HIV-associated central nervous system diseases in the recent combination antiretroviral therapy era. Eur J Neurol. 2011;18(3):527–34. https://doi.org/10.111 1/j.1468-1331.2010.03291.
31. Tan IL, Smith BR, von Geldern G, Mateen FJ, McArthur JC. HIV-associated opportunistic infections of the CNS. Lancet Neurol. 2012;11(7):605–17. https://doi.org/10.1016/S1474-4422(12)70098-4.
32. Walker NF, Scriven J, Meintjes G, Wilkinson RJ. Immune reconstitution inflammatory syndrome in HIV-infected patients. HIV AIDS (Auckl). 2015;7:49–64. https://doi.org/10.2147/HIV.S42328.
33. Müller M, Wandel S, Colebunders R, et al. Immune reconstitution inflammatory syndrome in patients starting antiretroviral therapy for HIV infection: a systematic review and meta-analysis. Lancet Infect Dis. 2010;10:251–61.
34. Lescure FX, Moulignier A, Savatovsky J, Amiel C, Carcelain G, Molina JM, Gallien S, Pacanovski J, Pialoux G, Adle-Biassette H, Gray F. CD8 encephalitis in HIV-infected patients receiving cART: a treatable entity. Clin Infect Dis. 2013;57(1):101–8. https://doi.org/10.1093/cid/cit175.
35. Gray F, Lescure FX, Adle-Biassette H, Polivka M, Gallien S, Pialoux G, Moulignier A. Encephalitis with infiltration by CD8⁺ lymphocytes in HIV patients receiving combination antiretroviral treatment. Brain Pathol. 2013;23(5):525–33. https://doi.org/10.1111/bpa.12038.
36. Moulignier A, Savatovsky J, Polivka M, Boutboul D, Depaz R, Lescure FX. CD8 T lymphocytes encephalitis mimicking brain tumor in HIV-1 infection. J Neurovirol. 2013;19(6):606–9. https://doi.org/10.1007/s13365-013-0217-3.
37. Morioka H, Yanagisawa N, Sasaki S, Sekiya N, Suganuma A, Imamura A, Ajisawa A, Kishida S. CD8 encephalitis caused by persistently detectable drug-resistant HIV. Intern Med. 2016;55(10):1383–6. https://doi.org/10.2169/internalmedicine.55.5783.
38. Salam S, Mihalova T, Ustianowski A, McKee D, Siripurapu R. Relapsing CD8⁺ encephalitis-looking for a solution. BMJ Case Rep. 2016. https://doi.org/10.1136/bcr-2016-214961.
39. Zarkali A, Gorgoraptis N, Miller R, John L, Merve A, Thust S, Jager R, Kullmann D, Swayne O. CD8⁺ encephalitis: a severe but treatable HIV-related acute encephalopathy. Pract Neurol. 2017;17(1):42–6. https://doi.org/10.1136/practneurol-2016-001483.
40. Moulignier A, Lescure FX, Savatovsky J, Campa P. CD8 transverse myelitis in a patient with HIV-1 infection. BMJ Case Rep. 2014. https://doi.org/10.1136/bcr-2013-201073.
41. Langford D, Letendre S. Editorial commentary: severe HIV-associated CD8⁺ T-cell encephalitis: is it the tip of the iceberg? Clin Infect Dis. 2013;57(1):109–11. https://doi.org/10.1093/cid/cit179.
42. Miller RF, Isaacson PG, Hall-Craggs M, Lucas S, Gray F, Scaravilli F, An SF. Cerebral CD8⁺ lymphocytosis in HIV-1 infected patients with immune restoration induced by HAART. Acta Neuropathol. 2004;108(1):17–23.

43. Venkataramana A, Pardo CA, McArthur JC, Kerr DA, Irani DN, Griffin JW, Burger P, Reich DS, Calabresi PA, Nath A. Immune reconstitution inflammatory syndrome in the CNS of HIV-infected patients. Neurology. 2006;67(3):383–8.
44. Langford TD, Letendre SL, Marcotte TD, Ellis RJ, McCutchan JA, Grant I, Mallory ME, Hansen LA, Archibald S, Jernigan T, Masliah E, HNRC Group. Severe, demyelinating leuko-encephalopathy in AIDS patients on antiretroviral therapy. AIDS. 2002;16(7):1019–29.
45. Petito CK, Torres-Muñoz JE, Zielger F, McCarthy M. Brain CD8+ and cytotoxic T lymphocytes are associated with, and may be specific for, human immunodeficiency virus type 1 encephalitis in patients with acquired immunodeficiency syndrome. J Neurovirol. 2006;12(4):272–83.

Challenges in the Management and Prevention of Japanese Encephalitis

11

Quanhathai Kaewpoowat, Linda Aurpibul, and Rommanee Chaiwarith

Introduction

Japanese encephalitis (JE) is the most common cause of vaccine-preventable encephalitis in the Asia-Pacific region [1, 2]. It is initially described as recurrent outbreaks of *summer encephalitis* in Japan during the late eighteenth to early nineteenth century [3–6] before its causative agent was first isolated in 1935 [7–9]. The JE virus is a small, single-stranded RNA enveloped agent of the genus *Flavivirus* [10, 11] that is the same genus with dengue virus (DENV), Zika virus, yellow fever virus, and West Nile virus [12, 13]. There are five different genotypes of JE virus. Genotype III was predominant prior to the vaccination era. However, recent studies revealed that genotype I has become the predominant type in some areas [14, 15] possibly related to climate change and geographic variations [16].

 Culex mosquitos are the main vectors of JE. Swine, especially piglets, and waddling birds are major amplifier hosts. Humans are "dead-end hosts," in that human-to-human transmission of JE via mosquitos is not possible because of the short duration and low levels of JE viremia in humans [17]. Most human JE infections do not result in clinical disease [18, 19]. The estimated ratio of symptomatic to asymptomatic infections ranges from 1:25 among previously nonimmune adults from

Q. Kaewpoowat (✉)
Division of Infectious Diseases and Tropical Medicine, Department of Medicine, Chiang Mai University, Chiang Mai, Thailand

Research Institute for Health Sciences, Chiang Mai University, Chiang Mai, Thailand
e-mail: quanhathai@rihes.org

L. Aurpibul
Research Institute for Health Sciences, Chiang Mai University, Chiang Mai, Thailand

R. Chaiwarith
Division of Infectious Diseases and Tropical Medicine, Maharaj Nakorn Chiang Mai Hospital, Chiang Mai University, Chiang Mai, Thailand

© Springer International Publishing AG, part of Springer Nature 2018
R. Hasbun (ed.), *Meningitis and Encephalitis*,
https://doi.org/10.1007/978-3-319-92678-0_11

non-endemic areas to 1:200–1:1000 in children in endemic areas [18, 20]. Neuroinvasive disease has been estimated to occur in 1:200 infections [19], with mortality up to 30% [20]. Among survivors, permanent neurologic, cognitive, and psychiatric sequelae were observed in 20–30% [20–22].

The World Health Organization (WHO) estimated in 2011 that 67,900 JE cases occur annually in endemic areas, yielding an estimated global incidence rate of 1.8/100,000 person-years [1, 23]. The incidence among children less than 15 years of age is estimated to be nine times higher than those of older age (5.4 vs. 0.6/100,000 person-years). Three billion of the world population are living in 24 Asian and the Western Pacific countries of JE at-risk area.

Management

Diagnosis

JE infection should be considered in patients presenting with acute encephalitis syndrome (AES) who live in or have a compatible travel history to JE-endemic areas [24]. Seizures and parkinsonian-like movement often occur in acute JE disease [25, 26]. Moreover, meningitis [27] and/or flaccid paralysis have also been observed [27–29]. Imaging studies of patients with JE disease may detect pathologic changes affecting the thalamus, basal ganglia, and midbrain [30], but are nonspecific. Laboratory findings, including cerebrospinal fluid (CSF) profiles, are similar to those found in other viral and some idiopathic encephalitis. The CSF opening pressure was found to be high in 50% of the patients. Seizure and high opening pressures >25 cmH$_2$O are the factors associated with poor clinical outcome [25, 26, 31].

The incubation period of JE infection is 4–14 days. Viremic phase and the presence of virus in CSF are short and usually absent by the onset of clinical symptoms [20, 32]. IgM in CSF and serum starts to appear soon after the clinical onset, followed by IgG in the serum [24]. The WHO *Manual for the Laboratory Diagnosis of Japanese Encephalitis Virus Infection*, published in 2007, recommends the following tests to confirm JE infection [24]:

1. Presence of JE IgM in CSF (preferred) or serum using JE ELISA.
2. Detection of JE virus by one or more of the following methods a) JE antigens detection in tissue by immunohistochemistry, OR b) JE viral isolation from serum, plasma, blood CSF or tissue, OR c) JE virus genome detection in serum, plasma, blood, CSF, or tissue by reverse transcriptase-polymerase chain reaction (RT-PCR) or equivalent test.
3. Fourfold rise of serum JE IgG, by hemagglutination inhibition (HI) or plaque reduction neutralization assay (PRNT), from acute and convalescent phases of illness. This should be done in parallel with other confirmatory tests.

Clinical studies among confirmed JE cases revealed that CSF IgM became detectable in 90% of patients within 4 days [33] and 100% by 7 days after onset of symptoms [34]. In serum, IgM turned positive slower. By day ninth after onset, 88%

had positive serum IgM [33]. However, the presence of acute-phase JE IgM alone cannot rule out alternative diagnoses for AES. Among 107 patients in Laos presenting with meningoencephalitis and 24 with acute meningitis who fulfilled the WHO criteria for diagnosis of JE infection, 12% of the former and 29% of the latter were ultimately diagnosed with other infections, most commonly cryptococcosis and scrub typhus (*Orientia tsutsugamushi*) infection [35]. Moreover, cross-reactivity is well recognized among various flavivirus infections [36]. The most challenging is distinguishing JE from DENV infection, which co-circulates with JE virus in hyperendemic areas and also shares antigenic epitopes with JE virus. Approximately 10% co-positivity of DENV IgM and JE virus IgM has been reported [37–39]. However, there was no definite consensus about how to differentiate true coinfection from cross-reactivity. Some suggest a diagnostic scheme prioritizing more sensitive tests such as viral genome detection, followed by assays for high neutralizing antibody [37, 38]. Assays for neutralizing antibodies against the DENV nonstructural protein 1 (NS1) and membrane proteins (prM) were claimed to enhance the sensitivity for detecting DENV infection [40] and thus if positive would tend to rule out JE infection. Nevertheless, the use of viral genomic detection and neutralizing antibody is restricted by limited availability and requires expertise and a long, labor-intensive period to perform. One group proposed diagnosing JE on the basis of high levels of IgM in CSF determined by routine JE ELISA [39].

Viral culture and detection of virus using methods equivalent to RT-PCR are highly specific, but sensitivity is poor [24]. Still, RT-PCR has been described as a useful tool in the early course of illness [41], particularly when IgM is negative, but clinical suspicion remains high [42]. More sensitive PCR techniques used for epidemiologic studies in mosquitoes and amplifying hosts are being investigated for clinical diagnosis [43, 44]. While JE virus was not found by RT-PCR from urine samples among 52 Chinese confirmed JE patients in 2013 [45], the report in 2017 using next-generation sequencing and viral metagenomics was able to detect JE virus in urine from 16-year-old Vietnamese male who presented with febrile illness, limb weakness, and seizure [46]. This advanced testing could be more sensitive and warrants further evaluation.

Treatment

In the absence of effective, JE-specific antiviral medications, supportive care is the sole therapy for JE disease, with the goal to anticipate and ameliorate its life-threatening complications. In the acute phase, these include aspiration, status epilepticus, increased intracranial pressure, and hypoglycemia [47]. For survivors of the acute phase, physical therapy, avoiding bedsores and contractures, and psychological therapy are indicated [20].

Several agents were studied in human without much success. Oral ribavirin, a broad-spectrum antiviral agent, was studied among 153 JE patients (6-month- to 15-year-olds) in India [48], but no mortality benefit was demonstrated. Non-antiviral therapeutic agents, such as interferon-alpha A [49], high-dose steroid [50], and intravenous immune globulin (IVIG) [51], have anecdotally been reported to ameliorate JE diseases. However, when interferon-alpha A [52] and high-dose steroids

[53] advanced to definitive randomized clinical trials (RCT) in humans, no clinical benefit for outcome mortality or morbidity was demonstrated. Slightly more promising agents were IVIG and minocycline. The compassionate off-label uses of IVIG for its antiviral/anti-inflammatory properties have been tried for flavivirus infections [54–57]. A small RCT among 22 children (aged 1–14 years) found IVIG from India greatly increased neutralizing antibody titers, induced no adverse safety signals, and was feasible for use in Nepal [58]. Although the study was not powered to compare clinical outcomes, an unexpected finding was complete recovery after 3–6 months for 45% in the IVIG group versus 18% in the placebo group (not statistically significant). Thus further study is warranted. Minocycline has been proposed as therapy because of its lipophilic nature, high concentration in CSF, and neuroprotective properties in vitro [59] and in an animal model [60]. A RCT of minocycline versus placebo among 281 Indian children and adults with clinically diagnosed JE did not reveal mortality benefit, but post hoc analysis of patients who survived beyond the first day of admission suggested a trend ($p = 0.090$) of better 3-month survival rate in those receiving minocycline [61]. However, only 10% (29 participants) had serologic confirmed JE diagnosis. Another smaller RCT that enrolled 44 JE-confirmed children reported that minocycline reduced days of fever, improved level of consciousness, and shortened duration of hospitalization but had no effect on mortality or other clinical outcomes [62].

Other potential therapeutic agents that aim to apply better understanding of JE virus structure and JE pathogenesis are in early in vitro and preclinical animal model studies of inhibition of viral fusion and/or replication, of reduction of inflammation to prevent neuronal damage, and of boosting host mechanisms to eliminate JE virus [63].

Prevention by Vaccination

There are four major categories of JE vaccines that have been extensively studied and utilized to prevent JE disease. All vaccines are derived from the JE genotype III virus. Several reports support that the vaccine induces cross-immunity against circulating JE virus including genotype I virus, an emerging dominant serotype [64, 65]. Still, the concern of vaccine effectiveness against serotype V [66] has emerged after the reports of disease outbreak in South Korea [67, 68]. Of note, there is no standardized JE neutralizing assay. Therefore, the comparison of immunogenicity across the studies must be done cautiously.

Mouse Brain-Derived Inactivated Vaccine (JE-MB)

JE-MB were grown in mouse brain cells and derived from the Nakayama and/or Beijing strains of JE virus [69–72]. It was first developed and licensed in Japan in 1954. In the United States, a JE-MB was available for travelers from 1983 through 1987 on an investigational basis [19], before it became licensed in the United States in 1992. **JE-MB** have been used in many countries for almost half century, during which efficacy of 90% or more has been demonstrated in preventing JE in endemic areas [73, 74]. **JE-MB** have been shown to induce good immune responses between both children in endemic area [70, 75–78] and adults from non-endemic area [79–82]. These **JE-MB** were manufactured by developing countries around the world and used extensively in the expanded immunization programs in endemic areas [83].

Among **JE-MB** adverse events following vaccination were acute disseminated encephalomyelitis (ADEM), which occurred in 1 case per 50,000–1,000,000 doses, while hypersensitivity reactions occurred in 18–64 per 10,000 [83]. Such adverse events seemed to happen more often among persons from non-endemic Western countries [83, 84]. Its main manufacturer, BIKEN (Research Foundation for Microbial Diseases of Osaka University, Japan), ceased production in 2005, and its last batch of vaccine expired in 2011. Administering booster doses of newer-generation JE vaccines to persons previously primed with **JE-MB** was found to be safe and able to induce good anamnestic responses [85–89]. Because of the intense dosing schedule and occasional serious side effects of **JE-MB**, the WHO recommends that they should be replaced by newer vaccine types [1]. However, local productions continue in countries unable to afford newer, safer vaccines.

Live Attenuated JE Virus Vaccines Using the SA-14-14-2 Strain (LAV-SA-14-14-2)

LAV-SA-14-14-2 uses the live, attenuated SA-14-14-2 strain, derived from the wild-type JE strain SA-14 [90, 91], which was first licensed in China in 1988 as CD.JEVAX® (Chengdu Institute of Biological Products, China). Since then, they have been widely used in China and other Asian countries, with over 700 million doses distributed [92] and administered to more than 120 million children [93]. A case-control study in China and Nepal indicated vaccine efficacy of 97–99% [94–96]. A 5-year follow-up study in Nepal estimated continuing efficacy of 96% [97].

In children and adults, **LAV-SA-14-14-2** induces good seroprotection rates [89, 98–100] and, conveniently, can be given concurrently with measles vaccine [101]. Safety surveillance during 30 days post-vaccination among 13,266 children found no differences compared to a control group [102]. Although a rare possible association with acute encephalitis was noted, 4 vaccinees within 2 weeks after vaccination [103] and 9 vaccinees in WHO report [1], this was not felt to be an unsafe signal as the number was extremely low compared to the number of distributed vaccines [92, 93].

Cell Culture-Derived Inactivated JE Vaccine (CC-JE)

CC-JE can be subclassified by the virus strain they use (SA-14-14-2 or Beijing-1 or Beijing-P3 or 821564XY strains) and by the tissue culture cell types in which they are grown; Vero cells, primary hamster kidney (PHK) cells, or other cells. The most common **CC-JE** around the world are those composed of an inactivated SA-14-14-2 virus strain, grown in Vero cells, and thus abbreviated as **JE-VC** in this chapter. IXIARO® and JESPECT® are differing brand names of the same **JE-VC** (Valneva Austria GmbH) which are licensed in 35 countries around the world [104, 105]. JEEV® is manufactured by Biological E (Hyderabad, India) available in South Asia with technology licensed from Valneva [104, 106]. IXIARO® is the only JE vaccine approved for use in the United States since 2009 [107]. Studies of this vaccine in children revealed excellent immunogenicity [108–110]. In adults in North America, Europe, and Australia, the responses were not inferior to **JE-MB** [111], with immunogenicity remaining high for up to 12 months [112]. These long-term immune responses were increased in **JE-VC** recipients who had previously been vaccinated with tick-borne encephalitis (TBE) vaccine [113, 114]. European **JE-VC** study of 200 elderly from 64–83 years of age (median 69) revealed that seroconversion rate was 65% [115] which was lower than the >95% found in a previous trial in adults of median age of 41 years [111]. Thus, a third dose was suggested for the elderly, in whom its safety profile had been acceptable in the two-dose primary series [115].

Another version of **CC-JE** was one made from the Beijing strain of JE virus grown in PHK cell culture. It was produced and used only in China for a limited period [116]. Its immunogenicity was found to be lower than for **JE-VC** and **JE-MB** [117]. KD-287 or ENCEVAC® (Chemo-Sero-Therapeutic Research Institute/Kaketsuken, Kumamoto, Japan), JEBIK®V (BIKEN, Japan), and TC-JEV (Boryung/Star-Bio, South Korea) are **JE-VC** commercially available in Asia. It was found non-inferior to **JE-MB** [118]. JENVAC® (Bharat Biotech, India) is another **CC-JE** variation using Kolar strain in Vero cell (JE virus 821564XY) [119, 120].

Adverse events following **JE-VC** in children were comparable to those of licensed vaccines (pneumococcal conjugate and hepatitis A vaccines) [121], in whom off-label use in travelers was well tolerated [122]. In adults, the common vaccine side effects were similar to those of **JE-MB** but with less local reactogenicity and hypersensitivity [111, 123]. Post-marketing surveillance on **JE-VC** safety in the United States found an overall rate of 15.2 adverse events per 100,000 doses distributed, with no fatalities [124]. Three episodes of serious neurologic symptoms (one encephalitis and two seizures) occurred in recipients of **JE-VC** who had received other vaccines concurrently.

Genetically Engineered JE Chimeric Virus Vaccine (JE-CV)

The prM and E proteins of the SA-14-14-2 JE virus grown in Vero cells were inserted by genetic engineering into a cDNA "backbone" of poxvirus [125] or the 17D strain of yellow fever virus [126], creating a live *chimera*. The one using poxvirus as a backbone ceased its development after the pilot study revealed low immunogenicity and more local reaction comparing to **JE-MB** [125]. IMOJEV® (Sanofi Pasteur, Lyon, France), the only **JE-CV** commercially available, was found to be non-inferior when compared to **JE-MB** among adults from non-JE-endemic areas, with seroconversion rates of up to 99% [127]. The immune response after a single dose of **JE-CV** was comparable to that of **LAV-SA-14-14-2** in RCTs of 274 children aged 12–24 months in Korea [128] and 300 children aged 9–18 months in Thailand [129, 130], with good safety profiles found in both trials. Studies of **JE-CV** children of 2- to 5-year-olds who had been primed with prior doses of other JE vaccine types found boosting with **JE-CV** to be safe and to still induce good immune responses [131–133]. Two studies for neutralizing antibody induced by **JE-CV** against both past and recent wild-type JE viruses circulating in Southeast Asia and India found high levels [64], lasting until the 5-year follow-up after a two-dose series [65].

Adverse reactions to **JE-CV** were significantly less frequent (68%) than after **JE-MB** (82%) in adults in non-endemic areas [127]. Further experience from post-marketing surveillance in Thailand of 10,000 healthy children of ages 9 months to <5 years who received **JE-CV** confirmed its safety [134].

Other Prevention Strategies

As with several other flaviviruses that threaten human health, the main prevention strategies for JE are (1) mosquito and environmental controls, (2) improved epidemiologic surveillance systems in endemic areas, and (3) immunization programs to vaccinate populations at risk.

Mosquito Bite Avoidance and Vector Controls

Recommended routine individual-level protective measures are bed nets, appropriate clothing, and repellants [135]. Environmental efforts to control mosquito vectors require a multidisciplinary approach, which is beyond the scope of this chapter. In short, these must overcome factors driving the emergence of JE such as population growth within the vicinity of poor sanity swine production and wet-rice paddy agriculture [136]. Classic strategies of insecticide use may no longer be as effective because JE vectors have developed resistance due to heavy use of pesticides in rice fields [137, 138]. Biological controls that are environmental-friendly are various [139]. They include plant-borne mosquitocides, repellents, and oviposition deterrents. Mosquito reproduction can also be interrupted by irradiated or chemically sterilized male mosquitos released to mate with females or endosymbiotic bacteria (*Wolbachia* spp.) that induces female sterility [139, 140]. Artificial swamps can lure mosquitoes, whose larvae are eaten by fish or killed by ingestion of the human-harmless bacteria *Bacillus thuringiensis* var. *israelensis*.

Although it is possible to reduce the virus-amplifying role of swine by JE vaccination of piglets, this control method has high cost and low immunogenicity due to passive transfer of maternal immunity [141]. South Korea has implemented this approach as national policy for 30 years; however, human JE outbreaks still emerged [142]. Of course, the control of wildlife that also serves as amplifying virus hosts is difficult, if not impossible. Poverty in most JE-endemic areas also limits improved hygienic practices in swine farming and the mechanization of irrigation practices that might also reduce vector populations.

Improved Epidemiologic Surveillance Systems

The WHO strongly urges JE surveillance in endemic areas to better characterize epidemiologic patterns of the disease and its burden, so that policymakers can compare the costs of prevention programs with their benefits [24]. Serologic surveys are recommended, as the use of solely clinical case definitions is poorly sensitive (65%; 95% CI, 56–73%) and poorly specific (39%; 95% CI, 30–48%) to identify or rule out true JE infections and noninfections, respectively [27]. Overall among the 24 JE at-risk countries in the world, national and/or sentinel surveillance programs for JE exist in 22 (92%) [2]. However, incomplete data and misclassification of JE cases continue to be the challenges leading to imprecise global burden estimation.

Immunization Programs

The use of some vaccines as described above to prevent JE has been shown to have a significant impact on decreasing its incidence in endemic areas [1, 143].

A 2016 survey by the WHO revealed that only 12 (50%) of 24 JE-endemic countries have the JE immunization programs in place [2]. Ten of these 12 countries have added JE vaccine to their routine national immunization programs for all children: Cambodia, China, Japan, Laos, Nepal, South Korea, Sri Lanka, Taiwan, Thailand, and Vietnam. The Philippines, Indonesia, and Myanmar plan to start the nationwide programs in late 2017 or early 2018. Immunization programs or campaigns limited to certain categories, locations, or events do exist. Australia implemented JE vaccination in areas with JE risk (the outer islands in the Torres Strait) [144]. Malaysia and India have programs to cover some of their sub-national jurisdictions. North Korea performed a vaccination campaign in 2016. Singapore decided not to implement routine JE vaccination because only sporadic JE cases are reported. This current patchwork of immunization programs to prevent JE remains a challenge to reducing the burden of the disease.

Special Populations

Travelers

Currently, the incidence of JE infection among travelers is estimated as <1 case per one million travelers to endemic countries [135, 145, 146]. Only 21 travelers with confirmed JE were reported to the US Centers for Disease Control and Prevention (CDC) during 1973–2015 [135]. Consistent with such low risk, a serologic survey in 2007–2010 among 363 short-term Australian travelers returning from Asia found no evidence of JE infection [146] and no case report through GeoSentinel Surveillance in 1997–2007 [147]. In contrast, one report estimated the attack rate of 1 per 400,000 among Swedish travelers visiting Thailand during 1994–2008 [148]. As might be expected, JE risk for travelers varies by visit duration, local destinations visited, activities engaged in, and the season of travel.

As with JE disease among endemic countries, JE in travelers is also devastating. Among 55 international JE-infected travelers reviewed for the period of 1973–2008, the fatality rate was 14%, and prolonged or permanent neuropsychiatric sequelae occurred in 44% of survivors [149]. One fatality (33%) occurred among three reported JE cases among US travelers in 2010–2012 [150]. Of course, such published rates of fatality and long-term morbidity are subject to underestimation, as less severe disease without sequelae may be less likely to be formally reported. In addition to travelers and expatriates at risk for JE, disease occurred among migrants from endemic areas that had never been vaccinated and returned to their JE-endemic homeland [151].

In addition to using personal protective measures to avoid mosquito bites, public health agencies advise expecting travelers and expatriate residents in JE-endemic areas to receive or consider JE vaccination, although with slightly varying recommendations and dosing (Table 11.1) [1, 135, 144, 152–155]. Despite public health recommendations of JE vaccination for travelers at risk, compliance by travelers and/or their physicians has been low (30%) [156]. The main reasons were listed such as physicians thought it was not indicated [156], travelers were not informed by their physicians about JE vaccine [157], and travelers declined because of the

Table 11.1 Japanese encephalitis (JE) vaccine recommendations for travelers from public health agencies

Public health agency: date	Vaccination indications for travelers	Vaccine types and dosing		Suggested timing of vaccination
World Health Organization Strategic Advisory Group of Experts (SAGE): February 2015	– Travel with extensive outdoor exposure (such as camping and hiking) during the transmission season in endemic countries or areas where farming involves irrigation by flooding	1° series	**CC-JE** 2 doses IM on d 0 and d 28 (0.25 mL/dose if age 2 m–2y, 0.5 mL/dose age ≥ 3y) or **JE-CV**, 0.5 mL IM once or **LAV-SA-14-14-2**, age ≥8 m 0.5 mL SC	Details not given
		Booster	**CC-JE** after >1 y with ongoing risk (age ≥17 y) **JE-CV**, 1–2 y after 1° dose age ≥9 m to <18 y. No booster for adults ≥18 y **LAV-SA-14-14-2**, not established	

(continued)

Table 11.1 (continued)

Public health agency: date	Vaccination indications for travelers	Vaccine types and dosing		Suggested timing of vaccination
United States Advisory Committee on Immunization Practices (ACIP): July 2017 update	– Travel ≥1 m in endemic areas during the JE virus transmission season – Travel <1 m to endemic areas during the JE virus transmission season, with travel outside urban areas and activities that increase the risk of JE virus exposure (e.g., substantial time or activities outdoors, accommodations without air conditioning, screens, or bed nets) – Travel to an area with an ongoing JE outbreak – Travel to endemic areas with uncertain specific destinations, activities, or duration of travel	**CC-JE (JE-VC**, IXIARO®**)**		Complete 2-dose 1° series ≥1 week before potential exposure
		1° series	2 doses IM on d 0 and d 28 (0.25 mL/dose if age 2 m-2 y, 0.5 mL/dose age ≥3 y)	
		Booster	After >1 y with ongoing risk (age ≥17 y)	
		Booster after previous **JE-MB**	New 2-dose 1° series of **CC-JE (JE-VC)**	
United Kingdom Public Health England: November 2016 update	– Travel ≥1 m to endemic areas during the transmission season in South Asia, Southeast Asia, and the Far East, especially if travel includes rural areas – Travel <1 m should be considered an indication if risk is sufficient, e.g., spending short periods in rice fields (where the mosquito vector breeds) or close to pig farms (a reservoir host for the virus)	**CC-JE (JE-VC**, IXIARO®**)**		Complete 2-dose 1° series ≥1 week before potential exposure
		1° series	Same as ACIP/USA	
		Booster	Adults at continuing risk, 12–24 m after 1° series (regardless of previous vaccine type)	

Table 11.1 (continued)

Public health agency: date	Vaccination indications for travelers	Vaccine types and dosing		Suggested timing of vaccination
Public Health Agency of Canada: January 2014 update	– Travel >30 d cumulatively in rural areas during the risk season or in urban areas known to be endemic or epidemic for JE – Long-term travelers or expatriates who, while based in urban areas, anticipate making intermittent short trips to rural areas of risk – Travel <30 d cumulatively in rural areas during the season of risk or in urban areas known to be endemic or epidemic for JE, if substantial outdoor activity anticipated or indoors if the area does not exclude mosquitoes, especially during the evening/night	**CC-JE (JE-VC, IXIARO®)**		Complete 2-dose 1° series 10 to 14 d week before potential exposure
		1° series	Same as ACIP/USA, except children indicated as off-label use	
		Booster	Same as ACIP/USA, except children indicated as off-label use	
		Alternative 1° dosing when time until exposure is short	2 doses same day by separate injections on separate limbs	
Australian Technical Advisory Group on Immunization (ATAGI): August 2017 update	– Travel ≥1 m in endemic areas in Asia and Papua New Guinea during the JE virus transmission season, including persons to be based in urban areas but are likely to visit endemic rural or agricultural areas. Also recommended to see US recommendation	1° series	**CC-JE (JE-VC, JESPECT®)**, same as ACIP/USA **JE-CV (IMOJEV®)**, same dosing as WHO	JESPECT® second dose at least 1 week prior to potential exposure IMOJEV® at least 14 days prior to potential exposure
		Booster	**CC-JE (JE-VC, JESPECT®)**, same as ACIP/USA **JE-CV (IMOJEV®)**, same dosing as the WHO	
		Booster after previous **JE-MB** as 1° series	Either **CC-JE (JE-VC)** or **JE-CV**	

1° primary, ***CC-JE*** inactivated tissue culture-grown JE virus vaccine, *IM* intramuscular, ***JE-CV*** genetically engineered JE chimeric JE vaccine, ***JE-MB*** mouse brain-grown inactivated JE virus vaccine, ***JE-VC*** Vero cell tissue culture-grown inactivated vaccines, ***LAV-SA-14-14-2*** live attenuated SA-14-14-2 JE virus vaccine, *m* month, *SC* subcutaneous, *y* year lack of concern about the disease [156] or the cost of vaccination [158]. IXIARO® costs ~US $120–150 per dose in Europe [159, 160] and ~US $250–450 in the United States (Internet survey in 2017). In endemic countries, the price of JE vaccine can be as low as US $16 for **LAV-SA-14-14-2** (CD.JEVAX™) or **JE-CV** (IMOJEV®) [161].

Other Special Populations

Clinical data are very limited on the use of JE vaccine in immunocompromised persons. **JE-MB** could be used safely in children with underlying diseases [162] and with HIV infection. Among HIV-positive children, immune responses to **JE-MB** were lower than in HIV negatives [163], especially among those with low CD4+ cell counts [164]. However, immune responses were comparable to HIV negatives if vaccination occurred after effective antiretroviral therapy [165, 166]. Low JE vaccine seroconversion rates (50%) were reported among 18 post-hematopoietic stem cell transplantation patients after a single dose of **LAV-SA-14-14-2** [167]. The WHO recommends inactivated **CC-JE** over live **LAV-SA-14-14-2** or **JE-CV** among travelers at JE risk who are immunocompromised or pregnant [1]. A report of 24 pregnant women who received **JE-VC** vaccine (IXIARO®), a subcategory of **CC-JE** vaccine, did not report any worrisome outcomes [1].

Another emerging group at risk of JE is the elderly in endemic countries. The incidence of disease in this age was noted to be rising in South Korea [168], Japan [169], and Taiwan [170], even though these countries implemented vaccination programs for over 40 years. The rise in incidence was believed to be the result of waning immunity—natural or by vaccination decades earlier—or increased vulnerability of the unvaccinated and never-infected adults. Study of strategies to prevent JE among the elderly group needs to be pursued.

Research Gaps and Future Issues to Address

A number of gaps in scientific knowledge and programmatic optimization are needed to improve both clinical care and prevention of JE:

- Standardizing the JE neutralization assay for better comparability of results between studies
- Improved sensitivity and specificity of diagnostic tests to confirm JE infection that would be affordable in endemic countries
- Research and development of specific antiviral drugs and other nonspecific medications or therapies to reduce the mortality and long-term neurologic sequelae of JE disease
- Understanding the significance of JE virus genotype and vaccine-induced immunity

- Cost-benefit and cost-effectiveness data on the use of JE vaccine in travelers
- Data on vaccine efficacy and safety, pathogenesis, and treatment strategies in special population, i.e., elderly, immunocompromised hosts, and pregnant women

Acknowledgment The authors acknowledge Dr. Bruce G. Weniger for his editorial advice and assistance.

Conflict of Interest The authors have no conflicts of interest to declare.

References

1. Japanese encephalitis vaccines: WHO position paper – February 2015. Wkly Epidemiol Rec. 2015;90:69–87.
2. Heffelfinger JD, Li X, Batmunkh N, Grabovac V, Diorditsa S, Liyanage JB, et al. Japanese encephalitis surveillance and immunization - Asia and Western Pacific Regions, 2016. MMWR Morb Mortal Wkly Rep. 2017;66:579–83. https://doi.org/10.15585/mmwr.mm6622a3.
3. Rosen L. The natural history of Japanese encephalitis virus. Annu Rev Microbiol. 1986;40:395–414. https://doi.org/10.1146/annurev.mi.40.100186.002143.
4. Miyake M. The pathology of Japanese encephalitis. Bull World Health Organ. 1964;30:153–60.
5. Solomon T, Ni H, Beasley DWC, Ekkelenkamp M, Cardosa MJ, Barrett ADT. Origin and evolution of Japanese encephalitis virus in southeast Asia. J Virol. 2003;77:3091–8. https://doi.org/10.1128/JVI.77.5.3091-3098.2003.
6. Lincoln AF, Sivertson SE. Acute phase of Japanese B encephalitis: two hundred and one cases in American soldiers, Korea, 1950. J Am Med Assoc. 1952;150:268–73. https://doi.org/10.1001/jama.1952.03680040010003.
7. Webster LT. Japanese B encephalitis virus: its differentiation from St. Louis encephalitis virus and relationship to louping ill virus. J Exp Med. 1938;67:609–18.
8. Lewis L, Taylor HG. Japanese B encephalitis; clinical observations in an outbreak on Okinawa Shima. Arch Neurol Psychiatry. 1947;57:430–63.
9. Sabin AB. Epidemic encephalitis in military personnel: isolation of Japanese B virus on Okinawa in 1945, serologic diagnosis, clinical manifestations, epidemiologic aspects and use of mouse brain vaccine. J Am Med Assoc. 1947;133:281–93. https://doi.org/10.1001/jama.1947.02880050001001.
10. Sumiyoshi H, Mori C, Fuke I, Morita K, Kuhara S, Kondou J, et al. Complete nucleotide sequence of the Japanese encephalitis virus genome RNA. Virology. 1987;161:497–510. https://doi.org/10.1016/0042-6822(87)90144-9.
11. Unni SK, Růžek D, Chhatbar C, Mishra R, Johri MK, Singh SK. Japanese encephalitis virus: from genome to infectome. Microbes Infect. 2011;13:312–21. https://doi.org/10.1016/j.micinf.2011.01.002.
12. Chambers TJ, Hahn CS, Galler R, Rice CM. Flavivirus genome organization, expression, and replication. Annu Rev Microbiol. 1990;44:649–88. https://doi.org/10.1146/annurev.mi.44.100190.003245.
13. Holbrook MR. Historical perspectives on flavivirus research. Viruses. 2017;9:E97. https://doi.org/10.3390/v9050097.
14. Han N, Adams J, Fang W, Liu S-Q, Rayner S. Investigation of the genotype III to genotype I shift in Japanese encephalitis virus and the impact on human cases. Virol Sin. 2015;30:277–89. https://doi.org/10.1007/s12250-015-3621-4.
15. Schuh AJ, Ward MJ, Brown AJL, Barrett ADT. Phylogeography of Japanese encephalitis virus: genotype is associated with climate. PLoS Negl Trop Dis. 2013;7:e2411. https://doi.org/10.1371/journal.pntd.0002411.

16. Le Flohic G, Porphyre V, Barbazan P, Gonzalez J-P. Review of climate, landscape, and viral genetics as drivers of the Japanese encephalitis virus ecology. PLoS Negl Trop Dis. 2013;7:e2208. https://doi.org/10.1371/journal.pntd.0002208.

17. Solomon T, Dung NM, Kneen R, Gainsborough M, Vaughn DW, Khanh VT. Japanese encephalitis. J Neurol Neurosurg Psychiatry. 2000;68:405–15. https://doi.org/10.1136/jnnp.68.4.405.

18. Misra UK, Kalita J. Overview: Japanese encephalitis. Prog Neurobiol. 2010;91:108–20. https://doi.org/10.1016/j.pneurobio.2010.01.008.

19. Inactivated Japanese encephalitis virus vaccine. Recommendations of the Advisory Committee on Immunization Practices (ACIP). MMWR Recomm Rep. 1993;42:1–15.

20. Solomon T. Flavivirus encephalitis. N Engl J Med. 2004;351:370–8. https://doi.org/10.1056/NEJMra030476.

21. Sarkari NBS, Thacker AK, Barthwal SP, Mishra VK, Prapann S, Srivastava D, et al. Japanese encephalitis (JE) part II: 14 years' follow-up of survivors. J Neurol. 2012;259:58–69. https://doi.org/10.1007/s00415-011-6131-9.

22. Ding D, Hong Z, Zhao S-J, Clemens JD, Zhou B, Wang B, et al. Long-term disability from acute childhood Japanese encephalitis in Shanghai, China. Am J Trop Med Hyg. 2007;77:528–33.

23. Campbell GL, Hills SL, Fischer M, Jacobson JA, Hoke CH, Hombach JM, et al. Estimated global incidence of Japanese encephalitis: a systematic review. Bull World Health Organ. 2011;89:766–74., 774A–774E. https://doi.org/10.2471/BLT.10.085233.

24. World Health Organization. Manual for the laboratory diagnosis of Japanese encephalitis virus infection. Geneva: WHO; 2007. http://www.who.int/immunization/monitoring_surveillance/burden/laboratory/JE/en/. Accessed 8 Mar 2017.

25. Solomon T, Dung NM, Kneen R, Thao LTT, Gainsborough M, Nisalak A, et al. Seizures and raised intracranial pressure in Vietnamese patients with Japanese encephalitis. Brain J Neurol. 2002;125:1084–93.

26. Sarkari NBS, Thacker AK, Barthwal SP, Mishra VK, Prapann S, Srivastava D, et al. Japanese encephalitis (JE). Part I: clinical profile of 1,282 adult acute cases of four epidemics. J Neurol. 2012;259:47–57. https://doi.org/10.1007/s00415-011-6118-6.

27. Solomon T, Thao TT, Lewthwaite P, Ooi MH, Kneen R, Dung NM, et al. A cohort study to assess the new WHO Japanese encephalitis surveillance standards. Bull World Health Organ. 2008;86:178–86.

28. Solomon T, Kneen R, Dung NM, Khanh VC, Thuy TT, Ha DQ, et al. Poliomyelitis-like illness due to Japanese encephalitis virus. Lancet. 1998;351:1094–7. https://doi.org/10.1016/S0140-6736(97)07509-0.

29. Chung C-C, Lee SS-J, Chen Y-S, Tsai H-C, Wann S-R, Kao C-H, et al. Acute flaccid paralysis as an unusual presenting symptom of Japanese encephalitis: a case report and review of the literature. Infection. 2007;35:30–2. https://doi.org/10.1007/s15010-007-6038-7.

30. Solomon IH, Milner DA. Histopathology of vaccine-preventable diseases. Histopathology. 2017;70:109–22. https://doi.org/10.1111/his.13057.

31. Griffiths MJ, Turtle L, Solomon T. Japanese encephalitis virus infection. Handb Clin Neurol. 2014;123:561–76. https://doi.org/10.1016/B978-0-444-53488-0.00026-2.

32. Kedarnath N, Prasad SR, Dandawate CN, Koshy AA, George S, Ghosh SN. Isolation of Japanese encephalitis & West Nile viruses from peripheral blood of encephalitis patients. Indian J Med Res. 1984;79:1–7.

33. Chanama S, Sukprasert W, Sa-ngasang A, A-nuegoonpipat A, Sangkitporn S, Kurane I, et al. Detection of Japanese encephalitis (JE) virus-specific IgM in cerebrospinal fluid and serum samples from JE patients. Jpn J Infect Dis. 2005;58:294–6.

34. Burke DS, Nisalak A, Ussery MA, Laorakpongse T, Chantavibul S. Kinetics of IgM and IgG responses to Japanese encephalitis virus in human serum and cerebrospinal fluid. J Infect Dis. 1985;151:1093–9.

35. Dubot-Pérès A, Sengvilaipaseuth O, Chanthongthip A, Newton PN, de Lamballerie X. How many patients with anti-JEV IgM in cerebrospinal fluid really have Japanese encephalitis? Lancet Infect Dis. 2015;15:1376–7. https://doi.org/10.1016/S1473-3099(15)00405-3.
36. Makino Y, Tadano M, Saito M, Maneekarn N, Sittisombut N, Sirisanthana V, et al. Studies on serological cross-reaction in sequential flavivirus infections. Microbiol Immunol. 1994;38:951–5.
37. Singh KP, Mishra G, Jain P, Pandey N, Nagar R, Gupta S, et al. Co-positivity of anti-dengue virus and anti-Japanese encephalitis virus IgM in endemic area: co-infection or cross reactivity? Asian Pac J Trop Med. 2014;7:124–9. https://doi.org/10.1016/S1995-7645(14)60007-9.
38. A-Nuegoonpipat A, Panthuyosri N, Anantapreecha S, Chanama S, Sa-Ngasang A, Sawanpanyalert P, et al. Cross-reactive IgM responses in patients with dengue or Japanese encephalitis. J Clin Virol. 2008;42:75–7. https://doi.org/10.1016/j.jcv.2007.10.030.
39. Garg RK, Malhotra HS, Gupta A, Kumar N, Jain A. Concurrent dengue virus and Japanese encephalitis virus infection of the brain: is it co-infection or co-detection? Infection. 2012;40:589–93. https://doi.org/10.1007/s15010-012-0284-z.
40. Gowri Sankar S, Balaji T, Venkatasubramani K, Thenmozhi V, Dhananjeyan KJ, Paramasivan R, et al. Dengue NS1 and prM antibodies increase the sensitivity of acute dengue diagnosis test and differentiate from Japanese encephalitis infection. J Immunol Methods. 2014;407:116–9. https://doi.org/10.1016/j.jim.2014.03.028.
41. Swami R, Ratho RK, Mishra B, Singh MP. Usefulness of RT-PCR for the diagnosis of Japanese encephalitis in clinical samples. Scand J Infect Dis. 2008;40:815–20. https://doi.org/10.1080/00365540802227102.
42. Saxena V, Mishra VK, Dhole TN. Evaluation of reverse-transcriptase PCR as a diagnostic tool to confirm Japanese encephalitis virus infection. Trans R Soc Trop Med Hyg. 2009;103:403–6. https://doi.org/10.1016/j.trstmh.2009.01.021.
43. Huang J-L, Lin H-T, Wang Y-M, Weng M-H, Ji D-D, Kuo M-D, et al. Sensitive and specific detection of strains of Japanese encephalitis virus using a one-step TaqMan RT-PCR technique. J Med Virol. 2004;74:589–96. https://doi.org/10.1002/jmv.20218.
44. Wu X, Lin H, Chen S, Xiao L, Yang M, An W, et al. Development and application of a reverse transcriptase droplet digital PCR (RT-ddPCR) for sensitive and rapid detection of Japanese encephalitis virus. J Virol Methods. 2017;248:166–71. https://doi.org/10.1016/j.jviromet.2017.06.015.
45. Zhao H, Wang Y-G, Deng Y-Q, Song K-Y, Li X-F, Wang H-J, et al. Japanese encephalitis virus RNA not detected in urine. Clin Infect Dis. 2013;57:157–8. https://doi.org/10.1093/cid/cit169.
46. Mai NTH, Phu NH, Nhu LNT, Hong NTT, Hanh NHH, Nguyet LA, et al. Central nervous system infection diagnosis by next-generation sequencing: a glimpse into the future? Open Forum Infect Dis. 2017;4:ofx046. https://doi.org/10.1093/ofid/ofx046.
47. Rao PN. Japanese encephalitis. Indian Pediatr. 2001;38:1252–64.
48. Kumar R, Tripathi P, Baranwal M, Singh S, Tripathi S, Banerjee G. Randomized, controlled trial of oral ribavirin for Japanese encephalitis in children in Uttar Pradesh, India. Clin Infect Dis. 2009;48:400–6. https://doi.org/10.1086/596309.
49. Harinasuta C, Nimmanitya S, Titsyakorn U. The effect of interferon-alpha A on two cases of Japanese encephalitis in Thailand. Southeast Asian J Trop Med Public Health. 1985;16:332–6.
50. Rose MR, Hughes SM, Gatus BJ. A case of Japanese B encephalitis imported into the United Kingdom. J Infect. 1983;6:261–5.
51. Caramello P, Canta F, Balbiano R, Lipani F, Ariaudo S, Agostini MD, et al. Role of intravenous immunoglobulin administration in Japanese encephalitis. Clin Infect Dis. 2006;43:1620–1. https://doi.org/10.1086/509644.
52. Solomon T, Dung NM, Wills B, Kneen R, Gainsborough M, Diet TV, et al. Interferon alfa-2a in Japanese encephalitis: a randomised double-blind placebo-controlled trial. Lancet. 2003;361:821–6.

53. Hoke CH, Vaughn DW, Nisalak A, Intralawan P, Poolsuppasit S, Jongsawas V, et al. Effect of high-dose dexamethasone on the outcome of acute encephalitis due to Japanese encephalitis virus. J Infect Dis. 1992;165:631–7.

54. Shimoni Z, Niven MJ, Pitlick S, Bulvik S. Treatment of West Nile virus encephalitis with intravenous immunoglobulin. Emerg Infect Dis. 2001;7:759. https://doi.org/10.3201/eid0704.010432.

55. Rhee C, Eaton EF, Concepcion W, Blackburn BG. West Nile virus encephalitis acquired via liver transplantation and clinical response to intravenous immunoglobulin: case report and review of the literature. Transpl Infect Dis. 2011;13:312–7. https://doi.org/10.1111/j.1399-3062.2010.00595.x.

56. Rajapakse S. Intravenous immunoglobulins in the treatment of dengue illness. Trans R Soc Trop Med Hyg. 2009;103:867–70. https://doi.org/10.1016/j.trstmh.2008.12.011.

57. Růžek D, Dobler G, Niller HH. May early intervention with high dose intravenous immuno-globulin pose a potentially successful treatment for severe cases of tick-borne encephalitis? BMC Infect Dis. 2013;13:306. https://doi.org/10.1186/1471-2334-13-306.

58. Rayamajhi A, Nightingale S, Bhatta NK, Singh R, Ledger E, Bista KP, et al. A prelimi-nary randomized double blind placebo-controlled trial of intravenous immunoglobulin for Japanese encephalitis in Nepal. PLoS One. 2015;10:e0122608. https://doi.org/10.1371/journal.pone.0122608.

59. Dutta K, Mishra MK, Nazmi A, Kumawat KL, Basu A. Minocycline differentially modulates macrophage mediated peripheral immune response following Japanese encephalitis virus infection. Immunobiology. 2010;215:884–93. https://doi.org/10.1016/j.imbio.2009.12.003.

60. Das S, Dutta K, Kumawat KL, Ghoshal A, Adhya D, Basu A. Abrogated inflammatory response promotes neurogenesis in a murine model of Japanese encephalitis. PLoS One. 2011;6:e17225. https://doi.org/10.1371/journal.pone.0017225.

61. Kumar R, Basu A, Sinha S, Das M, Tripathi P, Jain A, et al. Role of oral Minocycline in acute encephalitis syndrome in India - a randomized controlled trial. BMC Infect Dis. 2016;16:67. https://doi.org/10.1186/s12879-016-1385-6.

62. Singh AK, Mehta A, Kushwaha KP, Pandey AK, Mittal M, Sharma B, et al. Minocycline trial in Japanese encephalitis: a double blind, randomized placebo study. Int J Pediatr Res. 2016;3:371–5.

63. Basu A, Dutta K. Recent advances in Japanese encephalitis. F1000Res. 2017;6:259. https://doi.org/10.12688/f1000research.9561.1.

64. Bonaparte M, Dweik B, Feroldi E, Meric C, Bouckenooghe A, Hildreth S, et al. Immune response to live-attenuated Japanese encephalitis vaccine (JE-CV) neutralizes Japanese encephalitis virus isolates from South-East Asia and India. BMC Infect Dis. 2014;14:156. https://doi.org/10.1186/1471-2334-14-156.

65. Feroldi E, Boaz M, Yoksan S, Chokephaibulkit K, Thisyakorn U, Pancharoen C, et al. Persistence of wild-type Japanese encephalitis virus strains cross-neutralization 5 years after JE-CV immunization. J Infect Dis. 2017;215:221–7. https://doi.org/10.1093/infdis/jiw533.

66. Cao L, Fu S, Gao X, Li M, Cui S, Li X, et al. Low protective efficacy of the current Japanese encephalitis vaccine against the emerging genotype 5 Japanese encephalitis virus. PLoS Negl Trop Dis. 2016;10:e0004686. https://doi.org/10.1371/journal.pntd.0004686.

67. Takhampunya R, Kim H-C, Tippayachai B, Kengluecha A, Klein TA, Lee W-J, et al. Emergence of Japanese encephalitis virus genotype V in the Republic of Korea. Virol J. 2011;8:449. https://doi.org/10.1186/1743-422X-8-449.

68. Kim H, Cha G-W, Jeong YE, Lee W-G, Chang KS, Roh JY, et al. Detection of Japanese encephalitis virus genotype V in Culex orientalis and Culex pipiens (Diptera: Culicidae) in Korea. PLoS One. 2015;10:e0116547. https://doi.org/10.1371/journal.pone.0116547.

69. Hegde NR, Gore MM. Japanese encephalitis vaccines: immunogenicity, protective efficacy, effectiveness, and impact on the burden of disease. Hum Vaccin Immunother. 2017;0:1–18. https://doi.org/10.1080/21645515.2017.1285472.

70. Nimmannitya S, Hutamai S, Kalayanarooj S, Rojanasuphot S. A field study on Nakayama and Beijing strains of Japanese encephalitis vaccines. Southeast Asian J Trop Med Public Health. 1995;26:689–93.

71. Kurane I, Takasaki T. Immunogenicity and protective efficacy of the current inactivated Japanese encephalitis vaccine against different Japanese encephalitis virus strains. Vaccine. 2000;18(Suppl 2):33–5.

72. Yun S-I, Lee Y-M. Japanese encephalitis: the virus and vaccines. Hum Vaccin Immunother. 2014;10:263–79. https://doi.org/10.4161/hv.26902.

73. Hsu TC, Chow LP, Wei HY, Chen CL, Hsu ST. A controlled field trial for an evaluation of effectiveness of mouse-brain Japanese encephalitis vaccine. Taiwan Yi Xue Hui Za Zhi. 1971;70:55–62.

74. Hoke CH, Nisalak A, Sangawhipa N, Jatanasen S, Laorakapongse T, Innis BL, et al. Protection against Japanese encephalitis by inactivated vaccines. N Engl J Med. 1988;319:608–14. https://doi.org/10.1056/NEJM198809083191004.

75. Rojanasuphot S, Charoensuk O, Kitprayura D, Likityingvara C, Limpisthien S, Boonyindee S, et al. A field trial of Japanese encephalitis vaccine produced in Thailand. Southeast Asian J Trop Med Public Health. 1989;20:653–4.

76. Gowal D, Tahlan AK. Evaluation of effectiveness of mouse brain inactivated Japanese encephalitis vaccine produced in India. Indian J Med Res. 1995;102:267–71.

77. Muangchana C, Henprasertthae N, Nurach K, Theppang K, Yoocharoen P, Varinsathien P, et al. Effectiveness of mouse brain-derived inactivated Japanese encephalitis vaccine in Thai National Immunization Program: a case-control study. Vaccine. 2012;30:361–7. https://doi.org/10.1016/j.vaccine.2011.10.083.

78. Marks F, Nguyen TTY, Tran ND, Nguyen MH, Vu HH, Meyer CG, et al. Effectiveness of the Viet Nam produced, mouse brain-derived, inactivated Japanese encephalitis vaccine in Northern Viet Nam. PLoS Negl Trop Dis. 2012;6:e1952. https://doi.org/10.1371/journal.pntd.0001952.

79. Poland JD, Cropp CB, Craven RB, Monath TP. Evaluation of the potency and safety of inactivated Japanese encephalitis vaccine in US inhabitants. J Infect Dis. 1990;161:878–82.

80. Henderson A. Immunisation against Japanese encephalitis in Nepal: experience of 1152 subjects. J R Army Med Corps. 1984;130:188–91.

81. Defraites RF, Gambel JM, Hoke CH, Sanchez JL, Withers BG, Karabatsos N, et al. Japanese encephalitis vaccine (inactivated, BIKEN) in U.S. soldiers: immunogenicity and safety of vaccine administered in two dosing regimens. Am J Trop Med Hyg. 1999;61:288–93.

82. Sanchez JL, Hoke CH, McCown J, DeFraites RF, Takafuji ET, Diniega BM, et al. Further experience with Japanese encephalitis vaccine. Lancet. 1990;335:972–3.

83. Fischer M, Lindsey N, Staples JE, Hills S, Centers for Disease Control and Prevention (CDC). Japanese encephalitis vaccines: recommendations of the Advisory Committee on Immunization Practices (ACIP). MMWR Recomm Rep. 2010;59:1–27.

84. Plesner A-M. Allergic reactions to Japanese encephalitis vaccine. Immunol Allergy Clin North Am. 2003;23:665–97.

85. Erra EO, Askling HH, Rombo L, Riutta J, Vene S, Yoksan S, et al. A single dose of vero cell-derived Japanese encephalitis (JE) vaccine (Ixiaro) effectively boosts immunity in travelers primed with mouse brain-derived JE vaccines. Clin Infect Dis. 2012;55:825–34. https://doi.org/10.1093/cid/cis542.

86. Erra EO, Askling HH, Yoksan S, Rombo L, Riutta J, Vene S, et al. Cross-protection elicited by primary and booster vaccinations against Japanese encephalitis: a two-year follow-up study. Vaccine. 2013;32:119–23. https://doi.org/10.1016/j.vaccine.2013.10.055.

87. Woolpert T, Staples JE, Faix DJ, Nett RJ, Kosoy OI, Biggerstaff BJ, et al. Immunogenicity of one dose of Vero cell culture-derived Japanese encephalitis (JE) vaccine in adults previously vaccinated with mouse brain-derived JE vaccine. Vaccine. 2012;30:3090–6. https://doi.org/10.1016/j.vaccine.2012.02.063.

88. Wijesinghe PR, Abeysinghe MRN, Yoksan S, Yao Y, Zhou B, Zhang L, et al. Immunogenicity of live attenuated Japanese encephalitis SA 14-14-2 vaccine among Sri Lankan children with previous receipt of inactivated JE vaccine. Vaccine. 2016;34:5923–8. https://doi.org/10.1016/j.vaccine.2016.10.028.

89. Sohn YM, Park MS, Rho HO, Chandler LJ, Shope RE, Tsai TF. Primary and booster immune responses to SA14-14-2 Japanese encephalitis vaccine in Korean infants. Vaccine. 1999;17:2259–64.

90. Eckels KH, Yu YX, Dubois DR, Marchette NJ, Trent DW, Johnson AJ. Japanese encephalitis virus live-attenuated vaccine, Chinese strain SA14-14-2; adaptation to primary canine kidney cell cultures and preparation of a vaccine for human use. Vaccine. 1988;6:513–8.

91. Yu Y. Phenotypic and genotypic characteristics of Japanese encephalitis attenuated live vaccine virus SA14-14-2 and their stabilities. Vaccine. 2010;28:3635–41. https://doi.org/10.1016/j.vaccine.2010.02.105.

92. Ginsburg AS, Meghani A, Halstead SB, Yaich M. Use of the live attenuated Japanese Encephalitis vaccine SA 14-14-2 in children: a review of safety and tolerability studies. Hum Vaccin Immunother. 2017;13(10):2222–31. https://doi.org/10.1080/21645515.2017.1356496.

93. Halstead SB, Thomas SJ. Japanese encephalitis: new options for active immunization. Clin Infect Dis. 2010;50:1155–64. https://doi.org/10.1086/651271.

94. Hennessy S, Liu Z, Tsai TF, Strom BL, Wan CM, Liu HL, et al. Effectiveness of live-attenuated Japanese encephalitis vaccine (SA14-14-2): a case-control study. Lancet. 1996;347:1583–6.

95. Bista MB, Banerjee M, Shin SH, Tandan J, Kim MH, Sohn YM, et al. Efficacy of single-dose SA 14–14–2 vaccine against Japanese encephalitis: a case control study. Lancet. 2001;358:791–5. https://doi.org/10.1016/S0140-6736(01)05967-0.

96. Ohrr H, Tandan JB, Sohn YM, Shin SH, Pradhan DP, Halstead SB. Effect of single dose of SA 14-14-2 vaccine 1 year after immunization in Nepalese children with Japanese encephalitis: a case-control study. Lancet. 2005;366:1375–8. https://doi.org/10.1016/S0140-6736(05)67567-8.

97. Tandan JB, Ohrr H, Sohn YM, Yoksan S, Ji M, Nam CM, et al. Single dose of SA 14-14-2 vaccine provides long-term protection against Japanese encephalitis: a case-control study in Nepalese children 5 years after immunization. Vaccine. 2007;25:5041–5. https://doi.org/10.1016/j.vaccine.2007.04.052.

98. Khan SA, Kakati S, Dutta P, Chowdhury P, Borah J, Topno R, et al. Immunogenicity & safety of a single dose of live-attenuated Japanese encephalitis vaccine SA 14-14-2 in adults. Indian J Med Res. 2016;144:886–92. https://doi.org/10.4103/ijmr.IJMR_712_15.

99. Kwon HJ, Lee SY, Kim KH, Kim DS, Cha SH, Jo DS, et al. The immunogenicity and safety of the live-attenuated SA 14-14-2 Japanese encephalitis vaccine given with a two-dose primary schedule in children. J Korean Med Sci. 2015;30:612–6. https://doi.org/10.3346/jkms.2015.30.5.612.

100. Turtle L, Tatullo F, Bali T, Ravi V, Soni M, Chan S, et al. Cellular Immune Responses to Live Attenuated Japanese Encephalitis (JE) vaccine SA14-14-2 in adults in a JE/dengue co-endemic area. PLoS Negl Trop Dis. 2017;11:e0005263. https://doi.org/10.1371/journal.pntd.0005263.

101. Gatchalian S, Yao Y, Zhou B, Zhang L, Yoksan S, Kelly K, et al. Comparison of the immunogenicity and safety of measles vaccine administered alone or with live, attenuated Japanese encephalitis SA 14-14-2 vaccine in Philippine infants. Vaccine. 2008;26:2234–41. https://doi.org/10.1016/j.vaccine.2008.02.042.

102. Liu ZL, Hennessy S, Strom BL, Tsai TF, Wan CM, Tang SC, et al. Short-term safety of live attenuated Japanese encephalitis vaccine (SA14-14-2): results of a randomized trial with 26,239 subjects. J Infect Dis. 1997;176:1366–9.

103. Jia N, Zhao Q-M, Guo X-F, Cheng J-X, Wu C, Zuo S-Q, et al. Encephalitis temporally associated with live attenuated Japanese encephalitis vaccine: four case reports. BMC Infect Dis. 2011;11:344. https://doi.org/10.1186/1471-2334-11-344.

104. Japanese encephalitis vaccine – Valneva Products. http://www.valneva.com/en/products/japanese-encephalitis-vaccine. Accessed 4 Sep 2017.

105. Firbas C, Jilma B. Product reviews on the JE vaccine IXIARO. Hum Vaccin Immunother. 2015;11:411–20. https://doi.org/10.4161/21645515.2014.983412.

106. Centers for Disease Control and Prevention (CDC). Use of Japanese encephalitis vaccine in children: recommendations of the advisory committee on immunization practices, 2013. MMWR Morb Mortal Wkly Rep. 2013;62:898–900.

107. Research C for BE and. Approved Products - IXIARO. FDA. https://www.fda.gov/biologics-bloodvaccines/vaccines/approvedproducts/ucm179132.htm. Accessed 23 June 2017.
108. Kaltenböck A, Dubischar-Kastner K, Schuller E, Datla M, Klade CS, Kishore TSA. Immunogenicity and safety of IXIARO (IC51) in a Phase II study in healthy Indian children between 1 and 3 years of age. Vaccine. 2010;28:834–9. https://doi.org/10.1016/j.vaccine.2009.10.024.
109. Dubischar KL, Kadlecek V, Sablan B, Borja-Tabora CF, Gatchalian S, Eder-Lingelbach S, et al. Immunogenicity of the inactivated Japanese encephalitis virus vaccine IXIARO® n children from a Japanese encephalitis virus -endemic region. Pediatr Infect Dis J. 2017;36(9):898–904. https://doi.org/10.1097/INF.0000000000001615.
110. Paulke-Korinek M, Kollaritsch H, Kundi M, Zwazl I, Seidl-Friedrich C, Jelinek T. Persistence of antibodies six years after booster vaccination with inactivated vaccine against Japanese encephalitis. Vaccine. 2015;33:3600–4. https://doi.org/10.1016/j.vaccine.2015.05.037.
111. Tauber E, Kollaritsch H, Korinek M, Rendi-Wagner P, Jilma B, Firbas C, et al. Safety and immunogenicity of a Vero-cell-derived, inactivated Japanese encephalitis vaccine: a non-inferiority, phase III, randomised controlled trial. Lancet. 2007;370:1847–53. https://doi.org/10.1016/S0140-6736(07)61780-2.
112. Schuller E, Jilma B, Voicu V, Golor G, Kollaritsch H, Kaltenböck A, et al. Long-term immunogenicity of the new Vero cell-derived, inactivated Japanese encephalitis virus vaccine IC51 Six and 12 month results of a multicenter follow-up phase 3 study. Vaccine. 2008;26:4382–6. https://doi.org/10.1016/j.vaccine.2008.05.081.
113. Schuller E, Klade CS, Heinz FX, Kollaritsch H, Rendi-Wagner P, Jilma B, et al. Effect of pre-existing anti-tick-borne encephalitis virus immunity on neutralizing antibody response to the Vero cell-derived, inactivated Japanese encephalitis virus vaccine candidate IC51. Vaccine. 2008;26:6151–6. https://doi.org/10.1016/j.vaccine.2008.08.056.
114. Eder S, Dubischar-Kastner K, Firbas C, Jelinek T, Jilma B, Kaltenboeck A, et al. Long term immunity following a booster dose of the inactivated Japanese encephalitis vaccine IXIARO®, IC51. Vaccine. 2011;29:2607–12. https://doi.org/10.1016/j.vaccine.2011.01.058.
115. Cramer JP, Dubischar K, Eder S, Burchard GD, Jelinek T, Jilma B, et al. Immunogenicity and safety of the inactivated Japanese encephalitis vaccine IXIARO® in elderly subjects: open-label, uncontrolled, multi-center, phase 4 study. Vaccine. 2016;34:4579–85. https://doi.org/10.1016/j.vaccine.2016.07.029.
116. Li X, Ma S-J, Liu X, Jiang L-N, Zhou J-H, Xiong Y-Q, et al. Immunogenicity and safety of currently available Japanese encephalitis vaccines: a systematic review. Hum Vaccin Immunother. 2015;10:3579–93. https://doi.org/10.4161/21645515.2014.980197.
117. Wang S-Y, Cheng X-H, Li J-X, Li X-Y, Zhu F-C, Liu P. Comparing the immunogenicity and safety of 3 Japanese encephalitis vaccines in Asia-Pacific area: a systematic review and meta-analysis. Hum Vaccin Immunother. 2015;11:1418–25. https://doi.org/10.1080/21645515.2015.1011996.
118. Miyazaki C, Okada K, Ozaki T, Hirose M, Iribe K, Yokote H, et al. Phase III clinical trials comparing the immunogenicity and safety of the Vero cell-derived Japanese encephalitis vaccine Encevac with those of mouse brain-derived vaccine by using the Beijing-1 strain. Clin Vaccine Immunol. 2014;21:188–95. https://doi.org/10.1128/CVI.00377-13.
119. Indian Academy of Pediatrics, Advisory Committee on Vaccines and Immunization Practices (acvip), Vashishtha VM, Kalra A, Bose A, Choudhury P, Yewale VN, et al. Indian Academy of Pediatrics (IAP) recommended immunization schedule for children aged 0 through 18 years, India, 2013 and updates on immunization. Indian Pediatr. 2013;50:1095–108.
120. Aggarwal A, Garg N. Newer vaccines against mosquito-borne diseases. Indian J Pediatr. 2017;85(2):117–23. https://doi.org/10.1007/s12098-017-2383-4.
121. Dubischar KL, Kadlecek V, Sablan B, Borja-Tabora CF, Gatchalian S, Eder-Lingelbach S, et al. Safety of the inactivated Japanese encephalitis virus vaccine IXIARO® in children - an open-label, randomized, active-controlled, phase 3 study. Pediatr Infect Dis J. 2017;36(9):889–97. https://doi.org/10.1097/INF.0000000000001623.
122. Butler S, Sutter D, Maranich A. Tolerability of Japanese encephalitis vaccine in pediatric patients. Pediatr Infect Dis J. 2017;6:149–52. https://doi.org/10.1093/jpids/piw029.

123. Dubischar-Kastner K, Kaltenboeck A, Klingler A, Jilma B, Schuller E. Safety analysis of a Vero-cell culture derived Japanese encephalitis vaccine, IXIARO® (IC51), in 6 months of follow-up. Vaccine. 2010;28:6463–9. https://doi.org/10.1016/j.vaccine.2010.07.040.

124. Rabe IB, Miller ER, Fischer M, Hills SL. Adverse events following vaccination with an inactivated, Vero cell culture-derived Japanese encephalitis vaccine in the United States, 2009–2012. Vaccine. 2015;33:708–12. https://doi.org/10.1016/j.vaccine.2014.11.046.

125. Kanesa-thasan N, Smucny JJ, Hoke CH, Marks DH, Konishi E, Kurane I, et al. Safety and immunogenicity of NYVAC-JEV and ALVAC-JEV attenuated recombinant Japanese encephalitis virus--poxvirus vaccines in vaccinia-nonimmune and vaccinia-immune humans. Vaccine. 2000;19:483–91.

126. Chambers TJ, Nestorowicz A, Mason PW, Rice CM. Yellow fever/Japanese encephalitis chimeric viruses: construction and biological properties. J Virol. 1999;73:3095–101.

127. Torresi J, McCarthy K, Feroldi E, Méric C. Immunogenicity, safety and tolerability in adults of a new single-dose, live-attenuated vaccine against Japanese encephalitis: randomised controlled phase 3 trials. Vaccine. 2010;28:7993–8000. https://doi.org/10.1016/j.vaccine.2010.09.035.

128. Kim DS, Houillon G, Jang GC, Cha S-H, Choi S-H, Lee J, et al. A randomized study of the immunogenicity and safety of Japanese encephalitis chimeric virus vaccine (JE-CV) in comparison with SA14-14-2 vaccine in children in the Republic of Korea. Hum Vaccin Immunother. 2014;10:2656–63. https://doi.org/10.4161/hv.29743.

129. Feroldi E, Pancharoen C, Kosalaraksa P, Chokephaibulkit K, Boaz M, Meric C, et al. Primary immunization of infants and toddlers in Thailand with Japanese encephalitis chimeric virus vaccine in comparison with SA14-14-2: a randomized study of immunogenicity and safety. Pediatr Infect Dis J. 2014;33:643–9. https://doi.org/10.1097/INF.0000000000000276.

130. Kosalaraksa P, Watanaveeradej V, Pancharoen C, Capeding MR, Feroldi E, Bouckenooghe A. Long-term immunogenicity of a single dose of Japanese encephalitis chimeric virus vaccine in toddlers and booster response 5 years after primary immunization. Pediatr Infect Dis J. 2017;36:e108–13. https://doi.org/10.1097/INF.0000000000001494.

131. Chokephaibulkit K, Sirivichayakul C, Thisyakorn U, Sabchareon A, Pancharoen C, Bouckenooghe A, et al. Safety and immunogenicity of a single administration of live-attenuated Japanese encephalitis vaccine in previously primed 2- to 5-year-olds and naive 12- to 24-month-olds: multicenter randomized controlled trial. Pediatr Infect Dis J. 2010;29:1111–7. https://doi.org/10.1097/INF.0b013e3181f68e9c.

132. Janewongwirot P, Puthanakit T, Anugulruengkitt S, Jantarabenjakul W, Phasomsap C, Chumket S, et al. Immunogenicity of a Japanese encephalitis chimeric virus vaccine as a booster dose after primary vaccination with SA14-14-2 vaccine in Thai children. Vaccine. 2016;34:5279–83. https://doi.org/10.1016/j.vaccine.2016.09.005.

133. Sricharoenchai S, Lapphra K, Chuenkitmongkol S, Phongsamart W, Bouckenooghe A, Wittawatmongkol O, et al. Immunogenicity of a live attenuated chimeric Japanese encephalitis vaccine as a booster dose after primary vaccination with live attenuated SA14-14-2 vaccine: a phase IV study in Thai children. Pediatr Infect Dis J. 2017;36:e45–7. https://doi.org/10.1097/INF.0000000000001395.

134. Chotpitayasunondh T, Pruekprasert P, Puthanakit T, Pancharoen C, Tangsathapornpong A, Oberdorfer P, et al. Post-licensure, phase IV, safety study of a live attenuated Japanese encephalitis recombinant vaccine in children in Thailand. Vaccine. 2017;35:299–304. https://doi.org/10.1016/j.vaccine.2016.11.062.

135. Japanese encephalitis – Chapter 3 – 2018 Yellow Book | Travelers' Health | CDC. https://wwwnc.cdc.gov/travel/yellowbook/2018/infectious-diseases-related-to-travel/japanese-encephalitis. Accessed 13 June 2017.

136. Erlanger TE, Weiss S, Keiser J, Utzinger J, Wiedenmayer K. Past, present, and future of Japanese encephalitis. Emerg Infect Dis. 2009;15:1–7. https://doi.org/10.3201/eid1501.080311.

137. Dhiman S, Rabha B, Talukdar PK, Das NG, Yadav K, Baruah I, et al. DDT & deltamethrin resistance status of known Japanese encephalitis vectors in Assam, India. Indian J Med Res. 2013;138:988–94.
138. Karunaratne SH, Hemingway J. Insecticide resistance spectra and resistance mechanisms in populations of Japanese encephalitis vector mosquitoes, Culex tritaeniorhynchus and Cx. gelidus, in Sri Lanka. Med Vet Entomol. 2000;14:430–6.
139. Benelli G, Jeffries CL, Walker T. Biological control of mosquito vectors: past, present, and future. Insects. 2016;7:E52. https://doi.org/10.3390/insects7040052.
140. Jeffries CL, Walker T. The potential use of wolbachia-based mosquito biocontrol strategies for Japanese encephalitis. PLoS Negl Trop Dis. 2015;9:e0003576. https://doi.org/10.1371/journal.pntd.0003576.
141. Riley S, Leung GM, Ho LM, Cowling BJ. Transmission of Japanese encephalitis virus in Hong Kong. Hong Kong Med J. 2012;18(Suppl 2):45–6.
142. Mansfield KL, Hernández-Triana LM, Banyard AC, Fooks AR, Johnson N. Japanese encephalitis virus infection, diagnosis and control in domestic animals. Vet Microbiol. 2017;201:85–92. https://doi.org/10.1016/j.vetmic.2017.01.014.
143. World Health Organization SAGE Working Group on Japanese Encephalitis Vaccines. Background paper on Japanese encephalitis vaccines—SAGE working group. Geneva: World Health Organization; 2014. http://www.who.int/immunization/sage/meetings/2014/october/1_JE_Vaccine_Background_Paper.pdf?ua=. Accessed 7 Sep 2017.
144. Australian Government Department of Health. 4.8 Japanese encephalitis. 2017. http://www.immunise.health.gov.au/internet/immunise/publishing.nsf/Content/Handbook10-home~handbook10part4~handbook10-4-8. Accessed 7 Sep 2017.
145. Steffen R, Behrens RH, Hill DR, Greenaway C, Leder K. Vaccine-preventable travel health risks: what is the evidence—what are the gaps? J Travel Med. 2015;22:1–12. https://doi.org/10.1111/jtm.12171.
146. Ratnam I, Leder K, Black J, Biggs B-A, Matchett E, Padiglione A, et al. Low risk of Japanese encephalitis in short-term Australian travelers to Asia. J Travel Med. 2013;20:206–8. https://doi.org/10.1111/jtm.12019.
147. Boggild AK, Castelli F, Gautret P, Torresi J, von Sonnenburg F, Barnett ED, et al. Vaccine preventable diseases in returned international travelers: results from the GeoSentinel Surveillance Network. Vaccine. 2010;28:7389–95. https://doi.org/10.1016/j.vaccine.2010.09.009.
148. Buhl MR, Lindquist L. Japanese encephalitis in travelers: review of cases and seasonal risk. J Travel Med. 2009;16:217–9. https://doi.org/10.1111/j.1708-8305.2009.00333.x.
149. Hills SL, Griggs AC, Fischer M. Japanese encephalitis in travelers from non-endemic countries, 1973–2008. Am J Trop Med Hyg. 2010;82:930–6. https://doi.org/10.4269/ajtmh.2010.09-0676.
150. Hills SL, Stoltey J, Martínez D, Kim PY, Sheriff H, Zangeneh A, et al. A case series of three US adults with Japanese encephalitis, 2010–2012. J Travel Med. 2014;21:310–3. https://doi.org/10.1111/jtm.12127.
151. Centers for Disease Control and Prevention (CDC). Japanese encephalitis among three U.S. travelers returning from Asia, 2003–2008. MMWR Morb Mortal Wkly Rep. 2009;58:737–40.
152. WHO. International travel and health Chapter 6 Vaccine-preventable diseases and vaccines. Geneva: WHO; 2017. http://www.who.int/ith/en/. Accessed 25 June 2017.
153. Immunisation against infectious disease – GOV.UK. https://www.gov.uk/government/collections/immunisation-against-infectious-disease-the-green-book. Accessed 25 June 2017.
154. Canada PHA of, Canada PHA of. Page 11: Canadian immunization guide: part 4 – active vaccines. 2007. https://www.canada.ca/en/public-health/services/publications/healthy-living/canadian-immunization-guide-part-4-active-vaccines/page-11-japanese-encephalitis-vaccine.html. Accessed 25 June 2017.
155. Batchelor P, Petersen K. Japanese encephalitis: a review of clinical guidelines and vaccine availability in Asia. Trop Dis Travel Med Vaccines. 2015;1:11. https://doi.org/10.1186/s40794-015-0013-6.

156. Deshpande BR, Rao SR, Jentes ES, Hills SL, Fischer M, Gershman MD, et al. Use of Japanese encephalitis vaccine in US travel medicine practices in Global TravEpiNet. Am J Trop Med Hyg. 2014;91:694–8. https://doi.org/10.4269/ajtmh.14-0062.
157. Duffy MR, Reed C, Edelson PJ, Blumensaadt S, Crocker K, Griggs A, et al. A survey of US travelers to Asia to assess compliance with recommendations for the use of Japanese encephalitis vaccine. J Travel Med. 2013;20:165–70. https://doi.org/10.1111/jtm.12020.
158. Lammert SM, Rao SR, Jentes ES, Fairley JK, Erskine S, Walker AT, et al. Refusal of recommended travel-related vaccines among U.S. international travellers in Global TravEpiNet. J Travel Med. 2016;24:taw075. https://doi.org/10.1093/jtm/taw075.
159. Choices NHS. Japanese encephalitis – Prevention – NHS Choices 2016. http://www.nhs.uk/Conditions/Japanese-encephalitis/Pages/Whileyoureaway.aspx. Accessed 25 June 2017.
160. Tropical medical bureau prices I Travel vaccination prices. TMB – Trop Med Bur – Vaccin Health Inf Int Travel. http://www.tmb.ie/prices. Accessed 25 June 2017.
161. Thai Travel Clinic. Vaccine price list. Thai Travel Clin. https://www.thaitravelclinic.com/cost.html. Accessed 25 June 2017.
162. Yamada A, Imanishi J, Juang RF, Fukunaga T, Okuno Y, Tadano M, et al. Trial of inactivated Japanese encephalitis vaccine in children with underlying diseases. Vaccine. 1986;4:32–4.
163. Rojanasuphot S, Shaffer N, Chotpitayasunondh T, Phumiamorn S, Mock P, Chearskul S, et al. Response to JE vaccine among HIV-infected children, Bangkok, Thailand. Southeast Asian J Trop Med Public Health. 1998;29:443–50.
164. Chokephaibulkit K, Plipat N, Yoksan S, Phongsamart W, Lappra K, Chearskul P, et al. A comparative study of the serological response to Japanese encephalitis vaccine in HIV-infected and uninfected Thai children. Vaccine. 2010;28:3563–6. https://doi.org/10.1016/j.vaccine.2010.02.108.
165. Puthanakit T, Aurpibul L, Yoksan S, Sirisanthana T, Sirisanthana V. Japanese encephalitis vaccination in HIV-infected children with immune recovery after highly active antiretroviral therapy. Vaccine. 2007;25:8257–61. https://doi.org/10.1016/j.vaccine.2007.09.052.
166. Puthanakit T, Aurpibul L, Yoksan S, Sirisanthana T, Sirisanthana V. A 3-year follow-up of antibody response in HIV-infected children with immune recovery vaccinated with inactivated Japanese encephalitis vaccine. Vaccine. 2010;28:5900–2. https://doi.org/10.1016/j.vaccine.2010.06.048.
167. Pakakasama S, Wattanatitan S, Techasaensiri C, Yoksan S, Sirireung S, Hongeng S. Immunogenicity of a live-attenuated Japanese encephalitis vaccine in children and adolescents after hematopoietic stem cell transplantation. Bone Marrow Transplant. 2014;49:1307–9. https://doi.org/10.1038/bmt.2014.149.
168. Sunwoo J-S, Jung K-H, Lee S-T, Lee SK, Chu K. Reemergence of Japanese encephalitis in South Korea, 2010–2015. Emerg Infect Dis. 2016;22:1841–3. https://doi.org/10.3201/eid2210.160288.
169. Itoh K, Iwamoto K, Satoh Y, Fujita T, Takahashi K, Katano H, et al. Knowledge obtained from an elderly case of Japanese encephalitis. Intern Med. 2016;55:2487–90. https://doi.org/10.2169/internalmedicine.55.6646.
170. Chang Y-K, Chang H-L, Wu H-S, Chen K-T. Epidemiological features of Japanese encephalitis in Taiwan from 2000 to 2014. Am J Trop Med Hyg. 2017;96:382–8. https://doi.org/10.4269/ajtmh.16-0330.

Autoimmune Encephalitis

12

Arun Venkatesan and John C. Probasco

Introduction

Acute encephalitis is a rapidly progressive encephalopathy due to brain inflammation, progressive over the course of weeks, and associated with significant morbidity as well as care burden to patients, families, and society [1, 2]. Historically, the most frequently identified causes of acute encephalitis have been infectious; however over the past decade, an increasing number of autoimmune encephalitides have been described. A subset of these autoimmune encephalitides are paraneoplastic in that they occur physically and potentially temporally remote from a tumor. Paraneoplastic autoimmune encephalitis, like other paraneoplastic neurological syndromes, is often the by-product of the immunological response directed against a cancer, and the development of a paraneoplastic syndrome can herald the detection of cancer or its recurrence by years [3–5]. In contrast, primary autoimmune encephalitides have been described in the absence of detected cancer at diagnosis or in longitudinal clinical care, typically characterized by immune responses directed against cell surface proteins including neurotransmitter receptors, water channels, and ion channels [6].

The diagnosis of an autoimmune encephalitis carries import for not only the immediate care for a patient presenting with a rapidly progressive encephalopathy but also the detection and monitoring for occult malignancy when appropriate [7]. The diagnosis of autoimmune encephalitis can be challenging, prompting the recent development of consensus clinical criteria for autoimmune encephalitis to help providers better identify patients and to differentiate autoimmune encephalitis from other neurological and psychiatric disorders [6]. As described below, additional

A. Venkatesan (✉) · J. C. Probasco
Johns Hopkins Encephalitis Center, Division of Neuroimmunology and Neuroinfectious Diseases, Department of Neurology, Johns Hopkins University School of Medicine, Baltimore, MD, USA
e-mail: avenkat2@jhmi.edu

© Springer International Publishing AG, part of Springer Nature 2018
R. Hasbun (ed.), *Meningitis and Encephalitis*,
https://doi.org/10.1007/978-3-319-92678-0_12

Table 12.1 Challenges in the diagnosis and treatment of autoimmune encephalitis

Heterogeneity of clinical presentation
Limited utility of current radiographic methods for diagnosis and prognosis
False positives and negatives with autoantibody testing
Limited understanding of contribution of cellular autoimmunity and genetics
Lack of guidelines for escalation and duration of immunotherapy
Need for personalized therapeutic approaches
Inadequate understanding of long-term outcomes and sequelae

challenges arise when diagnosing and treating patients with autoimmune encephalitis, including syndrome recognition, antibody testing in the commercial or research laboratory setting, the interpretation of antibody test results, the utility of various diagnostic modalities, and the acute and chronic management of the autoimmune encephalitis and its sequelae (Table 12.1).

The field of autoimmune encephalitis has matured from syndrome recognition and description to the exploration of disease mechanisms, potential relationships of infectious and autoimmune encephalitides, the evaluation of treatment approaches and pharmaceuticals, and the potential for novel treatment approaches in the paradigm of precision medicine. In this chapter we explore the diagnostic and treatment challenges that face the neurologist caring for a patient with possible autoimmune encephalitis as well as future directions in diagnosis and care.

Diagnosis

Clinical Presentation

Encephalitis is a severe, debilitating inflammatory disorder of the brain, with varied possible etiologies of a rapidly progressive encephalopathy leading to a broad differential diagnosis (Table 12.2) and potentially extensive diagnostic evaluation [1, 6, 8].

Syndrome onset and tempo play important roles in differentiating acute encephalitis from more chronic neurodegenerative and psychiatric syndromes. In general, acute encephalitis is characterized by the development and progression of brain inflammation leading to a debilitating neurological disorder in a matter of weeks, usually less than 6 weeks [1, 6]. More specifically for autoimmune encephalitis, consensus clinical criteria require subacute onset with rapid progression of less than 3 months of working memory deficits (or short-term memory loss), altered mental status, or psychiatric symptoms [6]. Altered mental status is further defined as decreased or altered level of consciousness, lethargy, or personality change [6]. These symptoms may be accompanied by other neurological symptoms or examination findings, some of which have been associated with specific autoantibodies [4, 6, 9].

Table 12.2 Differential diagnosis of acute encephalitis [1, 6, 8]

CNS infections	Metabolic/mitochondrial disorders
Routinely assessed: HSV, VZV, enterovirus, cryptococcal, syphilis, HIV	Mitochondrial encephalomyopathy, lactic acidosis, and stroke-like episode syndrome
Immunocompromised host: CMV, HHV6/7, *Toxoplasma gondii, Mycobacterium tuberculosis*, West Nile virus	Urea cycle disorders
Geographic factors (e.g., malaria, trypanosomiasis, Japanese encephalitis virus, tick-borne encephalitis virus, dengue)	Reye syndrome (in children)
Seasonal (e.g., arbovirus)	*Rheumatologic disorders*
Exposure (e.g., bartonella, tick-borne disease testing, rabies testing, *Naegleria fowleri*)	Systemic lupus erythematosus
Encephalopathy due to systemic disease	Sarcoidosis
Sepsis	Behcet's
Organ failure (e.g., hepatic, renal/uremia, pulmonary/hypoxemia/hypercapnia)	Sjogren's syndrome
Electrolyte abnormalities (e.g., hypernatremia, hyponatremia, hypercalcemia)	*Cerebrovascular disease*
Endocrine (e.g., hyperthyroid/hypothyroid)	Ischemic stroke
Nutritional (e.g., Wernicke, B12 deficiency, niacin deficiency, folate deficiency)	Hemorrhagic stroke
Hyperviscosity syndrome	Venous sinus thrombosis
Drug toxicity	Posterior reversible encephalopathy syndrome (PRES)
Illicit drugs (e.g., ketamine)	*Cancer*
Neurotoxic effect of prescribed drugs (e.g., anticholinergics)	Central nervous system lymphoma
Seizures induced by drugs or medications	Brain metastases from systemic cancer
	Intravascular lymphoma
Idiosyncratic reaction (e.g., neuroleptic malignant syndrome)	Gliomatosis cerebri
Drug interaction (e.g., serotonergic syndrome)	*Epileptic disorders*
Drug withdrawal (e.g., alcohol, benzodiazepines, opiates)	Nonconvulsive status epilepticus
Creutzfeldt-Jakob disease	Febrile infection-related epilepsy syndrome (FIRES)
Kleine-Levin syndrome	Idiopathic hemiconvulsion hemiplegia and epilepsy (IHHE) syndrome

The subsequent evaluation of patients presenting with signs and symptoms consistent with autoimmune encephalitis should include a conventional neurological evaluation to assess for potential alternative etiologies as well as to investigate for supportive findings by standard diagnostic tests, including magnetic resonance imaging (MRI), cerebrospinal fluid (CSF), and electroencephalography (EEG) studies. The diagnosis of autoimmune encephalitis is clinical and not dependent on the detection of an autoantibody as at times autoantibody testing is not readily accessible, the results of autoantibody testing may take weeks to return, the failure to detect an autoantibody in the serum or CSF does not exclude an autoimmune encephalitis, and false-positive antibody assay results can occur. As early immuno-therapy appears to be associated with improved clinical outcome, the diagnostic evaluation is undertaken to support the diagnosis of autoimmune encephalitis while quickly clarifying the presence or absence of other etiologies, particularly infec-tious, to allow for rapid initiation of immunotherapy with treatment escalation as clinically indicated [10, 11].

Diagnostic Tests

As mentioned previously, the standard diagnostics used in the evaluation of patients with suspected autoimmune encephalitis include MRI of the brain, CSF assessment, and EEG [6]. The sensitivity and specificity of each of these standard diagnostics vary for autoimmune encephalitis in general and for specific autoantibody syndromes.

CSF assessment is of import in ruling out a number of infectious encephalitides, supporting a diagnosis of possible autoimmune encephalitis, and in diagnosing a specific autoantibody syndrome [6]. Routine CSF studies typically demonstrate a moderate lymphocytic predominant pleocytosis (≥ 5 WBC/mL), with normal glucose and potentially elevated CSF protein. The detection of intrathecal oligoclonal bands and an elevated serum to CSF immunoglobulin G (IgG) index indicate intrathecal antibody synthesis and are further supportive. It should be noted that a CSF pleocy-tosis may be transient, potentially only evident in the early stages of the encephalitis, as has been observed in anti-NMDA receptor (anti-NMDAR) encephalitis [6, 10, 12]. In addition, when evaluating patients for possible autoimmune encephalitis, it is recommended that autoantibody testing is sent from the CSF in addition to autoanti-body testing in the serum [6]. The reasons for this are manifold. First, in some syn-dromes (e.g., anti-NMDAR and anti-LGI1), CSF antibody testing has been demonstrated to be more sensitive than serum testing alone [10, 13]. In addition, multiple antibodies can be detected in the serum, potentially in addition to those detected in the CSF. In such cases, CSF antibodies are more likely pathologic, with a lower rate of false-positive and false-negative results compared to serum antibody testing [6].

EEG is of variable sensitivity in autoimmune encephalitis, with the most fre-quent findings being non-specific slowing and disorganized cortical activity [6, 12, 14]. Consensus criteria for the diagnosis of possible autoimmune encephalitis and definite limbic encephalitis include temporal slowing (either unilateral or bilateral) [6]. Patients with autoimmune encephalitis may be found to have electrographic seizures, potentially as nonconvulsive status epilepticus [14]. There have been descriptions of rare electrographic findings in specific autoimmune encephalitis syndromes, such as extreme delta brush in anti-NMDAR encephalitis which is noted in a minority of cases [15]. Patterns commonly associated with other neurological syndromes have been noted in cases of autoimmune encephalitis, such as periodic sharp wave complexes commonly described in Creutzfeldt-Jakob disease also observed in patients with autoimmune encephalitis with autoantibodies directed against the voltage-gated potassium channel complex [16].

Brain MRI is of variable sensitivity, for instance, being abnormal in 33–50% of patients with anti-NMDAR encephalitis. Depending on the syndrome, there can be abnormalities of the mesial temporal lobes, gray matter, and/or white matter on T2 sequences with subtle gadolinium enhancement. Some lesions may also appear consistent with demyelinating diseases. Findings by MRI may be subtle and transient, resolving spontaneously through the course of disease or with treatment [6, 10, 12].

Though currently included in the consensus criteria for *definite* autoimmune limbic encephalitis [6], FDG-PET may in the future prove to play an important role in the diagnostic evaluation of patients with *suspected* autoimmune encephalitis. Consensus criteria include hypermetabolism of the mesial temporal lobe in lieu of T2 hyperintensities on MRI as meeting the radiographic criterion for definite autoimmune limbic encephalitis [6]. This criterion is based on primarily qualitative observations of FDG-PET studies from small series of patients with a variety of autoantibody syndromes, chiefly anti-NMDA receptor and anti-LGI1 encephalitis. In a recent retrospective series applying semiquantitative techniques, brain FDG-PET/CT was observed to often be abnormal in patients with possible autoimmune encephalitis, most commonly demonstrating hypometabolism [17, 18]. Demonstration of abnormalities by brain FDG-PET/CT was also noted to be in weak agreement with detection of abnormalities on at least two of the routine diagnostic assessments (CSF analysis, brain MRI, and/or EEG), suggesting its potential utility in addition to these routine studies in the diagnosis of possible autoimmune encephalitis [17]. Some series have also found that FDG-PET may be more sensitive than brain MRI for abnormalities in autoimmune encephalitis [18]. Finally, characteristic metabolism patterns have been noted in some autoimmune encephalitides which have been found to resolve with patient clinical improvement, such as parieto-occipital hypometabolism and relative anterior hypermetabolism in anti-NMDAR encephalitis [18–20]. Much work remains to prospectively assess the utility of FDG-PET in the diagnosis and clinical monitoring of autoimmune encephalitis, including its differentiation from other causes of encephalitis (e.g., infectious encephalitides) and syndromes (e.g., psychiatric, drug-induced).

Several autoantibodies directed against neuronal targets have been described in autoimmune encephalitis, with patients at times presenting with additional neurological symptoms and signs suggestive of particular autoantibody syndromes (Table 12.3). The autoantibodies themselves may play a direct role in disease pathogenesis or may be markers of systemic immunoreactivity directed against the nervous system [4, 21, 22]. It is not uncommon for multiple autoantibodies to be detected in the serum. For instance, in a review over 550 seropositive patients evaluated for a paraneoplastic neurological syndrome at a tertiary medical center, nearly a third were found to have multiple autoantibodies [23]. The pattern of autoantibodies detected was suggestive of the cancer ultimately detected and was not specific for a particular

Table 12.3 Autoantibodies in autoimmune encephalitis [4, 6, 64]

	Syndrome and associated neurological findings	Other associated neurological syndromes	Frequency of cancer	Main cancer type
Antibodies against intracellular antigens				
Hu (ANNA1)	Limbic encephalitis	Brainstem encephalitis, encephalitis, subacute cerebellar degeneration, myelitis, sensory neuronopathy, autonomic neuropathy, peripheral neuropathy	>95%	Small-cell lung carcinoma
Amphiphysin	Limbic encephalitis	Stiff-person syndrome, encephalitis, subacute cerebellar degeneration, myelopathy, subacute sensory neuronopathy, peripheral neuropathy		Small-cell lung carcinoma, breast, thymoma
CV2/CRMP5	Limbic encephalitis	Encephalitis, chorea, subacute cerebellar degeneration, cranial neuropathies, uveitis, optic neuritis, retinopathy, myelopathy, subacute sensory neuronopathy, autonomic neuropathy, peripheral neuropathy		Small-cell lung carcinoma, uterine sarcoma
Ma2	Limbic encephalitis	Brainstem encephalitis, hypothalamic encephalitis, mesencephalic encephalitis, subacute cerebellar degeneration	>95%	Testicular seminoma
GAD 65 (65 kDa glutamic acid decarboxylase)	Limbic encephalitis	Stiff-person syndrome, cerebellar ataxia, epilepsy, brainstem encephalitis	25%	Thymoma, small-cell lung carcinoma
Antibodies against synaptic receptors				
NMDA receptor	Anti-NMDA receptor encephalitis	Anxiety, psychosis, epilepsy, extrapyramidal disorder, hypoventilation, central	Varies with age and sex	Ovarian teratoma
AMPA receptor	Limbic encephalitis	Epilepsy, nystagmus	65%	Thymoma, small-cell lung carcinoma
GABA-B receptor	Limbic encephalitis	Epilepsy, cerebellar ataxia	50%	Small-cell lung carcinoma

Table 12.3 (continued)

	Syndrome and associated neurological findings	Other associated neurological syndromes	Frequency of cancer	Main cancer type
GABA-A receptor	Encephalitis	Epilepsy, cerebellar ataxia	<5%	Thymoma
mGluR5	Encephalitis		70%	Hodgkin's lymphoma
Dopamine 2 receptor	Basal ganglia encephalitis	Sydenham chorea	0%	
Antibodies against ion channels and other cell-surface proteins				
LGI1 (leucine-rich glioma-inactivated 1)	Limbic encephalitis	Faciobrachial dystonic seizures, abnormal sleep behavior	5–10%	Thymoma
CASPR2 (contactin-associated protein 2)	Limbic encephalitis	Morvan syndrome, neuromyotonia	20–50%	Thymoma
DPPX (dipeptidyl-peptidase-like protein 6)	Encephalitis	Psychiatric symptoms, diarrhea tremor, nystagmus, hyperekplexia, ataxia, progressive encephalomyelitis with rigidity and myoclonus (PERM)	<10%	Lymphoma
MOG (myelin oligodendrocyte glycoprotein)	Acute disseminated encephalomyelitis	Neuromyelitis optica, optic neuritis, myelitis	0%	
Aquaporin 4	Encephalitis	Neuromyelitis optica, optic neuritis, myelitis	0%	

neurological syndrome [23]. In addition, autoantibodies have been detected in non-paraneoplastic, non-encephalitic syndromes, including Creutzfeldt-Jakob disease [24, 25]. Thus, in utilizing autoantibody testing in the serum alone, one runs the risk of detecting multiple autoantibodies, many of which are not involved in the pathogenesis of autoimmune encephalitis, leading to potential misdiagnosis. This issue of diminished specificity is compounded by the poorer sensitivity for serum autoantibody testing compared to autoantibody testing in the CSF [10, 13]. In light of these observations, current consensus recommendations include not only autoantibody testing in the serum but also concurrent testing in the CSF [6].

Intersection of Infection and Autoimmunity

As many as 10–25% of patients who experience an episode of herpes simplex encephalitis (HSE) will develop a relapse of neurologic symptoms weeks to months later in the absence of evidence of ongoing virus production [26]. Until recently the pathophysiology of these symptoms remained unclear and represented both a diagnostic and therapeutic challenge to clinicians. However, evidence has emerged that a number of these cases represent an autoimmune phenomenon in association with the development of antibodies to the NMDA receptor, thus representing a post-infectious autoimmune encephalitis. Indeed, such patients typically develop symptoms 4–6 weeks after HSE, have negative testing for herpes virus at the time of relapse, develop new enhancing or confluent lesions on brain MRI, demonstrate the presence of anti-NMDAR antibodies in the serum and/or CSF, and improve following the administration of immunotherapy [27, 28]. While an infection may lead to the generation of autoimmunity by a number of differing mechanisms including molecular mimicry, dysregulation of immune checkpoints, uncovering of cryptic neural epitopes, and bystander activation [28], the mechanisms by which HSE leads to the generation of anti-NMDAR antibodies remain to be discovered.

Identification of Autoantibodies

Autoantibody identification in autoimmune encephalitis is a rapidly emerging field that is typically based upon one or a combination of methodologies, including immunohistochemistry (IHC) on rodent brain sections, immunocytochemistry (ICC) of live primary neurons, and cell-based assays (CBA) where nonneural cells are transfected with an antigen of interest. Each of these methodologies has advantages and disadvantages, and together they can complement each other in the identification of autoantibodies. With ICC, for example, the tissue is typically from an adult animal and thus expresses mature (and likely relevant) antigens, various brain regions can be utilized, both cell surface and intracellular staining can be appreciated, and there is tremendous experience in interpretation of specific staining patterns [29]. Disadvantages are that the tissue is typically fixed in paraformaldehyde which even when done briefly may result in alteration of antigens and that cross-species differences between proteins may result in false negatives in some cases. ICC typically involves addition of serum or CSF to live primary rat hippocampal neurons such that the autoantibody only has access to the extracellular compartment, an advantage being specific detection of binding to extracellular epitopes. Disadvantages include the possibility that cultured hippocampal neurons may not express the range of antigens expressed in mature tissue, and that antigens expressed by other neuronal subtypes may not be found in hippocampal neurons, thus contributing to false negatives. Most CBAs utilize transfection of the antigen of interest into human embryonic kidney (HEK) cells, followed by either fixed or live staining utilizing either ICC or flow cytometry. Such methodologies theoretically allow for the precise detection of single autoantigens that serve as a target for patient autoantibodies [30, 31] and have been reported to have high sensitivity and specificity [30, 32, 33]. However, confounding factors include the potential need to express additional proteins to aid in targeting or localization of the antigen of interest to the cell surface, the potential for excitotoxicity in the setting of overexpression of ion channels, and subjectivity with scoring of ICC. Moreover, the need for *a priori* knowledge of the antigen of interest limits the potential for discovery of new auto-antigens by CBA [29].

Treatment

Treatment of patients with autoimmune encephalitis entails a three-part approach that addresses (1) the autoimmune syndrome with immunotherapy, (2) an underlying malignancy if detected, and (3) treatment of associated sequelae of the syndrome. As autoimmune encephalitis is rare, our understanding of disease mechanisms, expert opinion, case series, and a few prospective trials guides treatment selection. Important factors in treatment consideration are the autoantibody detected, patient comorbidities and sensitivities, and the phase of illness (Table 12.4).

In the acute setting, autoimmune encephalitides associated with autoantibodies directed at cell membrane proteins tend to respond well to antibody-directed therapies such as intravenous immunoglobulin and plasmapheresis. These treatments often follow or accompany courses of intravenous corticosteroids such as intravenous methylprednisolone. Second-line therapies used in the acute phase include rituximab and cyclophosphamide. Mycophenolate and azathioprine are typically used in the maintenance phase, as are rituximab, cyclophosphamide, corticosteroids, and intravenous immunoglobulin [34–36].

Table 12.4 Common therapies for autoimmune encephalitis. Modified from [65]

Therapies	Side effects
First line	
Intravenous methylprednisolone	Insomnia, psychiatric symptoms, hyperglycemia, electrolyte abnormalities, fluid retention, hypertension, peptic ulcer, Cushing syndrome, cataracts, infection, osteoporosis, avascular necrosis, Addisonian crisis in setting of rapid withdrawal
Intravenous immunoglobulin[a]	Headache, aseptic meningitis, thromboembolic events, acute renal failure, anaphylaxis in those IgA deficient
Plasmapheresis	Hypotension, electrolyte imbalance. With central line, infection, hemorrhage, thrombosis, pneumothorax
Second line	
Rituximab[a]	Allergic reaction, opportunistic infection, reactivation of tuberculosis or hepatitis B
Cyclophosphamide[a]	Nausea, vomiting, alopecia, mucositis, hemorrhagic cystitis, infertility, myelosuppression
Maintenance	
Mycophenolate mofetil	Diarrhea, nausea, vomiting, hypertension, peripheral edema, infections, myelosuppression, lymphoma, and other malignancies
Azathioprine	Diarrhea, nausea, vomiting, hypersensitivity reaction, alopecia, cytopenia, hepatotoxicity, lymphoma, infection

[a]Can be used in both acute and maintenance phases of treatment

In the case of autoimmune encephalitides associated with autoantibodies directed against intracellular antigens, immunomodulatory therapies such as plasmapheresis do not seem to be of benefit [9, 37]. Therapies directed at reducing the cell-mediated immune response, such as the cytotoxic agent cyclophosphamide and lymphocyte-specific medications such as mycophenolate, play an important role in mitigating the cytotoxic response and with hopes of minimizing the extent of consequent neuronal injury. The detection and treatment of an underlying cancer can have a dramatic clinical impact and play an important role in treatment. For instance, resection of detected ovarian teratomas has been considered as first-line treatment along with intravenous steroids, intravenous methylprednisolone, and plasmapheresis exchange in anti-NMDAR encephalitis [10]. Similarly, the chemotherapeutic medications used in the treatment of cancer have effects not only on the antigenic source, the cancer, but also immunosuppressive effects which can impact the immune response underlying the autoimmune encephalitis.

There are no guidelines of when is it appropriate to escalate from first- to second-line treatments, with administration of second-line agents typically utilized for cases of non-response or incomplete response to first-line therapies or for severe presentations of disease. In the largest series of anti-NMDAR encephalitis, the relapse rate for those treated with first-line therapy alone was 12%, while 10% of those treated with second-line therapy relapsed within the same time period [10]. There is mounting evidence for the use of rituximab as second-line immunotherapy in autoimmune encephalitis, regardless of antibody status, given reported tolerability and improved outcomes after first-line treatment [11, 38]. In addition, there is consideration for its use as a first-line agent, though prospective studies of this approach are lacking [6]. An additional therapeutic challenge revolves around duration of treatment. As with the decision to escalate treatments in autoimmune encephalitis, there are no guidelines as to how long to maintain such treatments. Goals of long-term immune treatment include cessation of neuroinflammation and attendant neurodegeneration, as well as limiting the risk of autoimmune relapse. While in many cases the ongoing neuroinflammation may subside over months, relapses can occur many years after the initial event [39]. A practical approach for patients with moderate to severe autoimmune encephalitis is to continue immunotherapy for 18–24 months with ongoing clinical and radiographic assessment of disease activity. Upon reaching a period of clinical stability, immune treatments can be gradually weaned with careful and frequent reassessment to determine whether treatment needs to be reinstituted.

Emerging Therapies

In patients who do not respond adequately to rituximab, tocilizumab, a monoclonal antibody against the interleukin-6 (IL-6) receptor, may hold promise. IL-6 is an important pro-inflammatory cytokine that has broad effects on multiple immune cells, and a number of recent efforts have focused on targeting the cytokine or its receptor to modulate inflammatory disease [40]. In a retrospective institutional cohort study of patients with autoimmune encephalitis initially treated with rituximab, tocilizumab resulted in better long-term outcomes compared to those given further rituximab or no subsequent treatment [41]. More recently, bortezomib, a proteasome inhibitor, was employed in patients with anti-NMDAR encephalitis, with the rationale that this drug can deplete plasma cells and potentially decrease levels of pathogenic autoantibodies. Four of five patients with treatment-refractory anti-NMDAR encephalitis treated with bortezomib were reported to show clinical improvement or disease remission and a corresponding fall in CSF antibody levels [42]. Another pro-inflammatory cytokine, interleukin-1 (IL-1), has also received recent attention as a potential therapeutic target, since levels of its antagonist are elevated in patients with a good outcome following encephalitis of infectious or autoimmune cause [43]. Indeed, a recent case report described the recovery of a patient with a chronic autoimmune meningoencephalitis following treatment with anakinra, an IL-1 receptor antagonist [44]. Notably, despite the growing number of potential therapeutic options, at the moment there is not enough evidence to inform a rationale treatment algorithm for those with autoimmune encephalitis refractory to conventional second-line agents.

Major Gaps

Despite the many advances described above, substantial gaps remain in our knowledge of diagnosis, treatment, and outcomes of autoimmune encephalitis. Here we discuss three such gaps: (1) arriving at an etiologic diagnosis for patients, (2) development of therapies based upon personalized medicine, and (3) achieving a more refined understanding of the sequelae of autoimmune encephalitis.

An Etiologic Diagnosis

Despite extensive testing for infectious and autoimmune conditions, up to 40% of all cases of acute encephalitis remain without an etiologic diagnosis [45, 46]. It is likely that some of these cases are accounted for by autoimmune conditions. Indeed, novel autoantibodies are being identified at a rapid clip via the methodologies mentioned above coupled with mass spectrometric identification of autoantigens [29]. However, screening techniques based upon rodent tissue may miss some human autoantigens, and thus the development of human protein-, cell-, or tissue-based platforms to identify novel autoantibodies is of importance. Protein display technologies such as phage immunoprecipitation sequencing (PhIP-Seq) can be utilized to identify binding between autoantibodies and large libraries of overlapping peptides that span most, if not all, of the human peptidome and have already been utilized to identify novel paraneoplastic autoantigens [47]. More recently, an in vitro translation platform termed parallel analysis of translated ORFs (PLATO) has been developed that enables translated proteins to remain bound to their mRNA. Thus, when autoantibody-antigen complexes are identified, the still attached mRNA allows for ready identification of the antigen of interest [48]. Notably, the approaches detailed above focus only on identification of autoantibodies, and it is becoming increasingly likely that additional novel autoantibodies will account for small proportions of disease. Disorders of cell-mediated immunity, which are not as readily identified as autoantibody-mediated disease, will likely account for a substantial proportion of undiagnosed autoimmune encephalitis cases. A combination of approaches, including careful clinical and immunophenotyping as well as immunogenetics, will be needed to elucidate these causes.

Toward Personalized Therapy

Current therapeutic paradigms for autoimmune encephalitis utilize broad strokes to impact the immune system and in so doing place patients at particular risk for opportunistic infections, malignancy, and systemic complications. Thus, a major challenge is to develop a more personalized approach to therapy based upon the specific pathogenic mechanism driving the disease process in each patient. There has been much interest in developing antigen-specific approaches that induce immune tolerance by targeting antigen-presenting cells (APCs) or T cells. For example, when an autoantigen is presented by an APC in the presence of low levels of co-stimulatory molecules and without additional activating stimuli, the T cell can be driven toward an anergic state that may at least transiently halt the autoimmune process. Engagement of additional negative signals between APCs and T cells can lead to death of T cells via clonal deletion or apoptosis, potentially resulting in longer-lived antigen-specific effects [49–51]. Current efforts are focused on cytokine-, cell-, and particle-based approaches as well as alternate antigen delivery methods (i.e., oral) that can cause specific reprogramming of lymphocytes either directly or through effects on APCs [49]. T cells can also be engineered to specifically detect and kill cells expressing a particular cell surface receptor [52, 53]. This technology, termed chimeric antigen receptor T cells (CAR-T), has been recently applied to a model of the autoimmune disease pemphigus vulgaris in which autoreactive antibodies target the protein desmoglien-3 (DSG3). CAR-T cells were found to selectively kill DSG3-reactive B cells, decrease autoreactive antibody titers, and prevent disease in this disorder of systemic autoimmunity [54]. It will be of interest to determine whether such approaches readily translate to disorders of CNS autoimmunity. Recent work on neuromyelitis optica (NMO), an autoimmune demyelinating disorder of the CNS, may also provide direction on novel specific therapies for autoimmune encephalitis. NMO is caused by binding of pathogenic autoantibodies to the aquaporin-4 (AQP4) water channel on astrocytes, resulting in complement-dependent cytotoxicity and antibody-dependent cell-mediated cytotoxicity. Mutation of the antibody to remove the pathogenic effector functions while maintaining tight binding to AQP4 resulted in a nonpathogenic antibody that competed with pathogenic antibodies for AQP4 binding, resulting in amelioration of lesion formation in a mouse model of disease [55]. Such approaches may be applicable to autoimmune encephalitis. Notably, methodologies that enable the identification and cloning of patient-specific autoantibodies in autoimmune encephalitis may facilitate the development of blocking antibodies as specific therapies [56].

Sequelae of Autoimmune Encephalitis

Following an episode of autoimmune encephalitis, patients experience a variety of neurocognitive sequelae and are at risk for seizures; however our understanding of the true impact of these is limited to case series and retrospective studies [57]. Not only are seizures a common initial presentation of autoimmune encephalitis, but many patients develop postencephalitis epilepsy [58, 59]. Antiepileptics are therefore commonly used both acutely and in the maintenance phase after the initial episode of encephalitis has resolved. In a subset of patients, antiepileptic medications alone were effective in controlling seizures [59], with consideration for antiepileptic selection based on patient-specific factors. Additionally, patients can experience long-term cognitive effects as a consequence of structural damage to underlying systems [60]. As such, patients may benefit from comprehensive rehabilitation services, with therapies tailored to specific patient deficits. Patients may also experience psychiatric sequelae such as psychosis and catatonia, both acutely as a part of the autoimmune encephalitis syndrome and chronically, necessitating psychiatric management. One point of caution is the use of antipsychotic medications in patients with anti-NMDAR encephalitis given observation of intolerance to these medications characterized by high temperature, mutism, coma, muscle rigidity, and rhabdomyolysis [61]. Finally, some of the treatments used may themselves have neurobehavioral side effects, such as steroid-induced encephalopathy or antiepileptic effects on concentration, memory, and mood [62, 63]. Future prospective studies of the long-term outcomes in patients with autoimmune encephalitis as well as sequelae of encephalitis and adverse effects of treatment are needed to help guide our care of patients as they recover as well as in counseling of patients and families regarding diagnosis, prognosis, and treatment selection.

References

1. Venkatesan A, Tunkel AR, Bloch KC, et al. Case definitions, diagnostic algorithms, and priorities in encephalitis: consensus statement of the international encephalitis consortium. Clin Infect Dis. 2013;57:1114–28.
2. Vora NM, Holman RC, Mehal JM, Steiner CA, Blanton J, Sejvar J. Burden of encephalitis-associated hospitalizations in the United States, 1998–2010. Neurology. 2014;82:443–51.
3. Darnell RB, Posner JB. Paraneoplastic syndromes involving the nervous system. N Engl J Med. 2003;349:1543–54.
4. Dalmau J, Rosenfeld MR. Paraneoplastic syndromes of the CNS. Lancet Neurol. 2008;7:327–40.
5. Tarin D. Update on clinical and mechanistic aspects of paraneoplastic syndromes. Cancer Metastasis Rev. 2013;32:707–21.
6. Graus F, Titulaer MJ, Balu R, et al. A clinical approach to diagnosis of autoimmune encephalitis. Lancet Neurol. 2016;15:391–404.
7. Titulaer MJ, Soffietti R, Dalmau J, et al. Screening for tumours in paraneoplastic syndromes: report of an EFNS task force. Eur J Neurol. 2011;18:19–e13.
8. Frontera JA. Metabolic encephalopathies in the critical care unit. Continuum. 2012;18:611–39.
9. McKeon A. Paraneoplastic and other autoimmune disorders of the central nervous system. Neurohospitalist. 2013;3:53–64.

10. Titulaer MJ, McCracken L, Gabilondo I, et al. Treatment and prognostic factors for long-term outcome in patients with anti-NMDA receptor encephalitis: an observational cohort study. Lancet Neurol. 2013;12:157–65.
11. Lee WJ, Lee ST, Byun JI, et al. Rituximab treatment for autoimmune limbic encephalitis in an institutional cohort. Neurology. 2016;86:1683–91.
12. Dalmau J, Lancaster E, Martinez-Hernandez E, Rosenfeld MR, Balice-Gordon R. Clinical experience and laboratory investigations in patients with anti-NMDAR encephalitis. Lancet Neurol. 2011;10:63–74.
13. Arino H, Armangue T, Petit-Pedrol M, et al. Anti-LGI1-associated cognitive impairment: presentation and long-term outcome. Neurology. 2016;87:759–65.
14. Johnson N, Henry C, Fessler AJ, Dalmau J. Anti-NMDA receptor encephalitis causing prolonged nonconvulsive status epilepticus. Neurology. 2010;75:1480–2.
15. Schmitt SE, Pargeon K, Frechette ES, Hirsch LJ, Dalmau J, Friedman D. Extreme delta brush: a unique EEG pattern in adults with anti-NMDA receptor encephalitis. Neurology. 2012;79:1094–100.
16. Savard M, Irani SR, Guillemette A, et al. Creutzfeldt-Jakob disease-like periodic sharp wave complexes in voltage-gated potassium channel-complex antibodies encephalitis: a case report. J Clin Neurophysiol. 2016;33:e1–4.
17. Probasco JC, Solnes L, Nalluri A, et al. Abnormal brain metabolism on FDG-PET/CT is a common early finding in autoimmune encephalitis. Neurol Neuroimmunol Neuroinflamm. 2017;4:e352.
18. Solnes LB, Jones KM, Rowe SP, et al. Diagnostic value of 18F-FDG PET/CT versus MRI in the setting of antibody specific autoimmune encephalitis. J Nucl Med. 2017;58:1307–13.
19. Leypoldt F, Buchert R, Kleiter I, et al. Fluorodeoxyglucose positron emission tomography in anti-N-methyl-D-aspartate receptor encephalitis: distinct pattern of disease. J Neurol Neurosurg Psychiatry. 2012;83:681–6.
20. Yuan J, Guan H, Zhou X, et al. Changing brain metabolism patterns in patients with ANMDARE: serial 18F-FDG PET/CT findings. Clin Nucl Med. 2016;41:366–70.
21. Dalmau J, Gleichman AJ, Hughes EG, et al. Anti-NMDA-receptor encephalitis: case series and analysis of the effects of antibodies. Lancet Neurol. 2008;7:1091–8.
22. McKeon A, Pittock SJ. Paraneoplastic encephalomyelopathies: pathology and mechanisms. Acta Neuropathol. 2011;122:381–400.
23. Pittock SJ, Kryzer TJ, Lennon VA. Paraneoplastic antibodies coexist and predict cancer, not neurological syndrome. Ann Neurol. 2004;56:715–9.
24. Kim B, Yoo P, Sutherland T, et al. LGI1 antibody encephalopathy overlapping with sporadic Creutzfeldt-Jakob disease. Neurol Neuroimmunol Neuroinflamm. 2016;3:e248.
25. Rossi M, Mead S, Collinge J, Rudge P, Vincent A. Neuronal antibodies in patients with suspected or confirmed sporadic Creutzfeldt-Jakob disease. J Neurol Neurosurg Psychiatry. 2015;86:692–4.
26. Sköldenberg B, Aurelius E, Hjalmarsson A, et al. Incidence and pathogenesis of clinical relapse after herpes simplex encephalitis in adults. J Neurol. 2006;253:163–70.
27. Prüss H, Finke C, Höltje M, et al. N-methyl-D-aspartate receptor antibodies in herpes simplex encephalitis. Ann Neurol. 2012;72:902–11.
28. Venkatesan A, Benavides DR. Autoimmune encephalitis and its relation to infection. Curr Neurol Neurosci Rep. 2015;15(3):3.
29. van Coevorden-Hameete MH, Titulaer MJ, Schreurs MW, de Graaff E, Sillevis Smitt PA, Hoogenraad CC. Detection and characterization of autoantibodies to neuronal cell-surface antigens in the central nervous system. Front Mol Neurosci. 2016;9:37.
30. Gresa-Arribas N, Titulaer MJ, Torrents A, et al. Antibody titres at diagnosis and during follow-up of anti-NMDA receptor encephalitis: a retrospective study. Lancet Neurol. 2014;13:167–77.
31. Ramberger M, Peschl P, Schanda K, et al. Comparison of diagnostic accuracy of microscopy and flow cytometry in evaluating N-methyl-D-aspartate receptor antibodies in serum using a live cell-based assay. PLoS One. 2015;10:e0122037.

32. Lancaster E, Lai M, Peng X, et al. Antibodies to the GABA(B) receptor in limbic encephalitis with seizures: case series and characterisation of the antigen. Lancet Neurol. 2010;9:67–76.
33. Höftberger R, van Sonderen A, Leypoldt F, et al. Encephalitis and AMPA receptor antibodies: novel findings in a case series of 22 patients. Neurology. 2015;84:2403–12.
34. Venkatesan A, Geocadin RG. Diagnosis and management of acute encephalitis: a practical approach. Neurol Clin Pract. 2014;4:206–15.
35. Lancaster E. The diagnosis and treatment of autoimmune encephalitis. J Clin Neurol. 2016;12:1–13.
36. Varley J, Taylor J, Irani SR. Autoantibody-mediated diseases of the CNS: structure, dysfunction and therapy. Neuropharmacology. 2017;132:71–82.
37. Didelot A, Honnorat J. Paraneoplastic disorders of the central and peripheral nervous systems. Handb Clin Neurol. 2014;121:1159–79.
38. Byun JI, Lee ST, Jung KH, et al. Effect of immunotherapy on seizure outcome in patients with autoimmune encephalitis: a prospective observational registry study. PLoS One. 2016;11:e0146455.
39. Gabilondo I, Saiz A, Galán L, et al. Analysis of relapses in anti-NMDAR encephalitis. Neurology. 2011;77:996–9.
40. Hunter CA, Jones SA. IL-6 as a keystone cytokine in health and disease. Nat Immunol. 2015;16:448–57.
41. Lee W-J, Lee S-T, Moon J, et al. Tocilizumab in autoimmune encephalitis refractory to rituximab: an institutional cohort study. Neurotherapeutics. 2016;13:824–32.
42. Scheibe F, Prüss H, Mengel AM, et al. Bortezomib for treatment of therapy-refractory anti-NMDA receptor encephalitis. Neurology. 2017;88:366–70.
43. Michael BD, Griffiths MJ, Granerod J, et al. The Interleukin-1 balance during encephalitis is associated with clinical severity, blood-brain barrier permeability, neuroimaging changes, and disease outcome. J Infect Dis. 2016;213:1651–60.
44. Novroski AR, Baldwin KJ. Chronic autoimmune meningoencephalitis and periodic fever syndrome treated with Anakinra. Case Rep Neurol. 2017;9:91–7.
45. Granerod J, Ambrose HE, Davies NW, et al. Causes of encephalitis and differences in their clinical presentations in England: a multicentre, population-based prospective study. Lancet Infect Dis. 2010;10:835–44.
46. Singh TD, Fugate JE, Rabinstein AA. The spectrum of acute encephalitis: causes, management, and predictors of outcome. Neurology. 2015;84:359–66.
47. Larman HB, Zhao Z, Laserson U, et al. Autoantigen discovery with a synthetic human peptidome. Nat Biotechnol. 2011;29:535–41.
48. Zhu J, Larman HB, Gao G, et al. Protein interaction discovery using parallel analysis of translated ORFs (PLATO). Nat Biotechnol. 2013;31:331–4.
49. Pearson RM, Casey LM, Hughes KR, Miller SD, Shea LD. In vivo reprogramming of immune cells: technologies for induction of antigen-specific tolerance. Adv Drug Deliv Rev. 2017;114:240–55.
50. Luo X, Miller SD, Shea LD. Immune tolerance for autoimmune disease and cell transplantation. Annu Rev Biomed Eng. 2016;18:181–205.
51. Schwartz RH. T cell anergy. Annu Rev Immunol. 2003;21:305–34.
52. Eshhar Z, Waks T, Gross G, Schindler DG. Specific activation and targeting of cytotoxic lymphocytes through chimeric single chains consisting of antibody-binding domains and the gamma or zeta subunits of the immunoglobulin and T-cell receptors. Proc Natl Acad Sci U S A. 1993;90:720–4.
53. Gross G, Eshhar Z. Endowing T cells with antibody specificity using chimeric T cell receptors. FASEB J. 1992;6:3370–8.
54. Ellebrecht CT, Bhoj VG, Nace A, et al. Reengineering chimeric antigen receptor T cells for targeted therapy of autoimmune disease. Science. 2016;353:179–84.
55. Tradtrantip L, Zhang H, Saadoun S, et al. Anti-aquaporin-4 monoclonal antibody blocker therapy for neuromyelitis optica. Ann Neurol. 2012;71:314–22.

56. Kreye J, Wenke NK, Chayka M, et al. Human cerebrospinal fluid monoclonal N-methyl-D-aspartate receptor autoantibodies are sufficient for encephalitis pathogenesis. Brain. 2016;139:2641–52.
57. Granerod J, Davies NW, Ramanuj PP, Easton A, Brown DW, Thomas SL. Increased rates of sequelae post-encephalitis in individuals attending primary care practices in the United Kingdom: a population-based retrospective cohort study. J Neurol. 2017;264:407–15.
58. Gaspard N, Foreman BP, Alvarez V, et al. New-onset refractory status epilepticus: Etiology, clinical features, and outcome. Neurology. 2015;85:1604–13.
59. Feyissa AM, Lopez Chiriboga AS, Britton JW. Antiepileptic drug therapy in patients with autoimmune epilepsy. Neurol Neuroimmunol Neuroinflamm. 2017;4:e353.
60. Finke C, Pruss H, Heine J, et al. Evaluation of cognitive deficits and structural hippocampal damage in encephalitis with Leucine-rich, Glioma-inactivated 1 antibodies. JAMA Neurol. 2017;74:50–9.
61. Lejuste F, Thomas L, Picard G, et al. Neuroleptic intolerance in patients with anti-NMDAR encephalitis. Neurol Neuroimmunol Neuroinflamm. 2016;3:e280.
62. Sacks O, Shulman M. Steroid dementia: an overlooked diagnosis? Neurology. 2005;64:707–9.
63. Kowski AB, Weissinger F, Gaus V, Fidzinski P, Losch F, Holtkamp M. Specific adverse effects of antiepileptic drugs—a true-to-life monotherapy study. Epilepsy Behav. 2016;54:150–7.
64. Iorio R, Lennon VA. Neural antigen-specific autoimmune disorders. Immunol Rev. 2012;248:104–21.
65. McKeon A. Immunotherapeutics for autoimmune encephalopathies and dementias. Curr Treat Options Neurol. 2013;15:723–37.

Neurosyphilis

13

Prathit A. Kulkarni and Jose A. Serpa

Introduction

Syphilis is a predominantly sexually transmitted infectious disease caused by the organism *Treponema pallidum* subspecies *pallidum*. Syphilis as a disease was first described in writing during the late 1400s in Europe [1]. The causative organism, *Treponema pallidum* (initially called *Spirochaeta pallida*), was not identified until the early twentieth century [2].

The concept of syphilis affecting the central nervous system was also described in the early twentieth century. For example, early studies demonstrated that between 30% and 70% of patients with secondary syphilis had cerebrospinal fluid (CSF) abnormalities [3]. More recent studies have shown similar findings [4, 5]. However, neurosyphilis is sometimes mistakenly thought of as "late" manifestation of syphilis or perhaps as a form of tertiary syphilis. While it is true that some forms of neurosyphilis do occur late in the course of disease, neurological symptoms and/or CSF abnormalities can be present during all stages of syphilis.

It is also important to note that the term "neurosyphilis" does not, on its own, signify a specific neurological syndrome. Rather, it only implies that the central nervous system (CNS) has been infected by *T. pallidum*. The range of neurological manifestations that might be produced by CNS infection is wide, as described later on. Also important is the fact that CNS infection by *T. pallidum* does not necessarily result in immediate neurological signs or symptoms, a condition called asymptomatic neurosyphilis.

P. A. Kulkarni · J. A. Serpa (✉)
Department of Medicine, Section of Infectious Diseases, Baylor College of Medicine, Houston, TX, USA
e-mail: Prathit.A.Kulkarni@uth.tmc.edu; Jose.A.Serpa@uth.tmc.edu

© Springer International Publishing AG, part of Springer Nature 2018
R. Hasbun (ed.), *Meningitis and Encephalitis*,
https://doi.org/10.1007/978-3-319-92678-0_13

Table 13.1 Definitions for terms related to clinical stages of syphilis

Term	Definition
Syphilis	Generic term that refers to infection with the organism *Treponema pallidum* at any stage with or without the presence of any clinical signs or symptoms
Early syphilis	Generally thought to encompass primary syphilis, secondary syphilis, and early latent syphilis
Late syphilis	Thought to represent late latent syphilis and tertiary syphilis
Primary syphilis	Initial stage of syphilis consisting of a genital chancre that appears at the site of inoculation approximately 10–90 days after acquisition of the infection [2]
Secondary syphilis	Second stage of syphilis resulting in a wide spectrum of symptoms, including fevers, malaise, lymphadenopathy, and rash (among myriad other possibilities)
Early latent syphilis	Evidence of infection due to *T. pallidum* as determined by serological testing but absence of signs or symptoms of clinical disease with infection having occurred within the prior 12 months [25]
Late latent syphilis	Evidence of infection due to *T. pallidum* as determined by serological testing but absence of signs or symptoms of clinical disease with infection having occurred more than 12 months prior [25]
Tertiary syphilis	Last stage of syphilis thought to occur approximately 5–30 years after initial infection with major forms being cardiovascular syphilis and non-CNS gummatous syphilis [2]
Neurosyphilis	Infection of the CNS due to *Treponema pallidum* can occur at any stage of syphilis
Early neurosyphilis	Neurosyphilis that occurs in the initial months to years after infection; thought to affect CSF, meninges, and vasculature more often and comprise the syndromes syphilis meningitis and meningovascular syphilis [3]
Late neurosyphilis	Neurosyphilis that occurs years to decades after initial infection; affects brain and spinal cord parenchyma more often; comprises the clinical syndromes general paresis (also known as syphilitic dementia or dementia paralytica) and tabes dorsalis [3]

Definitions/Terminology

The terminology surrounding different stages of syphilis and of neurosyphilis can be confusing. For the remainder of this chapter, it will be useful to define the terms that will be used in the interest of clarity; these terms are delineated in Table 13.1.

Clinical Presentation and Epidemiology

Natural History of Neurosyphilis

CNS invasion by spirochetes after initial infection can occur quickly. This initial invasion during the primary and secondary stages of syphilis can be asymptomatic or result in symptoms. If symptoms occur, they typically result in aseptic meningitis [6].

Whether or not asymptomatic neurosyphilis occurs during early syphilis, standard therapy for syphilis is thought to adequately prevent neurosyphilis. This was demonstrated in a number of studies performed during the 1950s and 1960s [7–12].

Although these studies were performed before the emergence of the HIV epidemic, a subsequent study in the 1990s that included more than 100 HIV-infected patients confirmed that enhanced therapy for early syphilis did not improve treatment outcomes despite detection of *T. pallidum* in CSF of ~25% of patients who were tested prior to therapy [5]. Ocular and otologic syphilis are most often a part of early neurosyphilis but can occur at any stage of the disease.

If a patient does not receive therapy during primary or secondary syphilis or if initial treatment is inadequate, spirochetes can replicate in the CNS and produce disease over time, resulting in meningovascular syphilis or forms of late neurosyphilis, including general paresis and tabes dorsalis [2].

As described in the terminology above, the term "early neurosyphilis" refers to disease which is thought to occur months to years after initial infection and most often results in syphilitic meningitis or meningovascular syphilis. It is important to note that the time frame of "early neurosyphilis" does not necessarily correspond directly to the time frame comprising "early syphilis." For example, in the case of meningovascular syphilis, symptoms developed an average of 7 years after initial infection [13, 14]. Late neurosyphilis is thought to occur many years to decades after initial infection. A useful illustration emphasizing these parallel timelines of the typical stages of syphilis and the progression of neurosyphilis is given in Fig. 13.1.

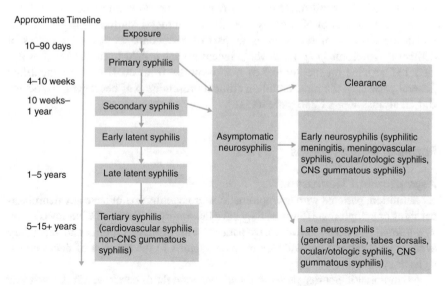

Fig. 13.1 This figure depicts the natural history and approximate timeline of untreated syphilis. Patients with primary and secondary syphilis can have asymptomatic neurosyphilis. The organism can be cleared from the CNS or can progress to early or late neurosyphilis. If asymptomatic neurosyphilis does not occur, the patient enters a phase, a latent infection which can progress to tertiary syphilis later on. It is important to note that asymptomatic neurosyphilis and early neurosyphilis can occur for up to years after initial infection

The relationship between HIV and neurosyphilis is complex and has led to different opinions about the management of syphilis and the need for lumbar puncture (LP) in this population. For example, in a study of 326 HIV-infected patients with syphilis, a peripheral CD4$^+$ cell count of ≤350 cells/µl was found to approximately triple the odds of neurosyphilis [15]. In another study of 180 patients with 231 episodes of a new diagnosis of syphilis, patients who had been on antiretroviral therapy prior to diagnosis had decreased the likelihood of having neurosyphilis (odds ratio 0.35) [16]. This study also confirmed the finding of approximately threefold increased odds of neurosyphilis when the CD4$^+$ count was ≤350 cells/microliter at the time of diagnosis.

Epidemiological Considerations

Syphilis became a reportable disease in the United States in 1941 [2]. Since that time, the incidence of syphilis had been declining overall and reached its nadir in the year 2000 [3]. However, since that time, the incidence of syphilis has been increasing [3].

It is generally thought that the incidence of "late neurosyphilis" has been declining over the last several decades [2, 3]. For example, tabes dorsalis in particular is extremely rarely diagnosed today, although precisely speaking, neurosyphilis itself is not a reportable condition; therefore, exact incidence rates are not available [2]. In addition, general paresis has become rare enough that the American Academy of Neurology does not recommend routine testing for syphilis (in the absence of risk factors) as part of a standard work-up for causes of dementia symptoms [17]. However, a recent review article from 2016 that evaluated 137 articles on the subject of neurosyphilis from 2010 to 2014 identified general paresis as the most common clinical presentation of neurosyphilis, occurring in almost 50% of 286 patients [18].

Forms of Neurosyphilis

Asymptomatic Neurosyphilis

By definition, patients with asymptomatic neurosyphilis do not have any neurological signs or symptoms. However, they have laboratory evidence of CNS invasion by *T. pallidum*. As noted above, many patients with primary syphilis and secondary syphilis have laboratory evidence of neurosyphilis in the absence of neurological signs or symptoms.

Asymptomatic neurosyphilis is sometimes thought to occur within the first few years of infection. However, it is important to note that asymptomatic neurosyphilis can be present later on. Patients with untreated or incompletely treated primary, secondary, or latent syphilis can harbor *T. pallidum* in the CNS for years, leading to late neurosyphilis in the future.

Early Neurosyphilis (Meningitis and Meningovascular Syphilis)

As mentioned above, early neurosyphilis tends to occur in the months to years following infection [3]. Early neurosyphilis is typically thought to comprise syphilitic meningitis and meningovascular syphilis.

Syphilitic meningitis most commonly occurs within 1 year of infection; however, meningitis can occur later as well [6]. Syphilitic meningitis resembles other forms of aseptic meningitis in its typical presentation [3]. In some instances, the spinal cord can also be involved, resulting in meningomyelitis or the so-called hyperplastic pachymeningitis [19]. In these cases, patients have typical symptoms of spinal cord pathology.

Meningovascular syphilis is typically thought of as a form of "early neurosyphilis" [2, 3]. The pathogenesis of meningovascular syphilis is inflammation of CNS vasculature, most often resulting in ischemia or infarction of the brain or spinal cord [3]. The clinical presentation will depend upon the particular neuroanatomical location of the ischemic event.

Late (Parenchymal) Neurosyphilis (General Paresis and Tabes Dorsalis)

Late neurosyphilis occurs years to decades after initial infection and is thought to result from the lack of or inadequate treatment at earlier stages of the disease [2, 3]. The main forms of late neurosyphilis are general paresis, also termed syphilitic dementia or dementia paralytica, and tabes dorsalis.

The term general paresis refers to the development of chronic neuropsychiatric symptoms. These symptoms can include personality changes, depressive symptoms, and psychotic symptoms. Most commonly, though, the disease manifests as progressive dementia with difficulties in judgment and memory, similar to other forms of progressive dementia. General paresis typically occurs anywhere from 2 to greater than 40 years after initial infection [2, 14, 20, 21]. One study identified a mean duration of infection prior to diagnosis of 10.5 years [21].

Tabes dorsalis, also known as locomotor ataxia, is a progressive form of late neurosyphilis that results in a variety of neurological signs and symptoms. These include electric pain, ataxia, paresthesias, loss of vibratory sensation and sensation to light touch, and pupillary abnormalities [3]. The pupillary abnormalities in tabes dorsalis reflect the so-called Argyll Robertson pupil, present in approximately half of patients with tabes dorsalis in one series [14]. The Argyll Robertson pupil does not constrict normally in response to light but does maintain response to accommodation. The electric pains described in the same series of cases of tabes dorsalis consisted of paroxysmal electric-type pain occurring in the face, back, and extremities. The pain lasted anywhere from several minutes up to several days.

CNS Gummatous Syphilis

Classically, "gummatous syphilis" is thought to be a tertiary form of the disease; this is typically the case with gummata that are present on the skin, bones, or viscera [2]. However, in the case of CNS gummatous syphilis, formation of gummata can occur at many different stages of neurosyphilis [3]. Gummata can arise from the meninges (most commonly the pia mater) or from the brain parenchyma itself. Gummata are well-circumscribed masses of granulomatous inflammation with lymphocytes and plasma cells with endarteritis and fibroblast and vascular proliferation; multinucleated giant cells are also present in some instances [22].

Ocular Syphilis

Ocular syphilis can occur at any stage of syphilis, but it is more commonly seen accompanying syphilitic meningitis. All parts of the eye may be affected. Various manifestations of ocular syphilis include optic neuritis, perineuritis (inflammation of the optic nerve sheath), episcleritis, interstitial keratitis, anterior uveitis, and posterior uveitis [2, 3]. Primary optic atrophy and retinal detachment can occur [2]. Anterior uveitis is often painful, while posterior uveitis is usually not [3].

Otologic Syphilis

Otologic syphilis, like ocular syphilis, can occur at any stage of syphilis. It most often manifests as hearing loss, either unilateral or bilateral. Symptoms such as vertigo and tinnitus can sometimes accompany hearing loss. Symptoms might sometimes be paroxysmal [23]. Otologic syphilis can occur in the presence or absence of syphilitic meningitis. In the presence of meningitis, cranial nerve VIII is thought to suffer inflammation, resulting in symptoms [2, 3]. In the absence of meningitis, there is probably osteitis of the temporal bone with long-term damage to the cochlea and labyrinth [2, 3].

Diagnosis

Diagnostic Criteria

The diagnosis of neurosyphilis can be straightforward in some instances but can be quite challenging in others. In particular, the diagnosis becomes more difficult when the CSF Venereal Disease Research Laboratory (VDRL) test is nonreactive. The CSF VDRL is considered to be highly specific for the diagnosis of neurosyphilis at any stage of the disease [2, 3, 24, 25]. However, its sensitivity is relatively low, ranging between 30% and 70% [3]. Therefore, a negative CSF VDRL test does not rule out the diagnosis of neurosyphilis, a key point that cannot be overemphasized. The current CDC case definition for neurosyphilis is given in Table 13.2.

Of note, although not explicitly stated in the case definition, CDC also writes, "Among persons with HIV infection, CSF leukocyte count usually is elevated (>5 white blood cell count [WBC]/mm^3). Using a higher cutoff (>20 WBC/mm^3) might improve the specificity of neurosyphilis diagnosis" [24, 25]. Also, although not specifically a part of the case definition, it is also important to consider the utility of the CSF fluorescent treponemal antibody absorbed (FTA-ABS) test. According to CDC, the "CSF FTA-ABS test is less specific for neurosyphilis than the CSF-VDRL but is highly sensitive. Neurosyphilis is highly unlikely with a negative CSF FTA-ABS

Table 13.2 2015 CDC case definition for neurosyphilis (modified format) [57]

Confirmed case
Positive CSF VDRL
and
Either reactive serum nontreponemal test or reactive serum treponemal test
Probable case
Negative CSF VDRL
and
Either reactive serum nontreponemal test or reactive serum treponemal test
and
Elevated CSF protein (>50 mg/dL) or WBC count (>5 WBCs/mm^3)
and
Clinical signs or symptoms consistent with neurosyphilis without other known causes for these abnormalities

CSF cerebrospinal fluid, *VDRL* Venereal Disease Research Laboratory, *WBC* white blood cell

test, especially among persons with nonspecific neurologic signs and symptoms." This topic was extensively reviewed in an article from 2012 [26]. The performance of CSF treponemal-specific antibody tests was close to but not uniformly 100%. Therefore, the negative predictive value of CSF FTA-ABS should take into account pretest probability of disease before being used as definitive evidence for ruling out neurosyphilis.

It should be noted that alternative diagnostic algorithms and criteria have been recommended by some experts [3]. These recommendations emphasize different diagnostic approaches for persons living with and without HIV; for patients living with HIV, factors such as CD4$^+$ count, HIV viral load, and CSF FTA-ABS are part of the diagnostic algorithm.

Role of Lumbar Puncture in Neurosyphilis

One of the major questions that should be asked for every patient diagnosed with syphilis is whether or not the patient should undergo CSF examination by means of LP.

In the 2015 CDC Sexually Transmitted Diseases Treatment Guidelines, the following approach is stated regarding this question: "unless clinical signs or symptoms of neurologic or ophthalmic involvement are present, routine CSF analysis is not recommended for persons who have primary or secondary syphilis" [24, 25]. Regarding latent syphilis, "Persons who receive a diagnosis of latent syphilis and have neurologic signs and symptoms… should be evaluated for neurosyphilis" [24, 25]. Contrary to this, all patients with tertiary syphilis (cardiovascular syphilis or gummatous syphilis) "should receive a CSF examination before therapy is initiated," regardless of the presence or absence of symptoms [24, 25]. In addition, a "CSF examination should be performed in all instances of ocular syphilis, even in the absence of clinical neurologic findings" [24, 25]. Regarding otologic syphilis, it might be reasonable to perform a CSF examination when otologic syphilis is suspected (and no other neurological signs or symptoms are present), although this issue has not been systematically studied. Of note, some experts recommend considering LP if the serum RPR is ≥1:32 [3].

With regard to HIV in particular, the question of which HIV-infected patients should undergo CSF examination is less straightforward and more controversial. The reason for this is that there is some evidence that HIV-infected patients have a higher risk of developing neurosyphilis as compared to HIV-uninfected patients, as discussed above. In addition, there is some evidence of higher rates of relapse and failure of treatment for neurosyphilis. For example, 4 out of 12 patients with AIDS and new diagnosis of neurosyphilis in a study from 1989 had been previously treated for syphilis [27]. In addition, increased reports of early neurosyphilis in HIV-infected patients emerged in the 1980s around the same time the HIV epidemic was unfolding [28]. With regard to failure of treatment for neurosyphilis, in a prospective study from 2004, the hazard ratio for HIV-infected patients to normalize CSF VDRL was 0.4 [29]. On the other hand, a large study conducted by CDC in the early 1990s demonstrated that enhanced therapy for early syphilis did not result in improved outcomes, regardless of HIV coinfection [5].

According to CDC guidelines, criteria for performing LP for HIV-infected patients with primary, secondary, or latent syphilis are no different than for HIV-uninfected patients. Other experts recommend different testing strategies for patients living with HIV [3].

Diagnosis of Ocular Syphilis

Another important diagnostic consideration is the diagnosis of ocular syphilis. In a situation where concomitant meningitis exists, the presence of abnormal eye findings can likely be more easily attributed to syphilis. However, in patients with anterior or posterior uveitis but no other neurological signs or symptoms, and an unremarkable CSF examination, a diagnosis of ocular syphilis would be very difficult to confirm. Routine dark-field examination or PCR testing for *T. pallidum* of vitreous or aqueous fluid typically does not occur in clinical practice. The point, therefore, is that the diagnosis of ocular syphilis, particularly in the absence of concomitant clinical meningitis or CSF abnormalities, requires a high index of clinical suspicion and the ability to connect serological testing with abnormal eye findings.

Diagnosis of Otologic Syphilis

Similar to ocular syphilis, the diagnosis of otologic syphilis might be obvious in a patient with syphilitic meningitis and concomitant hearing loss. However, in patients without meningitis, the diagnosis will by necessity be indirect; it might involve osteitis and vasculitis of the cochleovestibular system and temporal bone resulting in sensorineural hearing loss in conjunction with positive serological tests for syphilis. One likely will not be able to demonstrate direct evidence of infection in the involved tissue, a point that has been raised by some authors [30].

Role of Neuroimaging

Neuroimaging is not specifically required for the diagnosis of neurosyphilis. However, it can provide helpful adjunctive information in different circumstances. In the case of syphilitic meningitis, neuroimaging can demonstrate meningeal or CSF enhancement [31, 32]. With meningovascular syphilis, because the disease results in ischemia and infarction, evidence of these findings can be seen on neuroimaging [31, 33]. CNS gummatous syphilis can be seen on neuroimaging in the form of space-occupying lesions.

In general paresis, neuroimaging most often shows diffuse cerebral atrophy; other variable findings might also be seen [33]. In tabes dorsalis, spinal imaging can show increased signal intensity in the cord.

Treatment Regimens and Other Management Considerations

Intravenous penicillin remains the standard of care for the treatment of all forms of neurosyphilis, including asymptomatic neurosyphilis, ocular syphilis, and otologic syphilis.

In the second half of the twentieth century, the recognition of the treponemicidal effect of penicillin led to the widespread use of long-acting penicillin formulations such as intramuscular benzathine penicillin G (BPG) for the treatment of all stages of syphilis. However, not long after, case reports started documenting its inadequacy to treat cases of neurosyphilis [34–36]. The failure to treat neurosyphilis was probably associated with the low concentration of penicillin achieved in the central nervous system (CSF) of patients treated with these drug formulations.

Accepted treponemicidal concentrations of penicillin are approximately 0.018 µg/mL in both serum and CSF [37]. Although patients with neurosyphilis treated with intramuscular BPG showed adequate treponemicidal levels of penicillin in serum, the concentration of penicillin in CSF was remarkably low. In contrast, the majority of those patients who received intravenous aqueous crystalline penicillin G achieved adequate treponemicidal levels in CSF [38, 39]. For instance, an observational study evaluating different penicillin regimens found that patients treated with intravenous aqueous crystalline penicillin G at 4 million units every 4 h for 10 days consistently achieved CSF penicillin concentrations above the treponemicidal level [40]. This finding was further validated in a subsequent study [41].

No clinical trial that specifically confirms the superiority of aqueous crystalline penicillin G over BPG for the treatment of neurosyphilis has ever been conducted. Thus, the recommendation of using intravenous aqueous penicillin G for the treatment of neurosyphilis is derived from pharmacokinetic and observational data [42].

An alternative treatment regimen was described by Dunlop et al. They administered a combination of intramuscular procaine penicillin G 0.6 million units daily plus oral probenecid 500 mg every 6 h to 38 patients with neurosyphilis. All patients achieved treponemicidal concentrations of penicillin in serum and CSF [43]; however, subsequent studies suggested that this regimen might lead to subtherapeutic concentrations of penicillin in CSF of some patients. For instance, Goh et al. found that 6 out of 11 patients who received intramuscular procaine penicillin G and oral probenecid did not reach treponemicidal concentrations of penicillin in CSF [44]. In a similar study, van der Valk et al. observed a failure to achieve treponemicidal levels of penicillin in four out of ten patients with neurosyphilis who were treated with intramuscular procaine penicillin G and oral probenecid [45].

Another potential alternative regimen for treatment of neurosyphilis is ceftriaxone, given its ability to concentrate in CSF. Ceftriaxone might also be considered safe in patients with non-immediate-type penicillin allergies. Though the evidence to support its recommendation is limited. Ceftriaxone has been demonstrated to be active against syphilis in animal models [46]. Case reports and case series have also described successful outcomes in patients with neurosyphilis, including those coinfected with HIV, who received intravenous ceftriaxone 1–2 g daily for 10–14 days [47–50].

Doxycycline at doses of 200 mg twice daily has been demonstrated to penetrate the CSF of patients with neurosyphilis [51]. This regimen given for 21–28 days has been reported in small case series to lead to improvement in CSF parameters [51, 52]. However, the paucity of clinical data to support this regimen precludes its recommendation.

Current guidelines published by the Centers for Diseases Control and Prevention recommend the use of intravenous aqueous crystalline penicillin G as the first choice for the treatment of neurosyphilis [25]. Intramuscular procaine penicillin G with the addition of oral probenecid is considered an alternative (Table 13.3). Additionally, after completing treatment for neurosyphilis, some experts recommend administering intramuscular injections of BPG 2.4 million units weekly for

Table 13.3 Recommended regimens for treatment of neurosyphilis

First-line therapy	Dose and duration
Aqueous crystalline penicillin G	18–24 million units IV per day administered as
	3–4 million units IV every 4 h or continuous infusion for 10–14 days
Alternative regimen	
Procaine penicillin G plus oral probenecid	2.4 million units IM daily plus probenecid 500 mg PO administered
	four times a day for 10–14 days
For penicillin-allergic patients	
Ceftriaxone (non-immediate-type reactions)	2 g IV or IM daily for 10–14 days
Penicillin desensitization followed by first-line therapy	

up to 3 weeks [25]. Patients living with HIV and diagnosed with neurosyphilis should receive the same regimens as their non-HIV counterparts.

For penicillin-allergic patients, the use of intravenous or intramuscular ceftriaxone might be considered given the low likelihood of cross-reaction between penicillin and ceftriaxone. Other options involve formal penicillin allergy testing or a penicillin desensitization protocol in collaboration with an allergy specialist.

Treatment of neurosyphilis in pregnant women must be intravenous aqueous crystalline penicillin G. If a pregnant woman with neurosyphilis is allergic to penicillin, then penicillin desensitization should be performed. No other treatment is recommended in this setting.

Prognosis

CDC guidelines recommend monitoring treatment response in patients treated for neurosyphilis [25]. Experts suggest performing follow-up CSF studies every 3–6 months until CSF laboratory abnormalities, including VDRL titer, WBC count, and protein level, have resolved [53, 54]. Most patients experience a decrease in CSF WBC count by 6 months, a fourfold decrease in CSF VDRL titers by 1 year, and complete normalization of all CSF parameters by 2 years after treatment.

In a cohort study of patients living with HIV, the use of highly active antiretroviral therapy for more than 6 months after treatment of neurosyphilis showed a probable association with a lower rate of treatment failure [16].

In general, the clinical prognosis depends on the type of neurosyphilis. Overall, patients with syphilitic meningitis or gummata have a good prognosis after completing treatment with intravenous aqueous crystalline penicillin G. In contrast, patients with syphilis-associated dementia or tabes dorsalis will most likely experience persistent cognitive and sensory deficits, respectively. Similarly, patients with meningovascular neurosyphilis will usually experience residual neurological deficits from cerebrovascular complications [55].

Prevention

Because syphilis is predominantly a sexually transmitted infection, prevention of the infection understandably relies upon measures routinely taken to decrease the incidence of sexually transmitted diseases. These measures might include patient education, provision of condoms, and implementation of safe sex practices by patients. Patient education can include everything from counseling during a patient visit to broad public health campaigns and strategies that target the general public.

Prevention of neurosyphilis in particular is helped by screening for and early detection of syphilis. Early detection allows for prompt diagnosis and early treatment, thereby hopefully preventing symptomatic neurosyphilis from occurring. Current guidelines suggest that the following groups of patients should be routinely screened for syphilis [56]:

- Pregnant women (all patients at first prenatal visit and early in the third trimester and at delivery if at high risk)
- Men who have sex with men (at least annually if sexually active and every 3–6 months if at increased risk)
- Persons with HIV (for sexually active patients, at first evaluation and at least annually thereafter; more frequent screening could be needed depending upon individual risk and local epidemiology)

Future Areas of Research

Although significant progress has been made in the diagnosis and treatment of neurosyphilis, there are many areas of uncertainty that are yet to be elucidated.

For instance, the diagnosis of neurosyphilis continues to be challenging for clinicians. Although neurosyphilis may be suggested by the presence of one or more neurological syndromes, some patients may lack neurological symptoms (asymptomatic neurosyphilis). The diagnosis of neurosyphilis is confirmed with a lumbar puncture demonstrating a positive VDRL in CSF; however, this finding is not present in all patients, as discussed earlier. Some authors have proposed the use of other CSF findings including pleocytosis or an elevated protein level, to make a diagnosis of neurosyphilis; however, these abnormalities are nonspecific. Better diagnostic markers are needed to confirm the presence of CNS infection due to *T. pallidum*.

Another area of ambiguity is when to proceed with a diagnostic evaluation for neurosyphilis. In addition to performing LP on patients diagnosed with syphilis by serological methods who have neurological signs or symptoms, it is uncertain what other group or groups of patients would benefit from CSF examination. Some experts have recommended basing this decision on certain clinical and laboratory parameters. In our opinion, further studies, ideally collaborative multicenter cohort studies, should be conducted to validate previously proposed epidemiologic risk factors and laboratory markers for neurosyphilis.

Another area that deserves additional attention is the need for better prognostic tools. Currently, the response to the treatment of neurosyphilis is assessed by serial lumbar punctures until normalization of CSF parameters has occurred. Long-term follow-up studies are needed in order to confirm the use of these CSF markers for this purpose and to refine standards that confidently establish cure of the infection.

References

1. Farhi D, Dupin N. Origins of syphilis and management in the immunocompetent patient: facts and controversies. Clin Dermatol. 2010;28:533–8.
2. Radolf JD, Tramont EC, Salazar JC. Syphilis (*Treponema pallidum*). In: Bennett JE, Dolin R, Blaser MJ, editors. Mandell, Douglas, and Bennett's principles and practice of infectious diseases. Philadelphia: Elsevier; 2015. p. 2684–709.
3. Marra CM. Neurosyphilis. In: Scheld WM, Whitley RJ, Marra CM, editors. Infections of the central nervous system; 2014. p. 659–73.

4. Lukehart SA, Hook EW III, Baker-Zander SA, Collier AC, Critchlow CW, Handsfield HH. Invasion of the central nervous system by *Treponema pallidum*: implications for diagnosis and treatment. Ann Intern Med. 1988;109:855–62.

5. Rolfs RT, Joesoef MR, Hendershot EF, et al. A randomized trial of enhanced therapy for early syphilis in patients with and without human immunodeficiency virus infection. The Syphilis and HIV Study Group. N Engl J Med. 1997;337:307–14.

6. Merritt HH, Moore M. Acute syphilitic meningitis. Medicine (Baltimore). 1935;14:119–83.

7. Fernando WL. Cerebrospinal fluid findings after treatment of early syphilis with penicillin. Brit J Vener Dis. 1965;41:168–9.

8. Fernando WL. Cerebrospinal fluid findings after treatment of early syphilis with penicillin: a further series of 80 cases. Br J Vener Dis. 1968;44:134–5.

9. Chargin L, Sobel N, Vandow J, Rosenthal T. The long term results of the treatment. Acta Derm Venereol. 1958;38:168–72.

10. Perdrup A. Penicillin treatment of early syphilis. A follow-up study of 213 patients observed for one to eleven years. Comparison between the effect of six and twelve million units. Acta Derm Venereol. 1960;40:340–57.

11. Hellerstrom S, Skog E. Outcome of penicillin therapy of syphilis. Results of treatment in 231 cases at different stages of the disease. Acta Derm Venereol. 1962;42:179–94.

12. Jefferiss FJG, Willcox RR. Treatment of early syphilis with penicillin alone. Br J Vener Dis. 1963;39:143–8.

13. Merritt HH. The early clinical and laboratory manifestations of syphilis of the central nervous system. N Engl J Med. 1940;223:446–50.

14. Merritt HH, Adams RD, Solomon HC. Neurosyphilis. New York: Oxford University Press; 1946.

15. Marra CM, Maxwell CL, Smith SL, et al. Cerebrospinal fluid abnormalities in patients with syphilis: association with clinical and laboratory features. J Infect Dis. 2004;189:369–76.

16. Ghanem KG, Moore RD, Rompalo AM, Erbelding EJ, Zenilman JM, KA G. Neurosyphilis in a clinical cohort of HIV-1-infected patients. AIDS. 2008;22:1145–51.

17. AAN guideline summary for clinicians: detection, diagnosis, and management of dementia. Accessed 8 Aug 2017.

18. Drago F, Merlo G, Ciccarese G, et al. Changes in neurosyphilis presentation: a survey on 286 patients. J Eur Acad Dermatol Venereol. 2016;30:1886–900.

19. Adams RD, Merritt HH. Meningeal and vascular syphilis of the spinal cord. Medicine (Baltimore). 1944;23:181–214.

20. Hahn RD, Webster B, Weickhardt G, et al. Penicillin treatment of general paresis (dementia paralytica). AMA Arch Neurol Psychiatry. 1959;81:557.

21. Dewhurst K. The neurosyphilitic psychoses today. A survey of 91 cases. Br J Psychiatry. 1969;115:31–8.

22. Fargen KM, Alvernia JE, Lin CS, Melgar M. Cerebral syphilitic gummata: a case presentation and analysis of 156 reported cases. Neurosurgery. 2009;64:568–75.

23. Pasricha JM, Read TR, Street AC. Otosyphilis: a cause of hearing loss in adults with HIV. Med J Aust. 2010;193:421–2.

24. National Survey of Family Growth. 2015. Accessed 4 Nov 2016. http://www.cdc.gov/nchs/nsfg/key_statistics/s.htm-sexualorientationandattraction.

25. Workowski KA, Bolan GA, Centers for Disease Control and Prevention. Sexually transmitted diseases treatment guidelines, 2015. MMWR Recomm Rep. 2015;64:1–137.

26. Harding AS, Ghanem KG. The performance of cerebrospinal fluid treponemal-specific antibody tests in neurosyphilis: a systematic review. Sex Transm Dis. 2012;39:291–7.

27. Katz DA, Berger JR. Neurosyphilis in acquired immunodeficiency syndrome. Arch Neurol. 1989;46(8):895.

28. Musher DM. Syphilis, neurosyphilis, penicillin, and AIDS. J Infect Dis. 1991;163(6):1201.

29. Marra CM, Maxwell CL, Tantalo L, et al. Normalization of cerebrospinal fluid abnormalities after neurosyphilis therapy: does HIV status matter? Clin Infect Dis. 2004;38:1001–6.

30. Pletcher SD, Cheung SW. Syphilis and otolaryngology. Otolaryngol Clin N Am. 2003;36:595–605.
31. Peng F, Hu X, Zhong X, et al. CT and MR findings in HIV-negative neurosyphilis. Eur J Radiol. 2008;66:1–6.
32. Good CD, Jager HR. Contrast enhancement of the cerebrospinal fluid on MRI in two cases of spirochaetal meningitis. Neuroradiology. 2000;42:448–50.
33. Nagappa M, Sinha S, Taly AB, et al. Neurosyphilis: MRI features and their phenotypic correlation in a cohort of 35 patients from a tertiary care university hospital. Neuroradiology. 2013;55:379–88.
34. Zenker PN, Rolfs RT. Treatment of syphilis, 1989. Rev Infect Dis. 1990;12(Suppl 6):S590–609.
35. Greene BM, Miller NR, Bynum TE. Failure of penicillin G benzathine in the treatment of neurosyphilis. Arch Intern Med. 1980;140(8):1117.
36. Smith CA, Kamp M, Olansky S, Price EV. Benzathine penicillin G in the treatment of syphilis. Bull World Health Organ. 1956;15:1087–96.
37. Idsoe O, Guthe T, Willcox RR. Penicillin in the treatment of syphilis. The experience of three decades. Bull World Health Organ. 1972;47:1–68.
38. Mohr JA, Griffiths W, Jackson R, Saadah H, Bird P, Riddle J. Neurosyphilis and penicillin levels in cerebrospinal fluid. JAMA. 1976;236:2208–9.
39. Frentz G, Nielsen PB, Espersen F, Czartoryski A, Aastrup H. Penicillin concentrations in blood and spinal fluid after a single intramuscular injection of penicillin G benzathine. Eur J Clin Microbiol. 1984;3:147–9.
40. Polnikorn N, Witoonpanich R, Vorachit M, Vejjajiva S, Vejjajiva A. Penicillin concentrations in cerebrospinal fluid after different treatment regimens for syphilis. Br J Vener Dis. 1980;56:363–7.
41. Schoth PE, Wolters EC. Penicillin concentrations in serum and CSF during high-dose intravenous treatment for neurosyphilis. Neurology. 1987;37:1214–6.
42. Willcox RR. Treatment of syphilis. Bull World Health Organ. 1981;59:655–63.
43. Dunlop EM, Al-Egaily SS, Houang ET. Production of treponemicidal concentration of penicillin in cerebrospinal fluid. Br Med J (Clin Res Ed). 1981;283:646.
44. Goh BT, Smith GW, Samarasinghe L, Singh V, Lim KS. Penicillin concentrations in serum and cerebrospinal fluid after intramuscular injection of aqueous procaine penicillin 0.6 MU with and without probenecid. Br J Vener Dis. 1984;60:371–3.
45. van der Valk PG, Kraai EJ, van Voorst Vader PC, Haaxma-Reiche H, Snijder JA. Penicillin concentrations in cerebrospinal fluid (CSF) during repository treatment regimen for syphilis. Genitourin Med. 1988;64:223–5.
46. Johnson RC, Bey RF, Wolgamot SJ. Comparison of the activities of ceftriaxone and penicillin G against experimentally induced syphilis in rabbits. Antimicrob Agents Chemother. 1982;21:984–9.
47. Hook EW 3rd, Baker-Zander SA, Moskovitz BL, Lukehart SA, Handsfield HH. Ceftriaxone therapy for asymptomatic neurosyphilis. Case report and western blot analysis of serum and cerebrospinal fluid IgG response to therapy. Sex Transm Dis. 1986;13:185–8.
48. Gentile JH, Viviani C, Sparo MD, Arduino RC. Syphilitic meningomyelitis treated with ceftriaxone: case report. Clin Infect Dis. 1998;26:528.
49. Marra CM, Boutin P, McArthur JC, et al. A pilot study evaluating ceftriaxone and penicillin G as treatment agents for neurosyphilis in human immunodeficiency virus-infected individuals. Clin Infect Dis. 2000;30:540–4.
50. Dowell ME, Ross PG, Musher DM, Cate TR, Baughn RE. Response of latent syphilis or neurosyphilis to ceftriaxone therapy in persons infected with human immunodeficiency virus. Am J Med. 1992;93:481–8.
51. Yim CW, Flynn NM, Fitzgerald FT. Penetration of oral doxycycline into the cerebrospinal fluid of patients with latent or neurosyphilis. Antimicrob Agents Chemother. 1985;28:347–8.
52. Kang-Birken SL, Castel U, Prichard JG. Oral doxycycline for treatment of neurosyphilis in two patients infected with human immunodeficiency virus. Pharmacotherapy. 2010;30:119e–22e.

53. Ghanem KG. REVIEW: neurosyphilis: a historical perspective and review. CNS Neurosci Ther. 2010;16:e157–68.
54. Marra CM. Update on neurosyphilis. Curr Infect Dis Rep. 2009;11:127–34.
55. Conde-Sendin MA, Amela-Peris R, Aladro-Benito Y, Maroto AA. Current clinical spectrum of neurosyphilis in immunocompetent patients. Eur Neurol. 2004;52:29–35.
56. Screening recommendations and considerations referenced in treatment guidelines and original sources. 2015. Accessed 25 Sept 2017. https://www.cdc.gov/std/tg2015/screening-recommendations.htm.
57. Syphilis (*Treponema pallidum*): 2014 case definition. 2014. Accessed 7 Aug 2017. https://wwwn.cdc.gov/nndss/conditions/syphilis/case-definition/2014/.

Neuroborreliosis

14

John J. Halperin

Introduction

The term neuroborreliosis is commonly used, particularly in Europe, to describe the neurologic manifestations of infection with the tick-borne spirochetes *Borrelia garinii* and *B. afzelii*. In the USA, it is used—though less consistently—to describe nervous system involvement with the closely related spirochete, *B. burgdorferi* sensu stricto, the agent of Lyme disease. The neurologic manifestations of this multisystem infection were first described in 1922—more than half a century before the introduction of the terms Lyme arthritis and Lyme disease and the characterization shortly thereafter of the closely related *borrelia* species responsible for these disorders in North America and Europe.

Although this chapter will focus on disorders caused by these microorganisms, it is important to recognize that the term is also used to describe nervous system involvement in relapsing fevers. These *borrelia* infections include two principle tick-borne spirochetes in the USA—*B. hermsii* and *B. turicatae*. *B. recurrentis*, a louse-borne spirochete, causes epidemic relapsing fever in the underdeveloped world. Recent additions to this family include *B. miyamotoi*, first identified in 1994 in the USA as the rare cause of a relapsing fever-like illness [1], and *B. mayonii*, an even more rare organism that causes a Lyme disease-like disorder [2]. Of these, *B. turicatae* is neurotropic, commonly causing meningitis but remarkably little nervous system damage or symptomatology [3]. To date *B. miyamotoi* has only been associated with nervous system involvement in immunocompromised individuals [4]. In light of this, this chapter will focus on nervous system involvement in Lyme disease and the closely related disorders occurring in Europe.

J. J. Halperin
Department of Neurosciences, Overlook Medical Center, Summit, NJ, USA

Sidney Kimmel Medical College of Thomas Jefferson University, Philadelphia, PA, USA
e-mail: john.halperin@atlantichealth.org

© Springer International Publishing AG, part of Springer Nature 2018
R. Hasbun (ed.), *Meningitis and Encephalitis*,
https://doi.org/10.1007/978-3-319-92678-0_14

Lyme disease has been the source of remarkable controversy—much of it related to misconceptions about what constitutes neurologic disease. Given that neurodegenerative disorders such as Alzheimer's dementia are among the most feared of all diagnoses, it would seem self-evident that diagnosis of potentially brain damaging disorders, particularly those thought to be incurable, should be accurate. However, the widespread lack of awareness that fluctuations in memory and cognitive function are quite commonplace, particularly in the setting of systemic inflammatory disease, and that this is not evidence of nervous system damage, is probably responsible for the vast majority of the controversy. Misconceptions about these infections' treatment responsiveness reinforce this fear. When patients experiencing such cognitive difficulties read on the Internet that this is due to a very difficult to treat spirochetal infection of the nervous system, their anxiety about the symptoms is compounded, only worsening their symptoms. Subjecting them to prolonged and inappropriate antibiotic therapy and its side effects further adds to their difficulties. And, almost paradoxically, this focus on these non-neurologic issues can lead to failure to recognize those disorders that truly are attributable to neuroborreliosis and therefore amenable to simple treatment.

Diagnosis

The three key requirements for the diagnosis of neuroborreliosis are first, likely exposure; second, recognition of clinical disorders that are likely to indicate this infection; and third, laboratory confirmation, as appropriate.

Exposure

Lyme disease is spread exclusively by bites of *Ixodes* (hard-shelled) ticks. While exposure to these ticks is necessary, it is equally important that the ticks carry the causative organisms. 90+% of all US cases [5] occur in 14 northeast and north central states, the area where large numbers of these ticks coexist with abundant infected reservoir hosts—primarily white footed field mice—that maintain the responsible spirochetes in the ecosystem. Even within this geographic area, local geography is important. Since ticks and field mice do poorly in urban environments, this is a disease of suburbs, exurbs, and rural areas. It is extraordinarily rare in individuals who never leave heavily urban areas.

Lyme disease is a zoonosis—an infection that bridges different species. Vector ticks hatch uninfected. If these uninfected larvae feed on an infected reservoir host—white-footed field mice can be spirochetemic for an extended period of time, apparently asymptomatically—the ingested spirochetes can then survive in the tick gut. The tick larva then matures into a nymph—still quite small, about the size of a period on a printed page—and seeks its second blood meal. Ingested blood then triggers proliferation of these spirochetes within the tick gut. They then migrate through the tick, including to its salivary glands. While attached, ticks inject saliva, containing anticoagulants and other compounds into the host to enable the required prolonged feeding. Once spirochetes reach their salivary glands, they can be injected into the host, potentially infecting the host. Since this spirochete proliferation and spread within the tick requires at least 24–48 h, prolonged tick attachment is required for infection to occur. The same sequence can occur during feeding by infected adult ticks. Since there are fewer adults than nymphs, and since adults are larger and more noticeable, they are less commonly the culprit. This then provides two opportunities to limit the risk of Lyme disease—avoiding tick habitats and, when this is unavoidable, frequent tick checks with removal of any that are attached, before prolonged feeding has occurred.

Signs and Symptoms

The symptoms associated with Lyme disease can be divided into those that are relatively specific and those that are completely non-specific. Fever, malaise, fatigue, cognitive slowing, and diffuse aches and pains can occur in innumerable infections and inflammatory states and are well exemplified by the side effects experienced by patients treated with interferons for multiple sclerosis or other diseases. Such symptoms lack any specificity for Lyme disease. At the other extreme, the characteristic skin rash, erythema migrans (EM), is virtually pathognomonic. This slowly expanding, often asymptomatic, erythroderm, occurring at the site of the tick bite, is observed in 90% of children [6] with Lyme disease. It is reported less frequently in adults, perhaps reflecting lack of an outside observer to notice these asymptomatic rashes on difficult to see parts of the body. Typically at least several inches in diameter, EM appears days after the bite—differentiating it from the transient and immediate reaction typically seen at the site of arthropod bites—which disappears in a few days. Over the course of days to weeks, EM can expand to be a foot or more in diameter. In the USA, it can become multifocal in up to a quarter of patients, something seen less commonly with European strains. Since EM occurs very early in infection, about half of patients will not yet have had time to develop a measurable antibody response— i.e., will be seronegative. Patients with potential exposure and this rash should be treated—without either obtaining or waiting for laboratory confirmation of the diagnosis.

Several other extra-neurologic manifestations should bring Lyme disease to mind in individuals with plausible exposure. Heart block—up to complete heart block requiring a temporary pacemaker—can occur in otherwise healthy young individuals, as can large joint arthritis. The latter typically affects a single large joint at a time, arising and subsiding spontaneously. Heart block (affecting perhaps 1% of patients) tends to occur quite early in infection, arthritis somewhat later. Neither is so specific to Lyme disease as to be syndromically diagnostic like EM; in both serologies should be positive.

Neurologic Signs and Symptoms

Neuroborreliosis—infection of the nervous system with *B. burgdorferi*, *B. garinii*, or *B. afzelii*—is identified in 12–15% of infected individuals. Clinically evident involvement usually occurs fairly early in infection, occasionally preceding sero-conversion. Polymerase chain reaction (PCR)-based studies further support the con-clusion that CNS invasion occurs early but also suggests it may be both asymptomatic and more frequent than is clinically apparent [7]—although whether this is clini-cally important is unclear. The original emphasis on a "classic triad' [8, 9] remains useful. Patients develop—either singly or in combination—lymphocytic meningitis, cranial neuritis, and painful radiculitis.

Meningeal inflammation, as reflected in a cerebrospinal fluid (CSF) pleocytosis, may be asymptomatic or may have the same headache, fever, and systemic symp-toms seen in viral meningitis—although symptom onset may be somewhat less abrupt than in viral meningitis. Since it is usually an early manifestation of infec-tion, it typically follows the same seasonality as tick bites and EM. As such it may occur earlier in summer than enteroviral meningitis. However, despite the develop-ment of algorithms trying to differentiate between viral and Lyme meningitis, these tend to be heavily driven by the co-occurrence of other manifestations such as cra-nial neuropathies [10]. In the absence of these more specific manifestations, differ-entiating Lyme from other summertime meningitides cannot be done reliably on clinical grounds alone.

While other nervous system manifestations similarly lack sufficient positive pre-dictive value to be considered diagnostic of Lyme disease, some should definitely raise the possibility. Of these, cranial neuropathy is probably the most common, particularly facial nerve paralysis. In adults, it is estimated that a quarter of facial nerve palsies occurring in non-winter months in endemic areas are attributable to Lyme disease [11, 12]—i.e., three quarters are not— so a presumptive diagnosis of Lyme disease would be inappropriate. While idiopathic facial nerve palsies are comparatively common, idiopathic bilateral involvement is unusual and should bring to mind Lyme disease, sarcoid, other basilar meningitides, as well as HIV and Guillain-Barre syndrome. Patients with Lyme disease can develop other combina-tions of multiple cranial neuropathies as well, which may occur simultaneously or sequentially. Although it would seem logical to assume that facial nerve involve-ment occurs in the inflamed subarachnoid space, a systematic review of one center's experience [13] found a CSF pleocytosis in only a minority of patients and clinical evidence of extra-axial involvement in many.

The third element of the triad is the one most frequently forgotten—painful radiculitis. As well described in the original case report by Garin and Bujadoux, patients can develop severe radicular pain—identical in character to that occur-ring with mechanical radiculopathies. Usually there is no history of a likely physical precipitant. Involvement can be truncal or in a limb. Although often described as occurring in the same dermatome as the initial tick bite, this is not a consistent observation [14]. Not unlike diabetic radiculopathies, this can be less anatomically limited than mechanical radiculopathies, with involvement of several adjacent dermatomes. Although localized pain is often a dominant symptom, muscle weakness and atrophy in the same nerve root distribution can occur as well. Some patients, particularly in Europe, develop spinal cord inflammation involving the same segmental level. While patients often have a co-occurring CSF pleocytosis, this is not invariable. Detailed neurophysiologic testing suggests that this radiculopathy is probably pathophysiologically a mononeuropathy multiplex—as are cranial neuropathies [15]. In light of this, it should not be surprising that plexopathies and individual mononeuropathies are described as well.

Over the years the spectrum of nervous system involvement in this infection has broadened. In children, it is not uncommon to see raised intracranial pressure (typically with or following meningitis) creating a pseudotumor-like picture. These children have headaches, visual obscurations, and papilledema and require treatment of their raised intracranial pressure in addition to antibiotics.

Rare patients, particularly those infected with European borrelia, develop CNS parenchymal inflammation. Although most commonly involving the spinal cord at the segmental level of the radiculopathy, rare patients develop inflammation of the brain, brainstem, or cerebellum, evident on brain imaging and neurologic examination [16], and with inflammatory CSF. Like all neuroborreliosis this has been antibiotic responsive, though as with all nervous system insults, some residua may remain, depending on the extent of pretreatment damage.

Finally, European patients with an unusual late cutaneous manifestation, acrodermatitis atrophicans (not seen with US borrelia strains), develop a more clinically diffuse polyneuropathy [17]. A similar condition has been described in US patients with long-standing untreated Lyme arthritis [18]—a state that rarely occurs today. Importantly neurophysiologic findings in these patients suggest a confluent mononeuropathy multiplex, implicating the same pathophysiologic process seen in the more acute presentations, as well as in virtually all experimentally infected rhesus macaque monkeys [19].

Neurobehavioral Phenomena

In early studies, primarily of individuals with prolonged, untreated Lyme arthritis, many patients described cognitive and memory difficulties that interfered with their daily functioning. Clinically similar to the "toxic metabolic encephalopathy" seen in innumerable other systemic inflammatory states, extensive evaluations led to the conclusion that this was only very rarely related to nervous system infection [20, 21]. Unfortunately, evidence to the contrary notwithstanding, some concluded both that this very common and non-specific syndrome was in and of itself diagnostic of Lyme disease and that it was due to nervous system infection. This in turn led to antibiotic treatment with ever more prolonged, complex, and inappropriate regimens. Although the pathophysiology of this disorder remains unclear, it has been well established that it does not respond to prolonged courses of antibiotics [22–25].

More recently this has led to the related construct of posttreatment Lyme disease syndrome—occurrence of the same symptoms in individuals previously treated for Lyme disease. While it is unclear if this is a biologically distinct entity, or merely represents anchoring bias in individuals who develop these non-specific symptoms, it is quite clear that this disorder is not linked to central nervous system (CNS) infection [26, 27]. In fact, the best predictor of which patients might have such symptoms is the presence of multiple comorbidities and of having prolonged symptoms prior to treatment—and not whether or not the nervous system was ever infected.

Laboratory Diagnosis

Despite frequent discussion of the limitations of laboratory diagnosis in Lyme disease, these are comparable to those in other infections. As with syphilis and some other spirochetal diseases, culture is impractical. Unlike *Treponema pallidum*, *borrelia* can be grown in vitro—but it requires special culture medium not typically available in most microbiology laboratories and prolonged incubation at temperatures lower than those used for other pathogens. Moreover, other than in EM, the bacterial load appears to be quite low in readily obtainable samples. Using either culture or PCR, *borrelia* can be identified in CSF of patients with Lyme meningitis in fewer than 20% of patients. As a result, diagnosis rests on demonstration of antibodies—in serum, CSF, or both.

While in most other infections we measure acute and convalescent antibody titers, in Lyme disease, the usual practice is to measure antibodies just once. In one widely cited study that concluded, based on laboratory testing, that the true incidence of Lyme disease is ten times that derived from reported cases meeting the CDC case definition [28], the assumption was that 85% of patients had just one serologic test. Since serologies can remain positive for an extended period of time after a resolved infection, this poses obvious diagnostic limitations—even before considering false positives. A true positive result at best means exposure and infection, past or present, not necessarily a current or relevant one. In contrast, very early in infection—as in any infection—patients may be seronegative, as it takes time for the host immune response to produce sufficient antibodies to be measurable in serum. In patients with EM, which develops within the first 30 days of infection, fewer than half have measurable serum antibody [29]. While this number is widely quoted as evidence of the insensitivity of serologic tests, this only impacts very early disease. Among patients with infection of more than 1–2 month's duration, serology is essentially always positive.

The challenge of eliminating false positives due to cross-reacting antibodies is shared by all serologic tests. In Lyme disease, some false positives—to syphilis and relapsing fevers, for instance—occur because the organisms are so similar that serology cannot differentiate among them. For syphilis, reaginic tests (RPR, VDRL) are useful as these are rarely positive in Lyme. For other borrelia, fortunately there is minimal epidemiologic overlap. Between the differences in clinical presentation

Table 14.1 Western blot criteria [35]

IgG (5 of 10)	IgM (2 of 3)
18 kD	23 kD
23 kD	39 kD
28 kD	41 kD
31 kD	
39 kD	
41 kD	
45 kD	
58 kD	
66 kD	
93 kD	

(relapsing fevers) and the different geographic distributions, differentiation among these infections is rarely difficult.

The more common difficulty is in patients with other inflammatory states where polyclonal B cell expansion creates multiple false-positive serologic results. Western blots were added specifically to address this issue. Observations in large numbers of individuals with and without Lyme disease showed that some immunoreactivities (bands) had high predictive value for a correct diagnosis while others did not. This led to a widespread consensus that the presence of two of three specified IgM bands or five of ten specified IgG bands was highly indicative of Lyme disease (past or present) (Table 14.1). Combining this in a two-tier approach with a screening ELISA, proceeding to a Western blot when serology was positive or borderline, resulted in high diagnostic specificity. Importantly, bands were not selected because they are unique to *B. burgdorferi*. Those used—and not used—were selected based on their statistical ability, in combination, to diagnose infection accurately. More recent work measuring antibodies to C6 (a highly conserved domain in *B. burgdorferi*) suggests that this is at least as accurate as whole cell sonicate ELISAs and may provide a substitute for either the ELISA or Western blot [30] in the two-tier approach [31].

When considering infection in the CNS, an additional diagnostic approach can be used. The CNS acts as an immunologically separate compartment. While a small amount of peripheral IgG filters into the CSF (<1% with an intact blood-brain barrier), the presence of infecting organisms within the CNS triggers in-migration of B cells, their proliferation, and then local production of specific antibodies. Comparing CSF to serum antibody concentrations, after adjusting for overall concentration of IgG in both fluids, allows demonstration of intrathecal antibody production (ITAb). This method appears to identify virtually all patients with Lyme meningitis. In European guidelines, the presence of demonstrable ITAb is required to diagnose definite neuroborreliosis [32]. Since Lyme disease may be limited to the peripheral nervous system, there should be no logical expectation that there would be ITAb in such individuals. That notwithstanding, at least a third of such patients may have concurrent meningitis. Consequently, ITAb is sufficient to diagnose nervous system infection, but not necessary.

Measurement of ITAb has several limitations. Issues with false positives are comparable to those with peripheral serologies. Cross-reactivity in neurosyphilis is common—but again reaginic tests in the CSF help differentiate between the two. Few other infections show cross-reactivity. Polyclonal B cell expansion is less of an issue and generally is adequately addressed by indexing CSF specific antibody to that in serum. The most challenging issue is that, as with peripheral serology, ITAb can remain elevated long after successful treatment—with studies showing this to occur as much as 10 years after effective treatment. As in neurosyphilis successful treatment is followed by a slow decline in CSF cells and protein. An additional marker, CXCL13, a B cell-attracting chemokine, shows promise as an additional marker of disease activity and may be useful if it becomes commercially available.

Treatment

Like all forms of Lyme disease, nervous system infection is responsive to antibiotic treatment—with the one additional consideration that the nervous system is less able to heal after damage has occurred. Hence particularly in those rare individuals with parenchymal CNS inflammation, there may be residual difficulty after infection is eliminated. In choosing treatment it is important to recall that it was because of CNS involvement that meningeal dose penicillin was first introduced, followed by ceftriaxone and cefotaxime. However subsequent work has shown that oral doxycycline is equally effective in Lyme meningitis, cranial neuropathy, radiculopathy, and other peripheral nerve involvement [33]. Most would still treat parenchymal CNS disease with parenteral ceftriaxone, but there are no data directly bearing on this—nor are there likely to be—given the rarity and seriousness of this disorder. Current treatment recommendations (Table 14.2) support both oral doxycycline and parenteral regimens for all but parenchymal CNS neuroborreliosis; it is likely updated recommendations will support oral doxycycline as the first line treatment for non-parenchymal neuroborreliosis. Although historically doxycycline has been proscribed for children 8 years of age and younger, recent studies [34] suggest that

Table 14.2 Treatment of neuroborreliosis; all for 2–4 weeks

	Adult	Pediatric (not to exceed adult dose)
Ceftriaxone	2 g IV/d	50–75 mg/kg/day IV
Cefotaxime	2 g IV q8 hours	150–200 mg/kg/day IV, in 3 divided doses
Penicillin G	3–4 MU IV q4 hours	200,000–400,000 U/kg/day IV in 6 divided doses
Or		
Doxycycline	100–200 mg PO BID	2 mg/kg/day PO BID[a]
Possible alternatives		
Amoxicillin	500 mg PO TID	50 mg/kg/day PO in 3 divided doses
Cefuroxime axetil	500 mg PO BID	30 mg/kg/day PO in 2 divided doses

[a]Although tetracycline may cause bone and dental staining in children 8 years of age or younger and is typically avoided, this does not appear to be the case with doxycycline. While doxycycline is not currently recommended for children under 8, this recommendation is likely to change, and current pediatric recommendations should be consulted

the dental staining that led to avoiding tetracycline in young children is not an issue with doxycycline. It is anticipated that upcoming recommendations from pediatric societies will no longer list this contraindication.

Conclusion

Neuroborreliosis, nervous system infection with *B. burgdorferi* sensu stricto, *B. garinii*, and *B. afzelii*, can be manifested as lymphocytic meningitis and/or various forms of mononeuropathy multiplex—including cranial neuropathies, radiculopathies, plexopathies, and rarely a confluent mononeuropathy multiplex. Rarely it involves the parenchymal CNS, most often affecting the spinal cord at the same level as radicular involvement. Treatment with 2–4 weeks of oral doxycycline is highly effective in peripheral nerve disease—including cranial neuropathy and radiculoneuropathy—and in meningitis. Parenteral antibiotics (2–4 weeks) are typically used—and are highly effective—in the rare patients with parenchymal CNS involvement. Lyme encephalopathy and posttreatment Lyme disease syndrome (if the latter exists) do not involve nervous system infection.

References

1. Krause PJ, Narasimhan S, Wormser GP, Rollend L, Fikrig E, Lepore T, et al. Human *Borrelia miyamotoi* infection in the United States. N Engl J Med. 2013;368(3):291–3.
2. Pritt BS, Mead PS, Johnson DK, Neitzel DF, Respicio-Kingry LB, Davis JP, et al. Identification of a novel pathogenic Borrelia species causing Lyme borreliosis with unusually high spirochaetaemia: a descriptive study. Lancet Infect Dis. 2016;16(5):556–64.
3. Gelderblom H, Londono D, Bai Y, Cabral ES, Quandt J, Hornung R, et al. High production of CXCL13 in blood and brain during persistent infection with the relapsing fever spirochete *Borrelia turicatae*. J Neuropathol Exp Neurol. 2007;66(3):208–17.
4. Boden K, Lobenstein S, Hermann B, Margos G, Fingerle V. Borrelia miyamotoi-associated neuroborreliosis in immunocompromised person. Emerg Infect Dis. 2016;22(9):1617–20.
5. Mead PS. Epidemiology of Lyme disease. Infect Dis Clin N Am. 2015;29(2):187–210.
6. Pediatric Lyme Disease Study Group, Gerber MA, Shapiro ED, Burke GS, Parcells VJ, Bell GL. Lyme disease in children in southeastern Connecticut. N Engl J Med. 1996;335(17):1270–4.
7. Luft BJ, Steinman CR, Neimark HC, Muralidhar B, Rush T, Finkel MF, et al. Invasion of the central nervous system by *Borrelia burgdorferi* in acute disseminated infection. JAMA. 1992;267(10):1364–7.
8. Garin C, Bujadoux A. Paralysie par les tiques. J Med Lyon. 1922;71:765–7.
9. Reik L Jr, Burgdorfer W, Donaldson JO. Neurologic abnormalities in Lyme disease without erythema chronicum migrans. Am J Med. 1986;81(1):73–8.
10. Garro AC, Rutman M, Simonsen K, Jaeger JL, Chapin K, Lockhart G. Prospective validation of a clinical prediction model for Lyme meningitis in children. Pediatrics. 2009;123(5):e829–34.
11. Halperin JJ, Golightly M. Lyme borreliosis in Bell's palsy. Long Island Neuroborreliosis Collaborative Study Group. Neurology. 1992;42(7):1268–70.
12. Bremell D, Hagberg L. Clinical characteristics and cerebrospinal fluid parameters in patients with peripheral facial palsy caused by Lyme neuroborreliosis compared with facial palsy of unknown origin (Bell's palsy). BMC Infect Dis. 2011;11:215.
13. Halperin JJ. Facial nerve palsy associated with Lyme disease. Muscle Nerve. 2003;28:516–7.
14. Ogrinc K, Lusa L, Lotric-Furlan S, Bogovic P, Stupica D, Cerar T, et al. Course and outcome of early European Lyme neuroborreliosis (Bannwarth syndrome): clinical and laboratory findings. Clin Infect Dis. 2016;63(3):346–53.

15. Halperin JJ, Luft BJ, Volkman DJ, Dattwyler RJ. Lyme neuroborreliosis—peripheral nervous system manifestations. Brain. 1990;113:1207–21.
16. Kalina P, Decker A, Kornel E, Halperin JJ. Lyme disease of the brainstem. Neuroradiology. 2005;47(12):903–7.
17. Hopf HC. Peripheral neuropathy in acrodermatitis chronica atrophicans (Herxheimer). J Neurol Neurosurg Psychiatry. 1975;38(5):452–8.
18. Halperin JJ, Little BW, Coyle PK, Dattwyler RJ. Lyme disease: cause of a treatable peripheral neuropathy. Neurology. 1987;37(11):1700–6.
19. England JD, Bohm RP, Roberts ED, Philipp MT. Mononeuropathy multiplex in rhesus monkeys with chronic Lyme disease. Ann Neurol. 1997;41(3):375–84.
20. Halperin JJ, Krupp LB, Golightly MG, Volkman DJ. Lyme borreliosis-associated encephalopathy. Neurology. 1990;40:1340–3.
21. Halperin JJ. Editorial commentary: neuroborreliosis: what is it, what isn't it? Clin Infect Dis. 2016;63(3):354–5.
22. Klempner MS, Hu LT, Evans J, Schmid CH, Johnson GM, Trevino RP, et al. Two controlled trials of antibiotic treatment in patients with persistent symptoms and a history of Lyme disease. N Engl J Med. 2001;345(2):85–92.
23. Krupp LB, Hyman LG, Grimson R, Coyle PK, Melville P, Ahnn S, et al. Study and treatment of post Lyme disease (STOP-LD): a randomized double masked clinical trial. Neurology. 2003;60(12):1923–30.
24. Fallon BA, Keilp JG, Corbera KM, Petkova E, Britton CB, Dwyer E, et al. A randomized, placebo-controlled trial of repeated IV antibiotic therapy for Lyme encephalopathy. Neurology. 2008;70:992–1003.
25. Berende A, ter Hofstede HJ, Vos FJ, van Middendorp H, Vogelaar ML, Tromp M, et al. Randomized trial of longer-term therapy for symptoms attributed to Lyme disease. N Engl J Med. 2016;374(13):1209–20.
26. Dersch R, Sommer H, Rauer S, Meerpohl JJ. Prevalence and spectrum of residual symptoms in Lyme neuroborreliosis after pharmacological treatment: a systematic review. J Neurol. 2016;263(1):17–24.
27. Wills AB, Spaulding AB, Adjemian J, Prevots DR, Turk SP, Williams C, et al. Long-term follow-up of patients with Lyme disease: longitudinal analysis of clinical and quality-of-life measures. Clin Infect Dis. 2016;62(12):1546–51.
28. Hinckley AF, Connally NP, Meek JI, Johnson BJ, Kemperman MM, Feldman KA, et al. Lyme disease testing by large commercial laboratories in the United States. Clin Infect Dis. 2014;59(5):676–81.
29. Nowakowski J, Schwartz I, Liveris D, Wang G, Aguero-Rosenfeld ME, Girao G, et al. Laboratory diagnostic techniques for patients with early Lyme disease associated with erythema migrans: a comparison of different techniques. Clin Infect Dis. 2001;33(12):2023–7.
30. Branda JA, Linskey K, Kim YA, Steere AC, Ferraro MJ. Two-tiered antibody testing for Lyme disease with use of 2 enzyme immunoassays, a whole-cell sonicate enzyme immunoassay followed by a VlsE C6 peptide enzyme immunoassay. Clin Infect Dis. 2011;53(6):541–7.
31. Branda JA, Strle K, Nigrovic LE, Lantos PM, Lepore TJ, Damle NS, et al. Evaluation of modified 2-tiered serodiagnostic testing algorithms for early Lyme disease. Clin Infect Dis. 2017;64(8):1074–80.
32. Mygland A, Ljostad U, Fingerle V, Rupprecht T, Schmutzhard E, Steiner I. EFNS guidelines on the diagnosis and management of European Lyme neuroborreliosis. Eur J Neurol. 2010;17(1):8–16. e1–4.
33. Halperin JJ, Shapiro ED, Logigian EL, Belman AL, Dotevall L, Wormser GP, et al. Practice parameter: treatment of nervous system Lyme disease. Neurology. 2007;69(1):91–102.
34. Todd SR, Dahlgren FS, Traeger MS, Beltran-Aguilar ED, Marianos DW, Hamilton C, et al. No visible dental staining in children treated with doxycycline for suspected Rocky Mountain spotted fever. J Pediatr. 2015;166(5):1246–51.
35. Dressler F, Ackermann R, Steere AC. Antibody responses to the three genomic groups of *Borrelia burgdorferi* in European Lyme borreliosis. J Infect Dis. 1994;169(2):313–8.

Emerging Causes of Encephalitis: Zika, Dengue, Chikungunya, and Beyond

Mario Luis Garcia de Figueiredo
and Luiz Tadeu Moraes Figueiredo

Zoonotic viruses account for 75% of emerging infectious diseases in the world [1]. Many of these zoonotic viruses are arthropod-borne viruses (arboviruses) that can be transmitted by mosquitoes, flies, and ticks [2]. Arboviral infections can produce disease in the central nervous system (CNS) with acute clinical manifestations, such as headache and nuchal rigidity suggestive of meningitis, seizures, mental confusion or coma in cases of encephalitis, and motor dysfunctions in limbs and sphincter dysfunction, related to myelitis. Arbovirus infections can also produce later manifestations in the CNS including Guillain-Barré syndrome and Parkinsonism. The *Flaviviridae* of *Flavivirus* genera Zika (ZIKV), the four types of dengue (DENV-1–4), and the *Togaviridae* of *Alphavirus* genera chikungunya (CHIKV) are all arboviruses that cause epidemics of acute febrile illnesses in tropical world and, eventually, are reported producing diseases of the CNS [3].

ZIKV and CHIKV from Africa and the four types of DENV from Southeastern Asia are viruses originally maintained in cycles involving nonhuman primates and mosquitoes of tree canopy that at some point adapted to new cycles involving humans and the anthropophilic mosquito *Aedes aegypti*. This African mosquito is anthropophilic and lives in cities at tropical countries worldwide completely adapted to the urban conditions [4]. Other arboviruses such as West Nile (WNV) from the Old World, Japanese encephalitis from Asia, and the Americas Saint Louis encephalitis (SLEV) and Rocio (ROCV) viruses are all *Flavivirus* phylogenetically grouped in the Japanese encephalitis complex, having birds as reservoirs

M. L. G. de Figueiredo
Laboratory of Virology, Department of Clinical Analysis, Toxicology and Food Sciences,
School of Pharmaceutical Sciences of Ribeirao Preto, University of Sao Paulo,
Ribeirao Preto, Sao Paulo, Brazil

L. T. M. Figueiredo (✉)
Virus Research Unit, School of Medicine of the University of Sao Paulo,
Ribeirao Preto, Sao Paulo, Brazil
e-mail: ltmfigue@fmrp.usp.br

and mosquitoes of the Culicinae subfamily as vectors [5, 6]. These viruses are commonly reported causing outbreaks or sporadic cases of meningoencephalitis. Another arbovirus that causes human infections of the CNS is the *Peribunyaviridae* of *Orthobunyavirus* genera, Oropouche (OROV). OROV causes outbreaks of acute febrile illness in the Amazon region and Central Plateau of Brazil and neighboring countries. The virus has a sylvatic cycle involving sloths (*Bradypus tridactylus*), nonhuman primates, and wild birds and *Ochlerotatus serratus*, *Coquillettidia venezuelensis*, as well as other mosquitoes as vectors. The virus adapted to an urban cycle involving man, transmitted by the hematophagous midge *Culicoides paraensis* [7].

Arboviruses of the *Flaviviridae* family in *Flavivirus* genera, WNV, JEV, ROCV, SLEV, DENV-1–4, and ZIKV, are enveloped, positive-sense, single-stranded RNA viruses [8]. Arboviruses of *Alphavirus* genera in the *Togaviridae* family, CHIKV, are enveloped with a genome of a single positive-sense strand RNA, and three structural proteins of these viruses are translated from a subgenomic mRNA [9]. Arboviruses of *Orthobunyavirus* genera in the *Peribunyaviridae* family such as OROV have three-segmented negative-stranded RNA linear genome [10, 11]. Flaviviruses, alphaviruses, and orthobunyaviruses, when infecting humans, can cause meningitis or meningoencephalitis.

Special capabilities are necessary for an arbovirus to infect the CNS. The pathogen, besides being virulent, has to defeat general cellular and humoral immune response, be able to cross the blood-brain barrier (BBB) or the choroid plexus, and when in nervous tissue, defeat the local host defense mechanisms [12, 13].

Genomic mutations can increase the virulence of flaviviruses, alphaviruses, and orthobunyaviruses. An artificial example of that has been seen in ROCV and WNV, two neurovirulent flaviviruses. A chimeric WNV containing prM-E genes of ROCV replicated in mammalian cells more efficiently than WNV or chimeric ROCV containing WNV prM-E genes. WNV containing ROCV prM-E genes was as virulent as ROCV in adult mice. Proteins prM and E of ROCV showed major virulence determinants and inhibited type I interferon response which could potentially enhance neurovirulence [14]. Glycosylation and amino acid changes of the envelope (E) and membrane (M) proteins of WNV and JEV viruses can also increase their neuroinvasive capacities [15, 16].

Innate and adaptive immune system responses to *Flavivirus* infection can prevent CNS invasion. Immune deficiencies related to age, diabetes mellitus, hypertension, or other chronic diseases increase risk of CNS disease in infections by SLEV and WNV. Infection of the CNS in individuals infected by JEV can be prevented by their normal immune systems. The maturation of defense mechanisms in adolescents can explain the decline of JEV neurological infections compared to children [17]. Activation of MAVS, IRF-3, and IRF-7 and production of type I IFN are able to control OROV replication and restrict tissue injury in mouse experimental model. In infections by OROV, IFN signaling in nonmyeloid cells, probably, contributes to the host defense [10].

Despite not completely understood, factors responsible for neuroinvasion in flaviviruses, alphaviruses, and orthobunyaviruses bypass the BBB by infecting endothelial cells and emerging their viral progenies at the opposite side, inside the CNS. Likewise, viruses can infect leukocytes that migrate to the CNS. Some viruses, after introduced by arthropod bite in subcutaneous tissue, migrate through peripheral axonium reaching the neuron in the CNS [14]. A study in a mouse model showed that OROV, after subcutaneous infection, accesses nervous receptor and neural routes, reaches the spinal cord, and ascends toward the brain producing little inflammation [18].

The local CNS inflammation produces brain edema and ischemia that damages nervous tissues. Blood cells migrate induced by chemokines produced after viral presence in the CNS, and it produces and/or aggravates inflammation. The importance of the impact of macrophages on the severity of the encephalitis has been clearly shown in a study on macrophage chemokines, CCR5 (CC-chemokine receptor 5) and MIP-1 (chemokine receptor that binds to macrophage inflammatory protein), using knockout mice to genes of these chemokines. The knockout animals, after infected with ROCV, survived longer to the meningoencephalitis and had reduced inflammation in the brain than wild-type (WT) mice infected with ROCV. Knockout mice also required a higher lethal dose of ROCV than wild-type mice [19].

In the CNS, the BBB, neurons, and glial and endothelial perivascular cells all have cell membrane receptors for infection by *Flavivirus* and other arboviruses [14]. In an experiment infecting Balb/C adult mice with ROCV, brain inflammatory changes were produced by immune response induced by Th1 and Th2 cytokines. ROCV encephalitis evolved with irreversible damage of nervous tissues due to neuronal degeneration and apoptosis [20]. Likewise, studies with WNV show that E, M, NS3, and NS4 (the last two are nonstructural) viral proteins elicit response from CD8 T cells in the CNS producing pro-inflammatory cytokines such as interferon (IFN), granzymes A and B, and perforins that lyse infected cells [21]. CD8 T cells also induce apoptosis of neural cells infected by WNV through the Fas ligand, CD40-CD 40 ligand, and tumor necrosis factor-related apoptosis-inducing ligand (TRAIL). This is an important measure to prevent persistence of the virus in the CNS [22]. Apoptosis also occurs in mice OROV-infected neurons. Besides that, CNS infection by OROV produces astrocyte activation and glial reaction [18].

Neurologic features of infections by *Flavivirus* start after 3–15 days of incubation period and usually succeed a nonspecific febrile illness. Neurologic manifestations depend on the affected part of the nervous system, resulting in meningitis, encephalitis, or myelitis [5]. In many cases of encephalitis, overlap reduced level of consciousness, seizures, and flaccid paralysis.

A ZIKV Asian strain from Polynesia has produced large outbreaks of acute febrile illness with rash and conjunctivitis in Brazil since 2015. However, during these outbreaks, reports of severe forms of Zika fever surprised the world. First, it was reported that ZIKV infections increased the number of cases of Guillain-Barré (GBS) muscle paralysis syndrome, a serious neurological disease caused by autoantibodies that damage axons of motor neurons as a consequence of a viral infection [23]. Furthermore, an increase in the incidence of fetal microcephaly was observed in the Northeast Region of Brazil, which was soon associated with maternal infection by ZIKV [24]. Congenital disease caused by ZIKV, having microcephaly as severe manifestation, resulted in an international concern followed by a research effort to obtain information on the different aspects of the disease [25].

Infections of the CNS by ZIKV not associated with congenital disease also occurred. A prospective study in Rio de Janeiro, Southeast of Brazil, among hospitalized adults analyzed 40 patients infected by ZIKV (15 women and 25 men; median age, 44 years) including 27 cases of GBS, 5 cases of encephalitis, 2 of transverse myelitis, and 1 with chronic demyelinating polyneuropathy. Nine patients were admitted to the intensive care unit, and among them, five required mechanical ventilation. After 3 months, two patients died (6%) including one with encephalitis [26]. In Ribeirão Preto, also in the Southeast of Brazil, a 2-year-old girl became ill in March 2016, during a ZIKV epidemic. The girl had a fever (up to 38.5 °C) for 8 days and a macular rash of extremities in the last 2 days. She also presented with irritability, weakness, myalgias, and dysuria. Finally, 9 days after the onset of illness, she developed ataxic gait with normal reflexes and a positive Babinski sign. The cerebrospinal fluid (CSF) had no cells but 6400 erythrocytes/mm^3, 102.6 mg/dl of protein, and 35 mg/dl of glucose. RT-PCR for ZIKV was positive in plasma and CSF. Magnetic resonance imaging (MRI) demonstrated rhombencephalitis with lesions in the vermix and left cerebellar hemisphere. The ataxic gait disappeared after 3 days, and the patient recovered without sequelae (unpublished data). A 36-year-old man heart transplant recipient from Ribeirão Preto was also reported to have ZIKV encephalitis. This patient presented with a 2-day history of high-grade fever, malaise, headache, and seizures that evolved with progressive hemodynamic instability, mental deterioration, and finally death. CSF had 58 leukocytes (100% lymphocytes)/mm^3 and 105.37 mg/dl of protein. MRI revealed extensive cortical encephalitis with image suggestive of necrosis of the brain parenchyma and vasogenic edema. ZIKV genome was detected in the CSF by reverse transcriptase polymerase chain reaction (RT-PCR) and also by immunohistochemistry, by immunofluorescence, and by electron microscopy of brain tissue. The amplicon of viral genome was sequenced confirming the ZIKV infection. A pseudotumoral form of ZIKV meningoencephalitis was confirmed at autopsy [27].

The incidence of encephalopathy in patients with dengue ranges between 0.5% and 6.2% [28]. In a study of 49 patients with lymphocytic meningitis in Manaus City, North of Brazil, four of them had dengue fever, with headache, myalgias, and arthralgias that evolved to neck stiffness and impaired consciousness that healed without sequelae. Based on viral genomes detected in the CSF by RT-PCR, three patients had DENV-2 and one had DENV-1 [29]. Another study reported 498 DENV-3 cases from Goiania City in the Brazilian Central Plateau, in 2005–2006. Nine patients had clinical features compatible with infection of the CNS, five women and four men, mostly teenagers and young adults. These patients had encephalopathy (presented seizures or paresis) or meningoencephalitis, and two of them died. Fatal cases were of a 15-year-old girl with meningoencephalitis, whose CSF had 76 leukocytes (80% mononuclear cells)/μL, 64 mg/dL of glucose, and 127 mg/dL of protein. Her computed tomography scans revealed sulci effacement and intracranial hypertension, and DENV-3 was detected in brain tissues collected at necropsy. The other fatal case was of a 41-year-old woman that 10 days after onset of disease had tonic-clonic seizures and acute liver failure. PCR tests of blood were positive for DENV-3, and lumbar puncture was contraindicated due to thrombocytopenia [30]. In Ribeirão Preto City, a 65-year-old woman had acute meningoencephalitis by DENV. After 4 days with headache, fever, myalgia, and vomiting, the patient started with myopathy, seizures, and decreased level of consciousness. CSF showed normal leukocyte count, 72–86 mg/dL of protein, and immunoglobulins M (IgM) and G (IgG) positive to dengue. Brain MRI revealed acute central pattern encephalitis affecting internal capsule and nuclei of the base [31].

An Asian genotype of CHIKV was introduced into the Americas through the Caribbean in December 2013, and the first autochthonous Brazilian cases were reported in September 2014 in the State of Amapá, in the North, and at the same time, another genotype of CHIKV, the East, Central, and South African and Asian strain (ECSA), was found in Bahia State at the Northeast of Brazil. CHIKV ECSA rapidly spread through other northeastern states causing outbreaks [32]. During these large-scale outbreaks, uncommon severe clinical features of CHIKV infection were observed such as meningitis, encephalitis, GBS, and retrobulbar neuritis [33]. Two cases of encephalitis by CHIKV were reported in the Ceará State, Northeast of Brazil. These were a 55- and a 74-year-old man. Both patients tested positive for anti-chikungunya IgM in their serum. The first patient had acute febrile illness and disorientation in time and space. His CSF had 61 cells (71% lymphocytes)/mm^3, 98 mg/dL of protein, and 62 mg/dL of glucose. His MRI showed acute bilateral encephalitis affecting the white matter in nuclei of the base and brainstem and also extending to the internal capsule and the cerebellum. The second patient had temporal and spatial disorientation with fluctuating level of consciousness, progressive lower extremity weakness, and diffuse areflexia. He had 90 leukocytes (91% lymphocytes)/mm^3 and a protein of 179 mg/dL in CSF. MRI showed acute encephalitis affecting extensive area including the central white matter and cerebellum [34]. Another case of encephalitis by CHIKV was reported in Recife City, also in the Northeast of Brazil, a 48-year-old woman with fever, headache, muscle aches, skin rash, and painful polyarthralgia with edema that progressed to temporary functional impairment. The patient also presented a persistent hyponatremia with a plasma osmolality below 275 mOsm/kg of H$_2$O, compatible with a syndrome of inappropriate antidiuretic hormone secretion (SIADH). The patient evolved to cognitive impairment and apraxia of speech and had 90 leukocytes/mm^3 and a protein 68 mg/dL in CSF. MRI showed acute encephalitis involving putamen and nuclei of the base bilaterally but discrete edema [35].

In 2002, in Cordoba, Argentina, a 61-year-old businessman with headache, fever with chills, nausea, vomiting, unstable gait, left hand tremors, and diplopia was admitted to a hospital. He was lethargic and had neck rigidity. His CSF revealed 18 leukocytes (80% lymphocytes)/mm^3, 87 mg/dL of protein, and 48 mg/dL of glucose. Meningeal signs evolved with frank cervical stiffness, positive Kerning sign, and photophobia. Lower extremities were spastic with bilateral Babinski sign. He had a wide-based gait and had dysdiadochokinesia. All symptoms disappeared after 5 days [36]. Diagnosis of infection was made using the hemagglutination inhibition test whose titers to SLEV increased between acute- (320) and convalescent-phase (1280) samples. A serological survey of horses from various regions of Brazil showed that 415 (55.1%) of the 753 studied horses were seropositive for flavivirus and, among them, monotypic reactions were observed to SLEV in 93 (12.3%). These results suggest SLEV is infecting horses in Southeast, Pantanal, and Northeast of Brazil [37]. In 2007, during a large DENV-3 epidemic, six patients were found infected by SLEV in the city of São José do Rio Preto, southeastern Brazil. SLEV genome was detected by RT-PCR in CSF of all six patients. From these, two children had acute febrile illness, one of them had facial palsy, and both were diagnosed with meningoencephalitis (the first cases of meningoencephalitis by SLEV reported in Brazil). Their CSFs showed 12 (100% lymphocytes) and 286 (60% lymphocytes) leukocytes/mm^3 and both survived [38]. Therefore, SLEV is endemic in South America infecting horses and also producing small human outbreaks and sporadic cases of meningitis and encephalitis, probably misdiagnosed as dengue or other viral diseases.

ROCV has produced an outbreak of encephalitis in the southern coast of São Paulo State in 1973–1978, with 1021 reported cases [39]. ROCV patients presented acutely with fever, headache, anorexia, nausea, vomiting, myalgia, and malaise. Encephalitis signs appeared later, including confusion, reflex disturbances, motor impairment, meningeal irritation, and cerebellar syndrome. Some patients presented convulsions. The disease produced sequelae such as visual, olfactory, and auditory disturbances, lack of motor coordination, equilibrium disturbance, swallowing difficulties, incontinence, and impaired memory in 20% of the survivors. The case fatality rate of this ROCV outbreak was 10% [40]. After this outbreak, serologic evidence of ROCV circulation in the original area as well as in other parts of Brazil have been reported, and public health authorities are always concerned about reappearance of ROCV outbreaks in Brazil [6]. A serological survey of horses from various Brazilian regions showed that 415 (55.1%) of the 753 studied horses were seropositive for flavivirus, and among them, a monotypic reaction to ROCV was found in 46 animals (6.1%). These results suggest that ROCV, or other closely related virus, is infecting horses in Southeast, Pantanal, and Northeast of Brazil [38]. Besides that, in 2010, testing 23 CSF samples from human patients from Manaus City by RT-PCR, amplicons of ROCV genome from two patients were amplified and sequenced. These were a 53-year-old man with seizures and abnormal conscientiousness and a 30-year-old woman with headache, vomiting, and signs of intracranial hypertension. Curiously, both had AIDS and the woman also had tuberculosis. CSFs showed 45 and 29 lymphocytic cells/mm^3, 153 and 328 protein mg/dl, and 48 and 56 mg/dl of glucose, respectively. Both survived after 20 days of hospitalization (unpublished data, 2010). Interestingly, these human cases occurred in the North of Brazil, more than 2000 km from where the virus was originally isolated. Serologic evidence in horses and the casual finding of human cases in Manaus show that ROCV circulates unrecognized in Brazil and possibly in other South American countries, producing human infections including those of the CNS, particularly affecting immunodeficient individuals, such as AIDS patients.

WNV is a pathogen from Africa and Asia that emerged in North America in 1999 and spread toward all the Americas. This virus causes a severe encephalitis in humans and in horses. In North America, WNV has caused dozens of thousands of clinical cases and some thousands of deaths of humans and horses [41]. WNV was isolated in Argentina, in 2006, from the brain of three horses [42]. A serologic survey to WNV including sera of 753 healthy horses from Central-West, Northeast, and Southeast Brazil showed 79 seropositive horses to WNV, and among them, 9 sera expressed WNV-specific neutralizing antibodies. Eight of these animals were from the western Pantanal region in the State of Mato Grosso do Sul, and one was from the State of Paraíba in the Northeast of Brazil [43]. Based on the virus introduction in Argentina as well as on the results of serologic surveys shown above, WNV has been introduced in Brazil, and it is probably spreading in the country based on a transmission network that involves mosquitoes, birds, and horses. The first human case of encephalitis by WNV in Brazil was reported in 2014. A 52-year-old agricultural worker man from Piauí State, Northeast of Brazil, presented an acute febrile illness with headache, neck pain, vomiting, diarrhea, abdominal pain, and severe muscle weakness. The patient evolved with a tonic-clonic seizure and confusional state. Physical exam revealed nuchal rigidity, bilateral facial palsy, flaccid symmetrical tetraparesis and abolished myotatic reflexes. CSF showed 14 leukocytes (85% lymphomonocytic cells)/mm^3, 274 mg/dl of protein, and 59 mg/dl of glucose. Diagnosis of WNV infection was made by serologic tests including positive neutralization test to the virus. MRI images were normal. The patient recovered partially and was not able to walk after discharge [44]. It is probable that other WNV infections have occurred unrecognized in Brazil, particularly in Northeast and Pantanal regions.

OROV has caused large outbreaks of acute febrile illness with sporadic cases of meningitis, in Amazon region and Central Plateau of Brazil as well as in Peru and other South American countries [7, 10]. In a study performed from 2005 to 2010 in Manaus City, in the Amazonas State, North Region of Brazil, CSF samples of 110 patients with meningoencephalitis were submitted to RT-PCR in order to identify infecting viruses. OROV was found in three CSF samples. Patients were a 20-year-old agricultural worker man, a 54-year-old fisherman man, and a 37-year-old domestic worker woman. All patients referred headache; one patient had dizziness, cloud vision, and Romberg sign; the second had fever, chills, and malaise; and the third had nausea, vomiting, and paraplegia. CSFs showed 6, 134, and 533 lymphocytic cells/mm^3; 40, 107, and 136 mg/dl of protein; and 40, 50, and 107 mg/dl of glucose, respectively. All patients survived after hospitalization. Interestingly, two of these patients had other diseases affecting the CNS or immune system; the first had neurocysticercosis and the last had AIDS [29].

A summary of reported infections of the central nervous system (CNS) caused by arboviruses in Brazil is shown in Table 15.1.

Table 15.1 Infections of the central nervous system (CNS) caused by arboviruses in Brazil

Arbovirus	Family, genera	Vector	Disease	Remarks
Dengue	*Flaviviridae, Flavivirus*	*Aedes aegypti*	Acute febrile illness and encephalopathy in 0.5–6.2% [28]	Infection of CNS related to serotypes, 1, 2, and 3 [30, 31]
Zika	*Flaviviridae, Flavivirus*	*Aedes aegypti*	Acute febrile illness, congenital and acquired infections of the CNS [24, 26]	Infection of CNS in a child and in an immune-depressed patient [27]
Rocio	*Flaviviridae, Flavivirus*	*Culex* mosquitoes	Encephalitis with 10% lethality [40]	Two cases of encephalitis in AIDS patients
Saint Louis encephalitis	*Flaviviridae, Flavivirus*	*Culex* mosquitoes	Acute febrile illness and encephalitis specially in elderly with 5–15% lethality [5]	Small outbreak of meningoencephalitis in the middle of a dengue outbreak [38]
West Nile	*Flaviviridae, Flavivirus*	*Culex* mosquitoes	Encephalitis	One case of encephalitis reported in Brazil [44]
Chikungunya	*Togaviridae, Alphavirus*	*Aedes aegypti*	Acute febrile illness and seldomly encephalopathy	Three cases of encephalitis reported in Brazil [34, 35]
Oropouche	*Peribunyaviridae, Orthobunyavirus* [11]	*Culicoides paraensis*	Acute febrile illness and eventually meningoencephalitis [7]	Three cases of meningoencephalitis reported in Manaus City, two patients had AIDS or neurocysticercosis [29]

Cases of encephalitis by DENV, ZIKV, and other flaviviruses show a central pattern affecting neurons in the substantia nigra nucleus, thalamus, cerebellum, and cerebral cortex, correlating with the neuroradiological findings in MRI, as shown in Fig. 15.1 [45, 46]. These infections, particularly in immunodeficient individuals can extend to other areas of the brain. CHIKV, an *Alphavirus*, also produces encephalitis affecting the white matter in nuclei of the base and brainstem, and it can extend to the internal capsule and the cerebellum, as shown in Fig. 15.1.

As final remarks on arboviruses producing infection of the CNS:

– There is no specific antiviral treatment for arboviruses that cause meningoencephalitis. The treatment seeks to reduce cerebral edema by avoiding excessive hydration and eventually using corticosteroids, in addition to providing supportive care.
– It is probable that serological diagnosis of ZIKV, ROCV, and SLEV infections may be confused with dengue due to cross-reactivity with this virus.
– Our data suggest that CNS invasion by ZIKV, ROCV, OROV, and probably other arboviruses could be facilitated by immunodeficiency or by prior damage of the

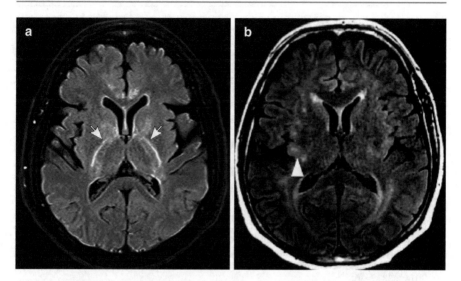

Fig. 15.1 (a) Magnetic resonance imaging (MRI) of a case of dengue encephalitis showing small areas of hyperintensity on T2/fluid attenuation inversion recovery (FLAIR), bilaterally, on the internal capsule (adapted of Queiroz et al. [31]); (b) MRI of a case of chikungunya encephalitis showing multiple supratentorial FLAIR hyperintense foci (arrowheads) distributed randomly in the white matter (adapted of Pereira et al. [34])

BBB. Arboviruses should be considered and tested in differential diagnosis of patients with CNS infections that have underlying diseases such as immunodeficiency or by prior neurologic pathologies.

References

1. Hubalek Z. Emerging human infectious diseases: anthroponoses, zoonoses, and sapronoses. Emerg Infect Dis. 2003;9:403–4.
2. Meltzer E. Arboviruses and viral hemorrhagic fevers (VHF). Infect Dis Clin N Am. 2012;26:479–96.
3. Figueiredo LTM. The recent arbovirus disease epidemic in Brazil. Rev Soc Bras Med Trop. 2015;48:233–4.
4. Patterson J, Sammon M, Garg M. Dengue, Zika and Chikungunya: emerging arboviruses in the new world. West J Emerg Med. 2016;17:671–9.
5. Solomon T. Flavivirus encephalitis. N Engl J Med. 2004;351:370–8.
6. Figueiredo LTM. The Brazilian flaviviruses. Microbes Infect. 2000;2:1643–9.
7. Vasconcelos HB, Nunes MR, Casseb LM, Carvalho VL, Pinto da Silva EV, Silva M, Casseb SM, Vasconcelos PF. Molecular epidemiology of Oropouche virus, Brazil. Emerg Infect Dis. 2016;17:800–6.
8. Brinton MA. Replication cycle and molecular biology of the West Nile virus. Viruses. 2013;6:13–53.
9. Jose J, Snyder JE, Kuhn RJ. A structural and functional perspective of alphavirus replication and assembly. Future Microbiol. 2009;4:837–56.
10. Proenca-Modena JL, Sesti-Costa R, Pinto AK, Richner JM, Lazear HM, Lucas T, Hyde JL, Diamond MS. Oropouche virus infection and pathogenesis are restricted by MAVS, IRF-3,

IRF-7, and type I interferon signaling pathways in nonmyeloid cells. J Virol. 2015;89(9):4720–37. https://doi.org/10.1128/JVI.00077-15.

11. Taxonomy—International Committee on Taxonomy of Viruses (ICTV). Virus taxonomy: 2016 release, Budapest, Hungary. 2016. https://talk.ictvonline.org/taxonomy.

12. Koyuncu OO, Hogue IB, Enquist LW. Virus infections in the nervous system. Cell Host Microbe. 2013;13:379–93.

13. Amarilla AA, Setoh YX, Periasamy P, Pali G, Figueiredo LT, Khromykh AA, Aquino VH. Chimeras between Rocio and West Nile viruses reveal the role for Rocio virus prM and E proteins in virulence and inhibition of type I interferon signaling. Sci Rep. 2017;7:44642.

14. Neal JW. Flaviviruses are neurotropic, but how do they invade the CNS? J Infect. 2014;69:203–15.

15. Shirato K, Miyosh H, iGoto A, Ako Y, Ueki T, Kariwa HA, Takashima I. Viral envelope protein glycosylation is a molecular determinant of neuro invasiveness of the New York strain of West Nile virus. J Gen Virol. 2004;85:3637–45.

16. Lee E, Lobbigs M. Mechanisms of virulence attenuation of glycosaminoglycan-binding variants of Japanese encephalitis virus and Murray Valley encephalitis virus. J Virol. 2002;76:4901–11.

17. Misra KM, Kalita J. Overview: Japanese encephalitis. Prog Neurobiol. 2010;91:108–20.

18. Santos RI, Bueno-Júnior LS, Ruggiero RN, Almeida MF, Silva ML, Paula FE, Correa VM, Arruda E. Spread of Oropouche virus into the central nervous system in mouse. Viruses. 2014;6:3827–36.

19. Chávez JH, França RFO, Oliveira CJ, Aquino MTP, Farias KJ, Machado PR, Yokosawa J, Silva JS, Fonseca BAL, Figueiredo LTM. CCR-5/MIP-1 alpha affect the pathogenesis of Rocio virus encephalitis in a mouse model. Am J Trop Med Hyg. 2013;89:1013–8.

20. Barros VD, Penharvel S, Forjaz J, Saggioro FP, Neder L, Figueiredo LTM. An experimental model of meningoencephalomyelitis by Rocio virus in Balb-C mice: hystopathology, inflammatory response and cytokine production. Am J Trop Med Hyg. 2011;85:363–73.

21. Shrestha B, Samuel MS, Diamond MS. CD8fl T cells require perforin to clear West Nile fever from infected neurons. J Virol. 2006;80:119–29.

22. Shresta B, Pinto AK, Green S, Bosch I, Diamond MS. CD8fl T cells use TRAIL to restrict West Nile virus pathogenesis by controlling infection in neurons. J Virol. 2012;86:8937–48.

23. Brazilian Ministry of Health. Dengue, Chikungunya, Zika, Syndrome of Guillain-Barré. 2016.

24. Butler D. Zika virus: Brazil's surge in small-headed babies questioned by report. Nature. 2016;530:13–4.

25. Macciocchi D, Lanini S, Vairo F, Zumla A, Figueiredo LTM, Lauria FN, Strada G, Brouqui P, Puro V, Krishna S, Kremsner P, Scognamiglio P, Köhler C, Nicastri E, Di Caro A, Cieri RM, Ioannidis JPA, Kobinger G, Burattini MN, Ippolito G. Short-term economic impact of the Zika virus outbreak. New Microbiol. 2016;39:287–9.

26. Silva IRF, Frontera JA, Filippis AMB, Nascimento OJM, RIO-GBS-ZIKV Research Group. Neurologic complications associated with the Zika virus in Brazilian adults. JAMA Neurol. 2017;74:1190–8.

27. Schwartzmann PV, Vilar FC, Takayanagui OM, Santos AC, Ayub-Ferreira SM, Ramalho LNZ, Neder L, Romeiro MF, Maia FGM, Tollardo AL, Zapata PM, Figueiredo LTM, Schmidt A, Simões MV. Zika virus associated encephalitis in immunocompromised patient. Mayo Clin Proc. 2017;92:460–6.

28. Misra UK, Kalita J, Syam UK, Dhole TN. Neurological manifestations of dengue virus infection. J Neurol Sci. 2006;244:117–22.

29. Bastos MS, Figueiredo LT, Naveca F, Figueiredo R, Oliveira CM, Gimaque JB, Assis K, Monte RL, Mourão MP. Infection of central nervous system by Oropouche Orthobunyavirus in three Brazilian patients. Am J Trop Med Hyg. 2012;86:732–5.

30. Tassara MP, Guilarde AO, Rocha BAM, Féres VCR, Martelli CMT. Neurological manifestations of dengue in Central Brazil. Rev Soc Bras Med Trop. 2017;50:379–82.

31. Queiroz RM, Prado RMA, Abud LG. Acute dengue encephalitis in a female Brazilian adult. Rev Soc Bras Med Trop. 2017;50:431.

32. Figueiredo MLG, Figueiredo LTM. Emerging alphaviruses in the Americas: Chikungunya and Mayaro. Rev Soc Bras Med Trop. 2014;47:677–83.
33. Figueiredo LTM. Chikungunya virus emerged in Brazil producing large outbreaks that revealed uncommon clinical features and fatalities. Rev Soc Bras Med Trop. 2017;50:583–4.
34. Pereira LP, Villas-Bôas R, Scott SSO, Nóbrega PR, Sobreira-Neto MA, Castro JDV, Cavalcante B, Braga-Neto P. Encephalitis associated with the chikungunya epidemic outbreak in Brazil: report of 2 cases with neuroimaging findings. Rev Soc Bras Med Trop. 2017;50:413–6.
35. Lucena-Silva N, Assunção MELSM, Ramos FAP, Azevedo F, Lessa Junior R, Cordeiro MT, Brito CAA. Encephalitis associated with inappropriate antidiuretic hormone secretion due to chikungunya infection in Recife, state of Pernambuco, Brazil. Rev Soc Bras Med Trop. 2017;50:417–22.
36. Spinsanti L, Basquiera AL, Bulacio S, Somale V, Kim CH, Ré V, Rabbat D, Zárate A, Zlocowski JC, Mayor CQ, Contigiani M, Palacio S. St. Louis encephalitis in Argentina: the first case reported in the last seventeen years. Emerg Infect Dis. 2003;9:271–3.
37. Silva JR, Romeiro MF, Sousa WM, Munhoz TD, Borges GP, Soares OAB, Campos CHC, Machado RZ, Silva MLCR, Faria JLM, Chávez JH, Figueiredo LTM. Serosurvey of Saint Louis encephalitis and Rocio viruses in horses of Brazil. Rev Soc Bras Med Trop. 2014;47:414–7.
38. Mondini A, Lázaro E, Cardeal ILS, Nunes SH, Moreira CC, Rahal P, Figueiredo LTM, Bronzoni RVM, Chiaravalloti Neto F, Nogueira ML. Saint Louis encephalitis virus, Brazil. Emerg Infect Dis. 2007;13:176–8.
39. Lopes OS, Coimbra TLM, Sacchetta LA, Calisher CH. Emergence of a new arbovirus disease in Brazil. 1. Isolation and characterization of the etiologic agent, Rocio virus. Am J Epidemiol. 1978;107:444–9.
40. Tiriba AC, Miziara AM, Lourenço R, Costa CRB, Cota CS, Pinto GH. Encefalite humana primária epidêmica por arbovirus observada no litoral sul do Estado de São Paulo. Rev Assoc Med Bras. 1976;22:415–20.
41. Roehrig JT. West Nile virus in the United States—a historical perspective. Viruses. 2013;5:3088–108.
42. Morales MA, Barrandeguy M, Fabbri C, Garcia JB, Vissani A, Trono K, Gutierrez G, Pigretti P, Menchaca H, Garrido N, Taylor N, Fernandez F, Levis S, Enría D. West Nile virus isolation from equines in Argentina, 2006. Emerg Infect Dis. 2006;12:1559–61.
43. Silva JR, Chávez JH, Munhoz TD, Borges GP, Soares OAB, Machado RZ, Valadão CAA, Silva MLCR, Faria JLM, Silva EE, Figueiredo LTM. Serologic survey for West Nile virus in Brazilian horses. Mem Inst Osvaldo Cruz. 2013;108:921–3.
44. Vieira MA, Romano AP, Borba AS, Silva EV, Chiang JO, Eulálio KD, Azevedo RS, Rodrigues SG, Almeida-Neto WS, Vasconcelos PF. West Nile virus encephalitis: the first human case recorded in Brazil. Am J Trop Med Hyg. 2015;93:377–9.
45. Bosanko CM, Gilroy J, Wang A-M, Sanders WS, Dulai M, Wilson J, Blum K. West Nile virus encephalitis involving the substantia nigra. Arch Neurol. 2003;60:1448–52.
46. Knox J, Cowan RV, Dayle JS, Liqtermont MK, ArcherJS Burrow JN, et al. Murray Valley encephalitis; a review of clinical features diagnosis and treatment. Med J Aust. 2012;196:322–6.

Index

Printed in the United States
By Bookmasters